Medicines Management

We work with leading authors to develop the
strongest educational materials in nursing,
bringing cutting-edge thinking and best
learning practice to a global market.

Under a range of well-known imprints, including
Pearson Education, we craft high quality print and
electronic publications which help readers to understand
and apply their content, whether studying or at work.

To find out more about the complete range of our
publishing, please visit us on the World Wide Web at:
www.pearsoned.co.uk

Medicines Management

a nursing perspective

Sandra Crouch

Carol Chapelhow

Michael Crouch (Consultant Pharmacist)

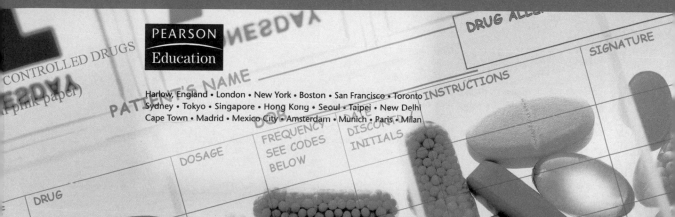

PEARSON
Education

Harlow, England • London • New York • Boston • San Francisco • Toronto
Sydney • Tokyo • Singapore • Hong Kong • Seoul • Taipei • New Delhi
Cape Town • Madrid • Mexico City • Amsterdam • Munich • Paris • Milan

Pearson Education Limited
Edinburgh Gate
Harlow
Essex CM20 2JE
England

and Associated Companies throughout the world

Visit us on the World Wide Web at:
www.pearsoned.co.uk

First published 2008
© Pearson Education Limited 2008

ISBN: 978-0-13-221734-7

British Library Cataloguing-in-Publication Data
A catalogue record for this book is available from the British Library

Library of Congress Cataloging-in-Publication Data
A catalog record for this book is available from the Library of Congress

Crouch, Sandra.
    Medicines management : a nursing perspective / Sandra Crouch, Carol Chapelhow,
Michael Crouch (consultant pharmacist).
        p. ; cm.
    Includes bibliographical references and index.
    ISBN 978-0-13-221734-7
    1. Pharmacology. 2. Nursing. I. Chapelhow, carol. II. Crouch, Michael. III. Title.
    [DNLM: 1. Drug Therapy--nursing--Great Britain. 2. Drug Monitoring--nursing--Great
Britain. 3. Medication Errors--prevention & control--Great Britain. 4. Nurse's
Role--Great Britain. WY 100 C952m 2008]
    RM300.C74 2008
    615'.1--dc22

                                                                        2008026902

10 9 8 7 6 5 4 3 2 1
12 11 10 09 08

Typeset in 9/12.5 Interstate Light by 30
Printed by Ashford Colour Press Ltd., Gosport

The publisher's policy is to use paper manufactured from sustainable forests.

Contents

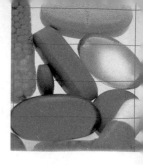

Chapter 10 Coronary heart disease:

an adult male with hyperlipidaemia, who has an acute myocardial infarction and develops heart failure

Chapter 11 A man with acute intestinal obstruction

Chapter 12 Epilepsy:

Chapter 13: Alzheimer's disease:

Chapter 14 Diabetes mellitus:

an adult with type 2 diabetes, depression and hypothyroidism 379

Chapter 15 Asthma:

a young man with asthma, eczema and Down's syndrome who develops pneumonia 407

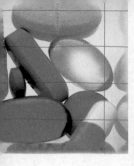

Guided tour

Learning outcomes and **Chapter at a glance** boxes provide an overview of the topics covered and summarise what you should have learnt by the end of each chapter.

72

This implies an underpinning knowledge and skills base related to medicines. In order to understand the effect (or lack of) that a drug or medicine is having on a particular patient, we need to understand how the medicine exerts its effects. We cannot know all information about all medicines in use today, but we should have knowledge about the commonly used medicines and the core medicines given to patients within the patient care context in which we are working, whether hospital-based, in patients' homes or in residential care.

Learning outcomes

By the end of this chapter you should be able to:
✔ Describe the process of drug development
✔ Identify and explain some of the terminology used when discussing drugs and medicines
✔ Explain how drugs exert their effects on the body
✔ Outline how drugs reach their target sites
✔ List the routes by which medicines are administered
✔ Identify some formulations of medicines in common usage.

Chapter at a glance

This chapter will introduce some of the essential underpinning information:

Sources of information
Terminology
Understanding pharmacology
Drug development
Aims of drug treatment
Pharmacodynamics
Pharmacokinetics
Adverse drug reactions and drug interactions
Routes of administration
Preparations
Quick reminder
References

Various boxed features including **Nursing implications, Nursing knowledge** and **Personal and professional development** link theory to practice and show you how to apply what you have learnt to your own experience.

196

There is a suggestion that the anti-inflammatory effect of corticosteroids can help shrink a tumour by reducing any accompanying inflammation. One of the effects of treatment by corticosteroids is euphoria, enhancing the sense of wellbeing of the patient, which can also result in an increase in appetite (Whittaker, 2004).

Nursing implications Pain management

Cancer pain is described as 'a complex chronic pain with multiple causes' (Dickman, 2007a). It is likely to be accompanied by depression and anxiety. For these reasons, approaches to pain relief should involve providing information and reassurance as well as analgesia. Using a combination of analgesics and non-pharmacological approaches is thought to be the most effective approach.

Nursing knowledge Approaches to pain relief

WHO (1986) recommends that pain relief should be given 'by the clock'; in other words, pain relief should be managed by administering pain relief at regular intervals to prevent the need for the patient to experience pain.

Breakthrough pain

Cancer often presents as continuous pain with incidents of more serious pain. This breakthrough pain is 'an exacerbation of pain that occurs despite relatively stable and adequately controlled background pain' (Dickman, 2007a). Breakthrough pain can occur as a consequence of an action, such as coughing or having a wound dressed, or it may have no apparent cause. The rescue treatment for this type of pain should be based upon the characteristics of the pain, the existing treatment and the patient.

Personal and professional development 7.6
Nursing interventions

There are a range of approaches to pain management in cancer care. Try to identify some non-pharmacological approaches that may be used concurrently to relieve pain.
Answers can be found at the back of the book.

26

DO I UNDERSTAND WHAT I AM READING?

Getting to grips with any new subject discipline such as pharmacology (the study of drugs and their actions) can be daunting and difficult, besides being exciting and challenging. Often the process of studying a new discipline means having to learn a new language and this certainly applies to learning how to use information about medicines. Consider, for example, some of the terms used in this chapter. The language used comes from a variety of subject disciplines, including pharmacology, physiology and chemistry.

When a subject area has its own language, this is sometimes referred to as 'jargon' by those not familiar with the subject. Using the language immediately identifies those who understand the subject and therefore can be said to be 'inside the circle' and those who do not understand it and are therefore 'outside the circle'. A frequently used quote used to explain this is 'knowledge is power', attributed to Freire (1972), who was an influential thinker about education.

Personal and professional development 2.2
Using information

Take a moment to consider a recent patient encounter between a patient and a nurse or between a patient and a doctor. You might wish to reflect upon an example where you have consulted a nurse or doctor.

• What type of information was used? Did the discussion include a lot of medical terminology?
• Was there an attempt by the health professional to establish whether the patient understood?
• Was there an attempt to explain any of the jargon used?
• Was the health professional controlling the discussion, or was there an attempt to develop a partnership between the patient and the professional?
• Can we sum this up and identify who had the 'power' in this situation?

Related knowledge Sociology

An interesting and important sociological debate explores the power that is inherent in the use of such jargon, particularly that used by professional groups such as nurses and doctors. Although this debate will not be examined in this book, it is important that you understand how such power can influence relationships between patients/carers and healthcare professionals.

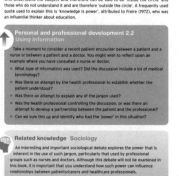

All areas of nursing are interconnected and the **Related knowledge boxes** show how your studies in anatomy & physiology, pathophysiology, sociology and legal aspects of nursing are highly relevant to medicines management.

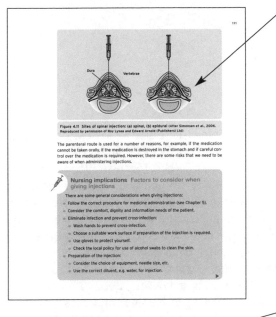

Figures are included to illustrate key concepts and processes, visually reinforcing your learning.

Essential terminology is highlighted in the text when it first appears, followed by a brief explanation of its meaning. There is also a Glossary of key terms at the end of the book.

In reality boxes highlight the tensions between theory and practice and show that your experience in practice could be slightly different to what you might expect.

Quick reminder sections recap and reinforce the key points to take away from each chapter.

References are included in all chapters and allow you to see the evidence base for the material covered.

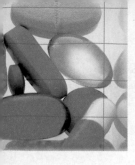

Introduction

This is a book we have wanted to write for some time. There are two key reasons for this; first, an overwhelming desire to help students understand complex information related to medicines and drugs in the context of the patient, and second, the frustration in accessing textbooks that present information in a factual way but don't go on to say 'what this means is ...' or 'this is because ...'. Yet on talking to colleagues they can often readily suggest 'the reason for that is ...'. Our teaching philosophy was the key driver for the approach that we've taken to the structure of this book, as it recognises that the reality of the world of work for novice nursing students is often bewildering. This is in common with all students, as many people can't always transfer learning from one context to another (Bransford *et al.*, 1989; Chapelhow *et al.*, 2005; Manias and Bullock, 2002). The nursing literature around teaching pharmacology to students of nursing reinforces this, as it identifies the difficulties that students have in applying theory to practice (King, 2004).

Also influencing this is one important change that has taken place in the education of student nurses; they now enter education via a variety of routes and often without knowledge of subjects such as chemistry and physiology. An understanding of science is essential for nursing students accessing nursing programmes. However, students often enter pre-registration programmes with 'little or no scientific background' (James *et al.*, 2002).

We also need to acknowledge that there are changes in care delivery and, therefore, inevitably in the delivery of medicines. Nurses' roles are changing, and changing quickly. In relation to medicines, the first major change was that of nurse prescribing. However, recent government initiatives such as Liberating the Talents (DH, 2002a), the NHS Plan (DH, 2000) and the change in junior doctors' working hours have meant that qualified nurses are expected to take on even more skills such as managing patient caseloads and running clinics, all of which imply the skill of diagnosis (DH, 2002b), as well as venepuncture and cannulation. Added to this we have differences in approaches to care, increased knowledge and technological advances, such as the Genome Project, which have added to the potential for changes in therapeutics.

Nurses and healthcare professionals are also delivering care to a more knowledgeable client/patient group. The government focus on the 'user' and increased access to information via the Internet have meant that clients rightly expect to be partners in their care, and may have more knowledge in specific areas than we do, and so are well able to be 'experts' in their care (DH, 2001). Couple this with the growing interest in complementary medicines, and it underlines the requirement for nurses not only to be knowledgeable, but also to possess a greater breadth of knowledge and skills than ever before.

Most pharmacology books written for nurses are very focused and provide comprehensive information about pharmacology, However, because of the points made above, we feel that writing a book that only provides information about medicines, however that is linked to care, will not provide nurses with the breadth of knowledge that they need. Nor will such a book enable nurses to cope with the other issues related to medicine administration, such as risk management. Contemporary care environments are busy and dynamic; this reality of care requires nurses to use a range of skills, which can be quite sophisticated. Much of contemporary nursing is what Chapelhow *et al.* (2005) describe as 'an insightful reaction to the moment' and so can be difficult to explain. Therefore, we need to equip new nurses with the skills to problem-solve, prioritise and make decisions whilst delivering care.

To provide all of this, within this book we offer a unique approach to learning about medicines. Unlike other such books, it uses patient scenarios to generate knowledge needs. The benefit of this approach to medicine administration is that it provides not only the pharmacological knowledge, such as how medicines work, but also other essential information, such as an exploration of a variety of influences that are often imperceptible. These influences range from the factors affecting concordance/adherence to covert prescribing, knowledge of which enables a nurse to provide safe, holistic and individualistic care.

The information provided in this book has been chosen carefully to reflect situations you, the student, will be most likely to meet in practice, created by using familiar patient scenarios. It includes medicines related to those patient conditions predicted by the Chief Nursing Officer as well as those that will be prevalent in the future (DH, 2002a,b; Welsh Institute for Health and Social Care, 1998), whilst reflecting developments such as National Service Frameworks (NSFs) and National Institute for Health and Clinical Excellence (NICE) guidelines. This choice is also based upon our own clinical experience as well as information gained from Prescribing Analysis and Cost (PACT) data and therefore will include, for example, analgesics, antibacterials and antihypertensives. Learning from case studies, or, as they are called in this book, patient scenarios, is a well-respected and robust method of learning used to teach all professionals, both students and graduates. From its roots in ancient Greece, where the method was used by Hippocrates, and still used to teach medicine today, the case study approach not only develops a broader understanding of medicines and their management but also helps the student to develop the ability of transferring skills and understandings from one situation to another. Many people find the skill of transferring their understanding difficult and can't always see how to transfer what they know and what they can do from one situation to another (Eraut *et al.*, 2000); Lave and Wenger, 1991; Vygotsky *et al.*, 1978; Wenger 1998). The patient scenarios we use in this book build the bridges that link all of the knowledge, understanding, attitudes and skill that an expert nurse uses in medicines management (Askew, 2003).

This book will, therefore, provide the reader with a model for learning about medicine management in practice, acknowledging pharmacological, professional, legal, ethical and sociopolitical issues and how these interrelate in practice.

FORMAT OF THE BOOK

This book is set out in various parts. Part 1 allows us to set the scene in relation to care and the type of drug/medicine information available, as well as to explore learning in practice. Chapter 1 will introduce the context of care delivery, acknowledging changes in epidemiological trends, changing needs of the consumer (patient/client) and changes in the nurse's role. Chapter 2 starts to identify what kind of information nurses need to understand medicines management and how this relates to patient care. Sources of information will be discussed, and several medicines will be used to demonstrate why we need to, and how we can, transfer knowledge about medicines to a range of patient situations, in order to understand treatments. Chapter 3 presents an overview of the complex skills required when administering medicines and discusses how these might be learnt. A more detailed justification for the approach used within this book to 'learning about medicines' is offered.

Part 2 introduces some of the important concepts and principles that are necessary to develop the understandings that relate to medicines management in practice. Chapters 4 and 5 start to identify the underpinning pharmacological and professional knowledge required by the nurse. Chapter 4 provides an overview of pharmacokinetics and pharmacodynamics, whilst Chapter 5 explores the related nursing responsibilities. Chapter 6 identifies some complementary medicines used by patients to prevent or treat illness.

Part 3 starts to apply the above principles to patient groups and conditions. Chapter 7 starts to look at categories of medicines; the breadth of medicines used for patients with cancer. We feel that this topic is worthy of an overview, so that the scope of medicines available can be identified. Chapter 8 takes an example of one group of patients – the older adult – to explore shared characteristics of a potentially vulnerable group from a physiological and social perspective, before focusing on the needs of individuals.

Part 4 begins to look at medicines management from the perspective of the individual patient/client. Chapters 9–15 present individual patient scenarios. These scenarios enable us to bring together not only the underpinning principles and general characteristics of some medicine groups but also individual patients' needs and responses. We tease out the difficulties inherent in practice when trying to work with patients, educating, advising and reassuring, but also attempting to explain some of the inconsistencies in therapeutic approaches that may be experienced in clinical practice.

Part 5 considers the question 'where next?' Chapter 16 investigates some of the current trends in drug/medicine development, whilst Chapter 17 explores two contemporary issues related to nursing roles and responsibilities.

HOW TO USE THIS BOOK

This book has been written for first-year student nurses undertaking the Foundation year of an adult-oriented pre-registration nursing programme, although we anticipate that it will be useful for all nursing students and newly qualified staff. The book is the first of its kind in that it provides the reader with a model for understanding medicine information and the implications of medicine administration in practice. Whilst other pharmacology books attempt to link theory to practice, this book takes a number of practice scenarios and teases out the information that the nurse will require. Thus, it not only uncovers pharmacological knowledge such as pharmacokinetics and pharmacodynamics, but also discusses the legal implications such as drug legislation, and the professional implications, such as Nursing and Midwifery Council guidance, adherence and consent. The book reveals the theory that underpins practice, which often in nursing appears almost invisible.

With this in mind, we have made this book as interactive as possible. Each chapter begins with learning outcomes so that you are very clear of the content and our expectations of what we feel you will learn by reading the chapter.

It might be that you will want to dip in and out of the book, choosing the part that is relevant to you at the time. The learning outcomes will help you identify this. However, because this book uses an integrative approach to pharmacology for nursing care, some key concepts and issues are to be found within the context of the patient scenarios rather than as stand-alone sections of information. This technique also allows us to revisit important concepts such as adherence/concordance and patient education from the individual patient perspective, so reinforcing the need for the development of skills such as problem-solving, decision-making and clinical judgement in response to differing situations.

A variety of features are used throughout the book:

- *Chapter at a glance:* This is an overview of the chapter content that reflects a range of perspectives, normal and altered physiology, medicines used, nursing implications, and patient and professional guidance/issues.

- *Essential terminology (definition of terms)*: Unfortunately, any discussion about pharmacology will generate unfamiliar terminology. There is a whole new language to learn when beginning nursing, whether related to conditions and diseases or specific to a subject such as physiology, as well as the terminology we use to describe specific aspects of care delivery such as routes of administration and equipment. These boxes provide a succinct definition not only to aid your understanding of the text but also to flag up any learning needs.

- *Related knowledge*: This gives an outline of the knowledge required to understand the discussion, which may be pharmacological or physiological or related to other disciplines such as psychology or sociology. This may also highlight an area of your knowledge base that may need further development.

- *Pharmacodynamics*: The study of drug actions.

- *Pharmacokinetics*: The study of drug actions within the body.

These two boxes provide information related to the specific medication under discussion in an attempt to apply general theory to specific examples.

- *In reality*: This reflects the differences and/or tensions between theory and practice that novice nurses can experience but find difficult to understand.
- *Quick reminder*: Chapter summaries are provided at the end of each chapter to enable a quick review of the information covered.
- *References*.
- *Glossary of terms*: Terms introduced for the first time appear with explanations at the end of the book.

There are also a range of interactive features:

- *Using pharmacological information - the nurse's role*: This is an opportunity to reflect upon the given information and to tease out the consequences of this information for the patient/client being discussed.
- *Nursing knowledge*: This identifies specific nursing knowledge/theory needed to understand the discussion.
- *Nursing implications*: It is important that pharmacological interventions are seen as only one aspect of care; pain relief, for example, can be enhanced by the careful moving and handling of a patient after surgery. Also, some pharmacological interventions such as chemotherapy may require supportive nursing interventions. These supporting nursing strategies not only help to remind you of this but also complete the picture, consistent with the delivery of holistic and individualised care.
- *Personal and professional development*: An essential part of any textbook for nurses, these activities involve you in linking theory to practice. They generate theory from practice related to your personal and ongoing learning needs. These activities become more complex and demanding as the book (and your knowledge and understanding) progresses.

CONCLUSION

Throughout this book, we introduce you to a way of learning about pharmacological interventions that involves not only knowledge about how drugs and medicines work but also the professional issues and patient factors that need to be taken into account to ensure safety and confidence for both you and the patient. You can then apply this approach to new situations, patient groups and clinical contexts as you continue in your nursing programme and then as a qualified nurse.

REFERENCES

Askew S (2003) Learning promotes health. *Education and Health* **21**, 68–71.

Bransford J D, Franks J J, Vye N J and Sherwood R D (1989) New approaches to instruction: because wisdom can't be told. In: Vosniadou S and Ortony A (eds) *Similarity and Analogical Reasoning*. Cambridge: Cambridge University Press.

Chapelhow C, Crouch S, Fisher M and Walsh A (2005) *Uncovering Skills for Practice*. Cheltenham: Nelson Thornes.

Department of Health (DH) (2000) *The NHS Plan: A Plan for Investment, a Plan for Reform*. London: The Stationery Office.

Department of Health (DH) (2001) *The Expert Patient: A New Approach to Chronic Disease Management for the 21st Century*. London: The Stationery Office.

Department of Health (DH) (2002a) *Liberating the Talents: Helping Primary Care Trusts and Nurses to Deliver the NHS Plan*. London: The Stationery Office.

Department of Health (DH) (2002b) *Developing Key Roles for Nurses and Midwives: A Guide for Managers*. London: The Stationery Office.

Eraut M, Alderton J, Cole G and Senker P (2000) Development of knowledge and skills at work. In:

Coffield F (ed.) *Differing Visions of a Learning Society*, Vol. 1. Bristol: Polity Press.

James J, Baker C and Swain H L (2002) *Principles of Science for Nurses*. Oxford: Blackwell Publishing.

King R L (2004) Nurses' perceptions of their pharmacology education needs. *Journal of Advanced Nursing* **45**, 393–400.

Lave J and Wenger E (1991) *Situated Learning: Legitimate Peripheral Participation*. Cambridge: Cambridge University Press.

Manias S and Bullock E (2002) The educational preparation of undergraduate nursing students in pharmacology: clinical nurses' perceptions and experiences of graduate nurses' medication knowledge. *International Journal of Nursing Studies* **39**, 773–784.

Vygotsky L S, Cole M, John-Steiner V, Scribner S and Souberman E (1978) *Mind in Society: Development of Higher Psychological Processes*, 14th edn. Harvard, MA: Harvard University Press.

Welsh Institute for Health and Social Care (1998) *Healthcare Futures 2010*. Pontypridd: UKCC Education Commission.

Wenger E (1998) *Communities of Practice, Learning, Meaning and Identity*. Cambridge: Cambridge University Press.

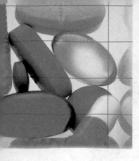

Acknowledgements

Our heartfelt thanks go to the many people who have helped and supported us in the writing of this book: the many students and clinical staff whose discussions have stimulated our further understandings of this complex area; our families and friends for helping us stick with it.

The continued love and support of our immediate families: they'll never appreciate how much this meant to us during the whole process.

There are also a number of colleagues who patiently listened and went the extra mile for us. We would particularly like to thank Peter Kerry, Chris Corkish, David Prior, Jane Douglas, Helen Pilkington and Peter Walsham, both for their expertise and for renewing our faith in ourselves and this project.

PUBLISHER'S ACKNOWEDGEMENTS

We would like to thank the reviewers for their comments:

Susan Anderson, University of Central Lancashire
Nicky Burns, University of Gloucestershire
Richelle Duffy, University of Derby
Jane Feetham, University of the West of England
Vincent Finn, University of Huddersfield
Jan Gill, Queen Margaret University Edinburgh
Gerri Kaufman, University of York
Jenny Kelly, University of East Anglia
Ehsan Khan, King's College London
John Ross, University of Bedfordshire
Katherine Sains, University of Essex
Martin Steggall, City University London
David Voegeli, University of Southampton

We are grateful to the following for permission to reproduce copyright material:

Figures 4.2 and 4.5 from *Applied Pharmacology: an introduction to pathophysiology and drug management for nurses and health care professionals* (Prosser, S., Worster, B., MacGregor, J., Dewar, K., Runyard, P. and Fegan 2002) © Elsevier 2002; Figures 4.4, 4.7, 4.8 and 4.11 from *Illustrated Pharmacology for Nurses* (Simonsen, T. *et al.*, illustrator Roy Lysaa 2006) published by Edward Arnold. Reproduced by permission of Roy Lysaa and Edward Arnold (Publishers) Ltd; Figure 4.6 from *Physiology for Nursing Practice* (Hinchliff, S.M., Montague, S.E. and Walton, R 1996) © Elsevier 1996; Figure 4.10 from *Pharmacology for Midwives* reproduced with permission of Palgrave Macmillan (Jordan, S. 2002); Figure 5.1 from nuth.nhs.uk; Figure 7.1 from *The Biology of Cancer* © John Wiley & Sons Limited. Reproduced with permission (Gabriel, J. 2004); Figure 7.2 from *The Biological Basis of Nursing: cancer*, (Blows, W.T. 2005) Routledge; Figure 7.4 from *Cancer Pain Relief* published by the World Health Organization 1986; Table 9.1 Overview of the characteristics and symptoms of osteoarthritis and rheumatoid arthritis from *Nursing Standard* 25 August 2004, Vol.18, No. 50 p.44, RCN Publishing Company; Figure 10.3 from *Physiology for Health Care and Nursing* (Kindlen, S. 2003) © Elsevier 2003; Figures 10.4, 10.5 and 10.6 and extract on pp. 478-9 from *Pharmacology and Medicines Management for Nurses* (Downie, G., Mackenzie, J. and Williams, A. 2003) © Elsevier 2003; Table 15.1 from *British Guideline on the Management of Asthma*, 2008, with permission from the British Thoracic Society; Figure 15.3 A Step Management Plan from the BTS/SIGN Asthma Guidelines 2005; Extract on p. 445 from *Death by Indifference* (Mencap, 2007); Table 17.1 from Reports in the NRLS database, The National Patient Safety Agency; Figure 17.2 The Prescribing Pyramid from *Nurse Prescribing Bulletin* (1999) Vol. 1, No. 1, National Prescribing Centre.

Extract on p. 30 from *Trounce's Clinical Pharmacology for Nurses* (Greenstein, B. and Gould, D. 2004); extract on p. 37 from *Oxford Handbook of Clinical Pharmacy*, By permission of Oxford University Press (Wiffen, P., Mitchell, M. and Snelling, M.N. 2007); extract on p. 297 from *Davidson's Principles and Practices of Medicine* 20th edition (Boon, N.A., Colledge, N.R., Walker, B.A. and Hunter, J.A.A. 2006) © Elsevier 2006; extract on p. 303 from *Annals of Emergency Medicine* (Gallagher, E,J., Esses, D., Lee, C., Lahn, M. and Bijur, P.E. 2006) © Elsevier 2006; extracts on p. 320 from *Pain: A Clinical Manual* (McCaffrey *et al.*, pp. 267-70, 50; 173-174, 54-56, 1999) © Elsevier 1999; extract on p. 347 from The Alzheimer's Society Real Lives Project; extract on pp. 348-9 from *Everyday Memory* (Magnussen, S. and Helstrup, T.) Psychology Press; extract on p. 350 Stages of dementia from *The Cambridge Examination for Mental Disorders of the Elderly: CAMDEX* 1st edition (Roth, M. Huppert, F.A., Tym, E., Mountjoy, C.Q., Diffident-Brown, A. and Shoesmith, D.J. 1988) Cambridge University Press; extract on p. 368 from *CG 34 Hypertension: management of hypertension in adults in primary care* (Quick Reference Guide) with permission from NICE; extract on p. 445 from *Death by indifference*, p. 20, with permission from Mencap.

In some instances we have been unable to trace the owners of copyright material, and we would appreciate any information that would enable us to do so.

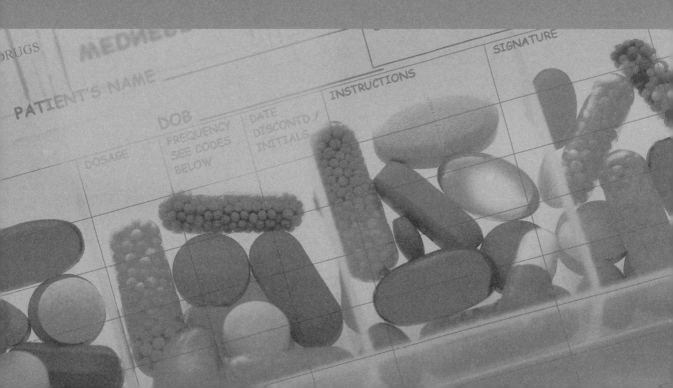

Part 1

Setting the scene

Chapter 1

The context of medicines management for adult nurses in today's NHS

A dult nurses working in the NHS have an increasing number of responsibilities in relation to prescribed medicines. Over the years these responsibilities have become more complex, with increasing amounts of time spent in fulfilling this role. One of the reasons for this is that healthcare is becoming ever more complex and frequently more expensive with our increasing understanding of how the body functions and technological advances. There have been calls for more effective medicines management to be recognised and addressed. Indeed, the Healthcare Commission (2007) highlighted research evidence in relation to hospital care when it stated that effective medicines management 'reduces lengths of stay and rates of re-admission'. Given this requirement, it is important to recognise the main factors that influence effective medicines management from a nursing perspective. As a result, this chapter explores the changing nature of care in the twenty-first century. The key issues that are examined are lifestyle factors, altering **demographics**, increased migration, **co-morbidity**, increasing public expectations, and the innovations and developing technology that affect us all in some way and that are influencing the shape of the role that adult nurses play in medicines management in today's NHS.

✔ Learning outcomes

By the end of this chapter you should be able to:

✔ Describe the key sociopolitical developments that have led to the developing role of the adult nurse

✔ Identify clinical situations that require medicines management skills

✔ Discuss the key nursing developments that have resulted from changes in the NHS

✔ Discuss how developing technology and innovations will demand increasingly sophisticated medicines management skills.

Chapter at a glance

Recent influences on health in the UK
Factors influencing the development of adult nursing
Cultural transformation in the NHS
The rise of self-medication
Complementary medicinal products
Over-the-counter medicines and their relevance to nursing
Changing role of the adult nurse
Continuing spread of non-medical prescribing
Developing technology and innovations
Adverse drug reactions
Impact of new knowledge and understanding on the nurse's role in medicines
    management
Changing medicine administration processes
Evidence-based practice
Quick reminder
References

RECENT INFLUENCES ON HEALTH IN THE UK

The demographic of the UK is changing. Increasing numbers of people are living longer, and consequently many of them are living with co-morbidities. Alongside this, large numbers of people from countries all over the world are working in the UK temporarily or migrating to the UK. Public attitudes have changed, and people now have greater expectations of the services and commodities that they buy and use; consequently, the expectations that individuals have about healthcare providers have changed too. In the first decade of the twenty-first century, we have lifestyles that are very different from the way people lived even 25 years ago. Much of this lifestyle change is a response to innovation and technology. For example, more of us use cars regularly rather than walk or cycle, few of us grow much of our own food, very few of us have jobs that are physically demanding, and many of us regularly take holidays in countries with a very high sun index or with endemic diseases such as salmonella, tuberculosis, human immunodeficiency virus (HIV)/acquired immunodeficiency syndrome (AIDS), malaria and typhoid. As a result of more accessible travel, the UK, along with many other European countries, probably has a much more multicultural population than it has ever had before. Throughout history, the UK has become home to a variety of immigrant populations. However, until recently, those who came in any number were predominantly from countries relatively close by, as travel for most of the world's population was both difficult and expensive. In the past 30 years or so, travel has become much easier and considerably cheaper. As a result, the UK supports large numbers of people from all over the world. Some of these people bring health problems with them, such as tuberculosis. Many others adopt a Western lifestyle, which increases their risk of metabolic syndrome, hypertension, diabetes, coronary heart disease and stroke.

All of these events, many of them quite small in themselves, have changed and continue to reshape healthcare both in the UK and in the rest of the industrialised world. An integral part of the provision of healthcare is the prescription of medicines, which, until recently, was purely in order to help treat and manage a variety of diseases and disorders.

The rationale for the medicines management strategy in the NHS

Today, however, healthcare professionals frequently prescribe medicines not only to treat and manage ill-health but also as a preventive measure or to enhance what used to be seen as lifestyle difficulties, such as obesity, erectile dysfunction and smoking cessation. Nothing in life is risk-free, however, and many people take both prescribed and non-prescribed medicines 'because it's believed that the benefits will outweigh the associated risks' (Healthcare Commission, 2007). It is important, therefore, that any risks of medicines are minimised as much as possible. This has resulted in the introduction of the policy of medicines management in the NHS, which is an essential part of a process that ensures not only that individual patient care is both successful and safe but also that the taxpayer gets value for money (Healthcare Commission, 2007).

The NHS will celebrate its sixtieth anniversary in July 2008. This anniversary may be used as an opportunity to reflect on and celebrate the organisation's successes, which are too numerous to list here. However, there is no doubt that the anniversary will be also used to highlight the NHS's failures in delivering healthcare to the people of the UK. Most of this criticism seems to be fuelled because of the early promises offered by the guiding principle so widely publicised when the NHS was first established: that everyone would receive all of their medical, dental and nursing care, free of charge, at the point of delivery. This seems to have encouraged the assumption that healthcare would be both comprehensive and universal, with unlimited healthcare free at the point of delivery. Unfortunately, for a variety of reasons, including lack of comprehension of what the true cost of such a service would be, increasing public demands and little recognition that medicine would advance in the way that it has, these founding principles have long been quietly abandoned by all of the UK governments since the establishing of the NHS (Klein, 2006; Ranade, 1997). From the 1940s to the 1960s most of the advances in the health of the population were not a direct result of the NHS but were due to a raft of social measures, such as improved housing and sanitation, clean running water, improved diet, better dental hygiene and immunisation and vaccination programmes. The years since the inception of the NHS have seen improving health. During this time, there have been many changes both in the NHS and in adult nursing: nowhere is this more evident than in what we think of today as medicines management. Certainly, even before the advent of the NHS, the administration of medicines was an important part of the adult nurse's role, particularly for nurses working in hospital wards and certain hospital departments such as accident and emergency (A&E). For nurses working in the community and attached to schools and workplaces, medicines management was a less important role, although these nurses did need a sound understanding of the medicines prescribed for their patients so that they could educate their patients. Although administration is a key part of the role of many adult nurses today, this role, along with many others, has changed and is still changing, and it can no longer be identified as the only role and responsibility that nurses have in relation to medicines management.

FACTORS INFLUENCING THE DEVELOPMENT OF ADULT NURSING

There is no doubt that the underlying knowledge and skill of adult nurses in the UK has changed considerably over the previous three centuries, and their values, beliefs, attitudes and images have changed too (Hallett, 2007). Hallett argues that nurses are now in what she calls the 'technocratic era'. This is because over the years nurses have taken on more procedural skills, such as venous **cannulation**, that were once perceived to be the skills that lay firmly within the discipline of medicine. Nursing cannot be separated from the society within which it operates, and UK society has altered markedly over recent decades. Today, some of the expectations that patients and healthcare professionals have about healthcare are very different from those of even just 25 years ago. There has been considerable social and cultural change during this time; there have also been a variety of political drivers that have influenced not only the way the NHS operates but also the development of nursing. These political changes appear to have been attempts to address the agendas of each of the more recent governments, challenging the power of the medical profession and attempting to contain the ever-rising cost of health services while at the same time attempting to increase the health of the population as a whole (Klein, 2006, 2007; Pollock, 2005; Ranade, 1997). These drivers have had a major influence on how adult nursing has developed, because in order to deliver these various agendas nurses and nursing have been key targets for many of these changes (DH, 2006a). The Department of Health (DH) has set up a strategy group whose sole purpose and remit is that of modernising nursing careers (DH, 2006b). This group recognises the changes that have happened to date and claims that it will propose further opportunities for change, which perhaps will be linked to the Knowledge and Skills Framework and the Agenda for Change. However, as discussed later in this chapter, both the Agenda for Change, which introduced new contracts for nurses and non-clinical staff in the NHS, and the other contractual changes brought in for medical consultants and GPs have come in for criticism (Buchan and Evans, 2007; Wanless *et al.*, 2007). Many of the developments and changes in the NHS that have happened over the past decade have been a result of a major political strategy taken when the Labour government was first elected to power in 1997 (DH, 1997). This strategy has been ongoing since then, and it has been announced that an internationally renowned, London-based surgeon, Lord Dazi, will lead another major review of the NHS, entitled 'Our NHS, Our Future'. This new vision for a twenty-first-century NHS will be 'a once-in-a-generation opportunity to ensure that a properly resourced NHS is clinically led, patient-centred and locally accountable' (Alan Johnson, Secretary of State, **www.ournhs.nhs.uk**.

This desire by the Labour Party to have a health service fit for the twenty-first-century was on its agenda from 1996, before they were elected to government in 1997, and has resulted in the NHS seeing regular major investment by UK taxpayers (DH, 2000). During this time, the UK's spending on health has increased each year and is now almost £100 billion per year (NHS Confederation, 2007), similar to that found in each of the countries in the European Union. This money seems to have been spent on improving access to and enhancing the quality of the services provided. This has resulted in major changes in the way the NHS is structured and the creation of some notable institutions, such as the National Institute for Health and Clinical Excellence (NICE) and the Healthcare Commission. The main aim of these changes was to bring about higher standards of care and a more consistent and equitable service. It was hoped that this would result in not only a more efficient service fit for the twenty-first century but also a move away from an NHS that was frequently criticised as being designed around the professionals (providers) rather than the patients (users) (Dixon, 2007; Klein, 2006, 2007; Pollock, 2005; Ranade, 1997). However, the transformation of the NHS from a public body that has long been seen by many as inefficient and ineffective to one that is accessible, proactive and truly patient-focused still seems to be very much in development and there are a number of challenges for the NHS that are yet to be addressed. Dixon (2007) suggests that there are three major challenges:

- maintaining the large and increasing numbers of people living with long-term conditions and reducing their reliance on expensive hospital care;
- encouraging people to safeguard their own health;
- a continued need to reconfigure services that will deliver both greater throughput and better value for money for the taxpayer.

CULTURAL TRANSFORMATION IN THE NHS

Much of the change that has happened since the Labour government came to power in 1997 has attempted to alter the culture of the NHS so that it is more responsive to patient needs, being patient-led rather than professionally led and providing more personalised care. It has also tried to empower patients to help them become both active and equal partners in their care (DH, 2001) rather than passive recipients of care (Playl and Keeley, 1998). The philosophy of encouraging patients to work in partnership with healthcare professionals endeavours to give back a sense of control to patients. This idea of empowerment has brought about the introduction of the Expert Patient Programme, with the aim of ensuring that individuals with long-term conditions see a real improvement in their quality of life brought about by understanding and managing their condition rather than having their condition manage them. Underlying this move towards making the service patient-centred is the need for the healthcare professional to have central to their practice a philosophy that considers:

- the patient as a person;
- the biopsychosocial perspective (which considers psychological, social and physical factors);
- the sharing of power and responsibility;
- therapeutic alliance (the healthcare professional working with the patient as an equal) (Mead and Bower, 2000).

Inherent in ensuring that this happens is the need for healthcare professionals to communicate effectively. Fundamental to effective communication is self-awareness: being comfortable with who you are, your attitudes, values, beliefs and culture (Leininger and McFarland, 2002). If the health beliefs of the patient differ greatly from those of the healthcare professional, then this may result in communication breakdown, causing frustration and confusion on both sides. Having knowledge and understanding of 'the self' ensures that the nurse is able not only to impart information to patients about their conditions but also to educate patients and their carers about how best to manage those conditions, including how to use and manage their medications. It also includes recognising how prescribed medicines fit with the potential that the patient may well self-medicate with over-the-counter (OTC) medicines. Teaching patients so that they have enough knowledge to manage their medicines successfully is a demanding development of the adult nurse's role.

THE RISE OF SELF-MEDICATION

Being able to select a nutritional or medicinal product off the shelf that you feel will make you healthier is extremely useful sometimes; for example, many people find it helpful to be able to walk into a shop and buy medicines that will support their motivation to stop smoking. On the other hand, whether certain probiotic drinks and 'superfoods' available OTC improve health is rather dubious. The manufacturers of such products claim that increasing the consumer's ability to self-medicate is a positive thing as it both empowers people and frees up healthcare professionals for more valuable work. However, the sceptical reader may consider this is a cynical drive by many pharmaceutical companies and manufacturers to increase the sales of their products by playing on consumers' fears of poor health. In recent years, the Department of Health has actively supported and promoted the increased use of self-medication by the general public. Many medicines have changed from being categorised as prescription-only medicines (POMs) to being pharmacy (P) or general sales list (GSL) medicines. For example, the statins, drugs used to lower blood cholesterol, which were previously POMs, have been reclassified as P medicines, so anyone can now buy them under the supervision of a pharmacist. A growing number and variety of medicines can be bought in pharmacies, supermarkets, general stores and petrol stations without a prescription. OTC medicines also include many vitamins and herbal preparations.

COMPLEMENTARY MEDICINAL PRODUCTS

When considering herbal medicines, vitamins and superfood supplements, we need to consider the many people who have moved to the UK from elsewhere, whether temporarily or permanently. Different people have different cultural understandings and philosophies of both health and healthcare. As a result, many people in the UK use herbs and medicines that previously were little known or used in this country. Knowledge about the cultural and philosophical backgrounds of our patients is becoming increasingly important for adult nurses. Patients have different backgrounds, experiences, values and beliefs. Understanding the cultural and philosophical context of a patient is relevant to medicines management, as these values and beliefs have the potential to influence a patient's concordance and persistence, while the patient's dietary habits may result in interactions with both traditional and herbal medicines.

Herbal medicines and vitamin and superfood supplements are part of what the Nursing and Midwifery Council (NMC) calls (2006) 'complementary medicinal products'.

OVER-THE-COUNTER MEDICINES AND THEIR RELEVANCE TO NURSING

It is often suggested that this ever-increasing market of medicines not only encourages people to self-care but also leads many people to believe that these medicines are generally safe because they are so freely available (Bond and Hannaford, 2003; Hughes *et al.*, 2002; Murcott, 2005). Encouraging people to accept some responsibility for the management of a variety of disorders and consequently become more self-sufficient is seen as a positive development (Aronson, 2004), although studies such as that of Hughes *et al.* (2002) have highlighted that most people have little understanding of their OTC purchases.

Nurses need to be aware of this increased use of OTC medicines and recognise that many of the individuals they care for may be taking OTC medicines. Nurses are required to be increasingly alert to self-medication, particularly during the assessment process, which means routinely enquiring at each assessment whether the patient takes any OTC medications. Patients often do not mention that they are taking OTC medicines because they consider them to be safe and free from side effects. Nurses may then notice the side effects or interactions of these OTCs but not recognise them as such because they are unaware that the patient is taking OTCs.

Many people are now buying medicines from other countries without prescription either when they travel abroad or over the Internet. There is currently little evidence available to show how frequently this happens. Nevertheless, it should always be considered by nurses and other healthcare professionals, as the patient may not realise that symptoms may be related to the use of these medicines.

All of these situations place a greater demand than ever before on the nurse to understand the principles underpinning medicines management. This means developing the skill of pharmacovigilance – being aware of side effects, adverse drug reactions, and potential interactions between medicines (prescribed and OTC), food and drink and other medicines. This does not mean that the nurse should learn these situations 'parrot fashion'. Indeed, trying to learn large amounts of information that may be used only infrequently is not only ineffective but also, from a medicines management perspective, dangerous. Instead, in unfamiliar situations, the nurse needs to know how to access appropriate information, interpret this information and then communicate it appropriately. Recognising how nurses can best manage this needs urgent consideration. Jordan *et al*. (2002) tried to develop a method to assist mental health nurses to reduce the side effects of medicines. Arnold (1998) demonstrated not only the subtle transformation that has been taking place in the role and responsibilities of the nurse towards medicines management but also the real potential for nurses to develop their role in relation to adverse drug reactions and side effects. Role change is nothing new for nurses: they have responded to a number of drivers for change over the years, particularly sociopolitical changes.

CHANGING ROLE OF THE ADULT NURSE

Beginning with the NHS Plan (DH, 2000), a number of DH White Papers have suggested improvements to bring the NHS into the twenty-first century. These plans have identified what the improved service should look like and what patients should expect from the new NHS. The working hours of junior doctors have been radically reduced to bring them into line with the rest of the workforce in the European Union based on the Working Time Directive and a need to introduce the changes to both pre-registration and postgraduate medical education that were proposed in the Calman Report (DH, 1993). It was also felt that the time had come for many of the roles of junior doctors and some more senior medical staff to be passed on to suitable trained nurses. Even as long ago as 1976, following the publication of the Breckenridge Report (Breckenridge, 1976), there was recognition that some nurses were more efficient than many junior doctors in the skill of cannulation. At the same time, changes to the availability of medicines were happening and improved access to medicines was being considered, particularly for patients with long-term conditions who made up the considerable numbers of individuals who fell through Jordan and Hughes' (1996) 'care gap'. As a result of these pressures, a variety of new nursing roles were created in order to achieve the results being demanded of the service. These roles were primarily organised around the ten key roles identified for adult nurses by the then Chief

Nursing Officer (DH, 2002). These roles, which are presented in more detail in Chapter 3 of this book, include diagnosing, prescribing, admitting and discharging patients and running clinics, and included skills that previously were viewed as those of the doctor. Although the new nursing role of prescribing has improved access to medicines for a large number of individuals, it is still considered a major challenge to the power and position of the doctor. These 'new' roles have also been the driver for the development of a strategy group within the DH, Modernising Nursing Careers, to examine the future role of the nurse in the NHS. This group has published its remit and aims, but at the time of writing this book the group's suggestions have not been published. At the same time, two King's Fund reports (Buchan and Evans, 2007; Wanless *et al.*, 2007) have put together rather damning criticism of the enormous costs of implementing Agenda for Change. Buchan and Evans (2007) also state how little NHS trusts have used the Knowledge and Skills Framework to match staff roles when moving staff on to the new pay bands of Agenda for Change. This, they claim, has resulted in both large pay rises and expensive implementation costs but very little overall attempt to ensure that all of the NHS staff change their culture and adopt twenty-first-century working practices. Consequently, Buchan and Evans' report concludes that, despite a large amount of taxpayers' money being spent, there has been no improvement in the service to the patient, despite the rhetoric that promised better patient outcomes. Wanless *et al.* (2007) reach the same conclusion but temper this slightly by suggesting that perhaps a little more time is needed to see any results. They also suggest that where service improvements have been seen, they tend to be piecemeal rather than national.

Unfortunately, it seems that the proposals of Modernising Nursing Careers will come at a time when the large amounts of 'modernisation monies' that have been made available over the past few years come to an end – 2008. What impact this will have is difficult to predict, but it is safe to assume that the nurse's role in medicines management will continue to develop given that Wanless *et al.* (2007) identified that between 2002 and 2006 the number of prescription items being dispensed increased by 25%. At the same time that these criticisms of the service provided by the NHS were published, the Secretary of State for Health announced that another review of the NHS was being undertaken. This review will consider the views of all healthcare professionals, all NHS staff and users of the service, with people being asked to input their views via a website. This review will be reported in 2008, in time to coincide with the sixtieth anniversary of the NHS (**www.ournhs.nhs.uk**). Whether and how this review will change the role of the nurse in relation to medicines management is difficult to predict at this time.

CONTINUING SPREAD OF NON-MEDICAL PRESCRIBING

It has become clear over time that the non-medical prescribing initiative gained impetus for implementation only once it was recognised that using non-medical prescribers could help to plug the gaps in the service by providing what is seen by some as a more efficient and cost-effective provision. Although it was recognised in the Cumberlege Report (DHSS, 1986) that there was a need for such a service, it took a number of years before nurse prescribing was implemented fully. Even today, when non-medical prescribing is thought to be fairly common, there are still only approximately 9000 nurses trained to be independent nurse prescribers and not all are practising (Home Office, 2007). The role that supplementary prescribing plays in the NHS today is frequently not recognised, however. In this situation, nurses and other healthcare professionals work within a clinical management plan that has previously been drawn up and agreed with an independent medical prescriber, a doctor. Compared with independent nurse prescribers, there are greater numbers of nurse supplementary prescribers, working mainly as nurse specialists. The main advantage of supplementary prescribing over independent nurse prescribing is that the former offers a wider range of medicines to patients to manage a broader range of medical conditions.

There has been a strong faction calling for nursing to recognise its holistic roots rather than acknowledging only its more 'scientific' activities such as pharmacological interventions and wound care (Hewitt-Taylor, 2002). The arrival of nurse prescribing has been a demanding change for nurses and seems to have led to improved outcomes for many patients. Not only can nurse prescribing be considered as a valuable strategy that gives better support to service users (Mullally, 2002), but it is also thought to increase the number of people who are adherent with prescribed medicines, which is consistent with current government initiatives (DH, 2002, 2006a; Healthcare Commission, 2007). However, Hewitt-Taylor's (2002) survey suggests that many nurses are concerned about taking responsibility for their prescribing decisions and many feel the need to be reassured that they have the required level of knowledge, understanding and skill to be truly accountable.

A number of commentators (McGavock, 2000; McKenna, 2005; Ramprogus, 2002; Rolfe, 1996) have identified how nursing in the NHS has continually been required to rise to the challenge of a number of political drivers rather than simply develop in the way that most other professions develop according to how the profession itself sees fit. Consequently, a number of new nursing roles have been introduced that extend the functions and skills of the registered nurse into realms that were once seen to be the hallowed ground of medicine, such as prescribing. These developments have caused a split within the nursing profession: many nurses support the new roles, but just as many argue that nursing risks losing its focus and that these developments may cause it to lose its identity (McKenna, 2005). As we mentioned earlier, the number of prescribing nurses is still small, but those that are now able to prescribe independently do so from the *British National Formulary* (BNF) and carry their own caseloads of patients in the same way that doctors do. However, few of these nurses have acquired either the status or the remuneration levels of doctors with similar levels of skill, expertise and experience.

DEVELOPING TECHNOLOGY AND INNOVATIONS

Although nurse prescribing has been one of the more controversial developments to change the role of the adult nurse in relation to medicines management, there are also other developments that are beginning to influence the practice of greater numbers of nurses.

At the same time that the nursing workforce is changing, technology is developing and transforming, often in groundbreaking ways that affect not only how patients are treated but also how their care is managed. One of the areas where this is being felt most is surgery. In all of the surgical specialties, many patients now have non-invasive or minimally invasive surgery, with the result that patient throughput is quicker, patients' recovery time both in the surgical unit and at home is quicker, and patients experience less pain and fewer complications. Many more people now survive major life-threatening events that would have been thought impossible even just a decade ago (DH, 2006a). As a consequence, more people are living with chronic long-term conditions, patients in hospital are frequently sicker and patients generally have briefer hospital stays than before (DH, 2006a). Meanwhile, many of the working environments where adult nurses practise are becoming increasingly technical and using more sophisticated equipment, and knowledge is advancing and information becoming easier to find. Many individuals are now able to access information much more easily. In addition, because an increasingly large proportion of the population has benefited from higher education, many people now have improved skills to critique the information that they find. Interestingly, however, many of the general public remain relatively ignorant about their anatomy and how their body works.

Innovations are also being seen more and more frequently in the area of drug development. New drugs and new ways of targeting existing drugs, such as monoclonal antibodies and inhaled insulin, are the results of pharmaceutical companies continually pushing at the boundaries of knowledge. Cynics suggest that large amounts of money are spent by many pharmaceutical companies on developing and marketing 'lifestyle drugs' aimed at Western consumers. Such drugs may be seen to provide a 'pill for every ill' so that many problems that were once perceived as a lifestyle problem, such as alcohol and drug dependence, obesity and impotence, are now being 'medicalised' (Aronson, 2002; Fitzpatrick, 2005; Illich, 2001; Porter, 2002) and seen as diseases; some go so far as to consider this 'disease-mongering' (Dean and Webb, 2007; Moynihan and Cassels, 2005; Moynihan *et al.* 2002; Payer, 1992). There is even development work under way to produce a medicine to overcome social phobia (Domes *et al.*, 2007). On the other hand, there is little evidence of any real philanthropy given that AIDS drugs are available to relatively few people in Africa, where most of the world's problems with HIV/AIDS lie.

Although this ethical debate is a relevant one for the nurse to consider, it is worth remembering that the development of new medicines and new delivery systems is extremely important to healthcare.

Technology and innovation are also being applied in other healthcare arenas that impact on the nurse's role generally and specifically related to medicines management. Technology is being developed to help manage patient safety more appropriately both from a prescribing and an administrative perspective. The NHS Connecting for Health project, which was tasked with introducing information technology (IT) across the NHS, has a number of strands, some being more advanced in their development than others. The electronic patient record (EPR), electronic prescribing (e-prescribing) and digital X-ray systems (picture archiving and communication systems – PACS) are some of the more advanced strands. Trials are also being carried out using Wireless Fidelity (Wi-Fi) in hospitals to ensure that the correct patient receives the correct operation, tests, treatments and medicines prescribed for them wherever they are in the hospital. Just as you can now access the Internet on your phone or laptop from a 'hotspot', so from strategically placed 'hotspots' patients can be scanned and identified and the pre-scribed surgery, treatment, test or medicines flagged up in some way (National Patient Safety Agency, 2007). There is currently debate over how the NHS can best utilise the rise of the new Web 2.0 links, which could give patients more control over the NHS services that they use.

Everyone in the UK now has the opportunity to have an account with NHS HealthSpace (**www.healthspace.nhs.uk**), which will eventually contain each individual's EPR. At the time of writing, access to your EPR is available only in those areas trialling the system, but all individuals can use NHS HealthSpace for a number of other things, such as booking the hospital of your choice for surgery. Access to EPRs will give users the opportunity to add their own information to enable them to manage their own health; this might include requesting health promotion strategies, text message alerts for appointments for cervical screening, or messages about safe alcohol use. EPRs could be used to help patients manage long-term conditions more effectively or share infor-mation with others.

Developments such as these offer exciting opportunities for nurses to offer individual medication education and for all healthcare professionals to learn about the effects of medications from the patient's perspective. This may help to reduce the number and frequency of adverse drug reactions by flagging up poor prescribing practice by doc-tors and facilitating improvements in concordance and persistence. Given that many people do not persist with taking medicines in the long term, this medium may present better opportunities to understand why.

ADVERSE DRUG REACTIONS

The development of a greater knowledge and understanding of human physiology, par-ticularly in the fields of genetics (the science of genes), proteomics (the science of proteins), neurology (the science of the nervous system) and endocrinology (the science of hormones) and how they are interrelated, is having a major impact on pharmacother-apeutics and is leading to an increased understanding of how many medicines work (e.g.

the discovery of the opioid receptors (Pert, 1999)). This increased knowledge is also highlighting why many people have adverse reactions to some medicines, and why some medicines have no effect in some people, for example those who carry a specific type of a particular gene that makes them resistant to asprin (Goodman *et al.*, 2007). This highlights the need for further research in this area and offers hope for the development of new, more targetable medicines that will travel directly to the site where they are required but will not act in other areas of the body. The latter is an important aim, particularly in the field of cancer treatments.

It has been suggested that nurses can use their understanding of proteomics and pharmacodynamics to observe more efficiently and effectively for adverse drug reactions (Pierce *et al.*, 2007). Proteins control the major processes in cells, and so understanding more fully how proteins work can help nurses to understand how drugs affect the body at a cellular level. Knowing how the physiological processes are affected by biochemical processes will lead to a greater understanding of how the organs of the body function. This will result in the development of a greater understanding of disease processes at a cellular level. Because a large number of drugs prescribed today are directed at proteins, and many drugs are distributed around the body attached to plasma proteins, drugs that are directed more clearly at specific proteins may result in more targeted treatment and more efficient distribution. Proteomics also hints at the possibilities of new drugs.

Nurses who develop an understanding of proteomics can use this skill to carve out a unique new nursing role in detecting and preventing the many adverse drug reactions that occur as a result of polypharmacy (prescribing multiple medicines for one individual) (Arnold, 1998; Pierce *et al.* 2007). The outcomes of adverse drug reactions not only have a financial cost for the NHS but also have a major effect on patients, their families and society in general too. The Audit Commission (2001) estimated that affected patients spent on average an extra 8.5 days in hospital as a result of adverse drug reactions.

The causes of adverse drug reactions are multifactorial (Arnold, 1998; Aronson and Ferner, 2003; Ioannidis *et al.*, 2004; NPSA, 2007; Pierce *et al.* 2007). Common factors include the following:

- Poor prescribing practices, such as prescribing medications that are known to interact with each other.
- Patient's susceptibility to a particular medicine.
- Patient's perceptions of the risks of using medicines.
- Prescriber's perceptions of the risks associated with prescribing particular medicines.
- Lack of healthcare professionals' education in medicines management.
- Medicalisation of health and so-called 'disease-mongering' by pharmaceutical companies (Aronson, 2002; Dean and Webb, 2007; Fitzpatrick, 2000; Illich, 2001; Moynihan and Cassels, 2005; Moynihan *et al.*, 2002; Payer, 1992; Porter, 2002).

Nurses are well placed to recognise and assess the effects of adverse drug reactions as they tend to be the healthcare professionals that spend most time with patients, often engaging with patients intimately (Arnold, 1998). By allying this with a greater understanding of pharmacodynamics, genomics and proteomics, some adult nurses could further develop and change their roles in the future.

IMPACT OF NEW KNOWLEDGE AND UNDERSTANDING ON THE NURSE'S ROLE IN MEDICINES MANAGEMENT

There is no doubt that all branches of nursing have undergone considerable change in the past two decades or so. For adult nurses, this has meant not only changes in the way that many NHS services are delivered but also the development of new roles and responsibilities, such as nurse specialists and nurse consultants. Advances in technology and a greater understanding of how the body works have greatly influenced the treatment and management of some diseases and disorders. This understanding has led not only to the development of new medicines – for example, the statins and the monoclonal antibodies – but also to a better understanding of how many medicines work. Consequently, in order to ensure safe and effective medicines management, nurses have to develop a much greater understanding of normal and disordered physiology, pharmacokinetics and pharmacodynamics, human behaviour, communication, learning and teaching than ever before. An example that demonstrates this clearly is related to the significant growth in the number of people who are classified as overweight or obese. This increase has been blamed on an increasing trend of poor diet and ever-decreasing individual levels of physical activity (European Union, 2007; Wanless et al., 2007).

 Related knowledge The implications of overweight and obese individuals for medicines management

Being overweight or obese is linked with increased morbidity and mortality. It is primarily associated with diseases such as hypertension (high blood pressure), diabetes, coronary heart disease, stroke, some cancers and many musculoskeletal disorders (European Union, 2007). Nurses must consider the potential implications of this from a medicines management perspective. For example, although intramuscular injections are not used commonly in the UK, one major point to consider when treating an overweight patient is whether an intramuscular injection using the standard 19-22 gauge (green) needle actually reaches the muscle from which the medicine is designed to be absorbed. Zaybak and colleagues' (2007) study, while having some limitations, demonstrates that using a standard 19-22 gauge needle for an intramuscular injection into the gluteal muscle of most overweight/obese people will mean that the medicine is injected into adipose tissue (fat) rather than the striated muscle into which it is meant to be deposited. This not only causes pain to the patient but also carries a risk of the patient developing a granuloma and/or a sterile abscess at the injection site (Zaybak *et al.*, 2007). Zaybak *et al.* suggest that nurses should exert their political role and lobby equipment manufacturers to produce needles more suited to the increased amounts of adipose tissue found in overweight and obese people. This example highlights the complexity of the nurse's role in relation to medicines management and the need to apply knowledge and understanding from a variety of disciplines.

It also draws attention to the need for more appropriate equipment. Using inappropriate equipment and maintaining ritualistic practices is an aspect of NHS nursing culture that has been challenged from time to time (Ford and Walsh, 1994; NPSA, 2007; Walsh, 1989; Woodhead, 2000).

Personal and professional development 1.1

Consider whether you would be comfortable lobbying equipment manufacturers to provide more suitable equipment. Is this part of a nurse's role?

In reality

At first thought it would seem that large amounts of adipose tissue in the body would have a considerable impact from a pharmacodynamic perspective, because lipid-soluble drugs are stored in fat cells. However, in reality, because of the lack of water in fat and its poor blood supply, this needs to be considered for relatively few drugs (Rang *et al.*, 2003). Indeed Rang *et al.* (2003) cite only thiopental (an intravenous anaesthetic), the benzodiazepines (tranquillisers) and the regular intake of a type of insecticide, xenobiotics, to be of concern to the prescriber from this perspective.

CHANGING MEDICINE ADMINISTRATION PRACTICES

In both NHS and private hospital wards and departments and in nursing homes, nurses repeatedly carry out the administration of medicines. This is such a time-consuming task for nurses that the Audit Commission (2001) estimated that 40% of ward nurses' time is spent carrying out medicine rounds using a medicine trolley. The administration of medicines has long been, and is likely to remain, a required competency for entry to nursing's professional register (Nursing and Midwifery Council, 2008); as a result, nurses must be not only competent but also confident about their knowledge and skills. It must be recognised, however, that the medicine round is far from being a routine task. Medicine administration is a complicated activity that carries a significant amount of risk, both for the patient and for the nurse (Kapborg, 1994). Carrying out one complex task that requires analysis and decision-making can absorb most of a nurse's available working memory, leaving little memory for other thinking (Sohn and Doane, 2003). It is often the expectation, however, that a nurse administering medicines also maintains the work of the ward. For example, the nurse administering medicines may be expected to take phone calls, deal with verbal enquiries unrelated to the medicines that they are administering, or help with some aspect of direct care for another patient. Unfortunately, many nurses in the UK have long been, and continue to be, socialised to ensure that some kind of service to patients continues whether safe for patients or not (Audit Commission, 2001; Ford and Walsh, 1994; Healthcare Commission, 2007; NPSA, 2004; Walsh, 1989). The National Patient Safety Agency (NPSA) (2004) has recognised that, in order to safeguard patients, medicine rounds, must not be interrupted by day-to-day activities. It has been suggested that hospital patients who are able to administer their own medicines should be enabled to do so. Despite this being one of the major recommendations of the Audit Commission report in 2001, by 2007 the Healthcare Commission (2007) reported that only 19.5% of the wards qualified to implement self-administration had done so. The risk of making a mistake increases dramatically when a nurse is unable to concentrate on the task in hand.

The DH (2004b) estimated that the financial impact of medication errors felt by NHS hospitals was between £200 million and £400 million per year. In addition to these financial costs, costs are also borne by patients, their familes, healthcare professionals and society in general. Medication errors increase the time spent in hospital, causing inconvenience and anxiety for patients and preventing other people from being admitted.

Although the administration of medicines is an important part of the role of many adult nurses, the causes of medication errors are complex and can also involve other healthcare professionals.

The reasons for medication errors are explored in more detail in Chapter 17. These reasons include:

● prescription errors;
● workload and staffing issues;
● environment;
● equipment;
● calculation difficulties.

EVIDENCE-BASED PRACTICE

All healthcare professionals in today's NHS are expected to base their care delivery on rigorous evidence rather than ritual or tradition. Nowhere is this more important than in medicines management. Today there is a wealth of evidence available for nurses to use to inform their medicine management skills. However, this presents some difficulties for many nurses:

- In order to be able to use evidence, nurses have to be able not only to discriminate between what may be conflicting evidence but also to evaluate the quality of the evidence.

- Although much of the evidence used by prescribers is derived from randomised controlled trials and is firmly rooted in the 'harder' scientific methods of quantitative research philosophy, there are also other sources of evidence derived from the 'softer' sciences of qualitative methodologies, such as seeking patients' views. Nurses must be familiar with using a wider base of evidence, retrieving and using information from a variety of sources in order to strengthen their clinical decision-making (Chapelhow *et al*. 2005).

- There is a need to reorganise the working day of the qualified nurse in order to allow 'protected time' to research the reliable and valid information that a nurse needs to ensure that their practice remains up-to-date.

We must also bear in mind that randomised controlled trials and users' experiences are not the only evidence that we can use. Many medicines have been used for centuries and much is known about their effects, even if we are unsure how or why they produce these effects. Much of this knowledge has been garnered by painstaking observation and documentation of these observations and sharing them for wider discussion and debate. Perhaps the use of recognised facilities such as NHS HealthSpace to support such debate would be invaluable for nurses to develop their role in medicines management. Being involved more intimately with individual patients would seem to present an ideal opportunity for the nurse to build on their understanding, so developing their knowledge and skills and enabling professional growth.

As we have seen, a number of factors are changing the roles and responsibilities of the adult nurse in medicines management. These factors include a greater understanding of how medicines work and how they interact not only with other medicines but also with food and drink; the introduction of new medicines and new medicine forms; the rise of self-medication; the impact of technology and innovation; and sociopolitical change. Not only has the role of the adult nurse changed, but it is also continuing to develop and probably will for the foreseeable future. However, the process of change may be easier for some people than for others. Many people across the nursing hierarchy are comfortable with their familiar routines and working practices and rarely challenge them. Although change is recognised to be a healthy dynamic of any organisation, there is little doubt that to some individuals daring to change working practices often means discomfort and uncertainty and consequently appears to makes the job more difficult. Trefino (1997) suggests that some nurses find this too uncomfortable and consequently cannot rise to the challenge.

Quick reminder

✔ In 2008 the NHS will have been in existence for 60 years. Although there is much in its history to be proud of, the NHS has many critics.

✔ Since the inception of the NHS, UK society has changed considerably. It has become more multicultural, and many people living in the UK have philosophies of health and healing that may not be the same as those underpinning mainstream Western medicine.

✔ Patients' expectations have changed to reflect the society in which the NHS operates.

✔ The role of the nurse in the NHS has changed rapidly over the past 10-15 years as nursing responds to a number of different drivers, including the political masters of the NHS, individuals' enthusiasm to provide an improved service and professional leadership.

✔ A number of strategies have been introduced in an attempt to address failing services and the varying delivery of services across the UK, including a variety of treatment guidelines such as National Service Frameworks.

✔ We have a greater understanding of how the body works, including recognition that the body and mind can no longer be regarded as separate entities.

✔ Pharmacological research has led to the development of many new drugs and families of drugs and to a greater understanding of how some drugs work at a cellular level.

✔ The 'information explosion' means that people are becoming increasingly more knowledgeable.

✔ Encouraging and supporting patient concordance and adherence is a key role of the nurse. Nurses must be able to engage in partnership with patients and to teach patients how to maximise the benefits of medicines prescribed for them. This means having a greater range of skills. Consequently, like other professionals, nurses are expected to engage in lifelong learning.

REFERENCES

Arnold G J (1998) Clinical recognition of adverse drug reactions: obstacles and opportunities for the nursing profession. *Journal of Nursing Care Quality* **13**, 2, 45-55.

Aronson J K (2002) When I use a word ... medicalisation. *British Medical Journal* **324**, 904.

Aronson J K (2004) Editor's view: over-the-counter medicines. *British Journal of Clinical Pharmacology* **3**, 231-234.

Aronson J K and Ferner R E (2003) Joining the DoTS: new approach to classifying adverse drug reactions. *British Medical Journal* **327**, 1222-1225.

Audit Commission (2001) *A Spoonful of Sugar: Medicines Management in NHS Hospitals*. Wetherby: Audit Commission Publications.

Bond C and Hannaford P (2003) Issues related to monitoring the safety of over-the-counter (OTC) medicines. *Drug Safety* **26**, 1065-1074.

Breckenridge A (1976) *Report of the Working Party on the Addition of Drugs to Intravenous Infusion Fluids*. London: Department of Health and Social Security

Buchan J and Evans D (2007) *Realising the Benefits? Assessing the Implementation of Agenda for Change*. London: King's Fund.

Chapelhow C, Crouch S, Fisher M and Walsh A (2005) *Uncovering Skills for Practice*. Cheltenham: Nelson Thornes.

Dean J W and Webb D J (2007) Disease mongering: a challenge for everyone involved in healthcare. *British Journal of Clinical Pharmacology* **64**, 122-124.

Department of Health (DH) (1993) *Hospital Doctors: Training for the Future*. London: HMSO.

Department of Health (DH) (1997) *The New NHS: Modern and Dependable* (CM 3807). London: The Stationery Office.

Department of Health (DH) (2000) *The NHS Plan: A Plan for Investment, A Plan for Reform*. London: The Stationery Office.

Department of Health (DH) (2001) *The Expert Patient: A New Approach to Chronic Disease Management for the 21st Century*. London: The Stationery Office.

Department of Health (DH) (2002) *Developing Key Roles for Nurses and Midwives: A Guide for Managers*. London: The Stationery Office.

Department of Health (DH) (2004a) *Improving Chronic Disease Management*. London: The Stationery Office.

Department of Health (DH) (2004b) *Building a Safer NHS for Patients: Improving Medication Safety*. London: The Stationery Office.

Department of Health (DH) (2006a) *Our Choice, Our Health, Our Say: A New Direction for Community Services*. **www.dh.gov.uk** (accessed 7 February 2006).

Department of Health (DH) (2006b) *Modernising Nursing Careers: Setting the Direction*. **www.dh.gov.uk/enPublicationsandstatistics/Publications/PublicationsPolicyandGuidance/DH_4138756**

Department of Health and Social Security (DHSS) (1986) *Neighbourhood Nursing: A Focus for Care. Report of the Community Nursing Review*. London: HMSO.

Dixon N (2007) *Health Challenges for New Labour Leadership*. London: King's Fund.

Domes G, Heinrichs, M, Michel A, Berger C and Herpetz S (2007) Oxytocin improves mind reading in humans. *Biological Psychiatry* **61**, 731-733.

European Union (2007) *A Strategy for Europe on Nutrition, Overweight and Obesity Related Health Issues*. **www.ec.europa.eu/health/**

Fitzpatrick M (2000) *The Tyranny of Health: Doctors and the Regulation of Lifestyle*. London: Routledge.

Fitzpatrick M (2005) Selling sickness: how drug companies are turning us all into patients (Review). *British Medical Journal* **331**, 701.

Ford P and Walsh M (1994) *New Rituals for Old: Nursing Through the Looking Glass*. Oxford: Butterworth Heinemann.

Goodman T, Sharma P and Ferro A (2007) The genetics of aspirin resistance. *International Journal of Clinical Practice* **61**, 826-834.

Hallett C (2007) Editorial: a gallop through history - nursing in social context. *Journal of Clinical Nursing* **16**, 429-430.

Healthcare Commission (2007) *The Best Medicine: The Management of Medicines in Acute and Specialist Trusts*. London: Commission for Healthcare Audit and Inspection.

Hewitt-Taylor J (2002) Evidence-based practice. *Nursing Standard* **17**, 47-52.

Home Office (2007) *Independent Prescribing of Controlled Drugs by Nurse and Pharmacist Independent Prescribers* (closed consultation).**www.homeoffice.gov.uk/documents/cons-2007-ind-pres?view=Binary**.

Hughes L, Whittlesea C and Luscombe D (2002) Patients' knowledge and perceptions of the side effects of OTC medication. *Journal of Clinical Pharmacy and Therapeutics* **27**, 243-248.

Illich I (2001) *Limits to Medicine: Medical Nemesis - The Expropriation of Health*. London: Marion Boyars Publishers.

Ioannidis J P, Evans S J, Gotzsche P C, O'Neill R T, Altman D G, Schultz K and Moher D (2004) Better reporting of harms in randomised controlled trials: and extension of the CONSORT statement. *Annals of Internal Medicine* **141**, 781-788.

Jordan S and Hughes D (1996) Bioscience knowledge and the health professions: has professional monopoly created a care gap? *Social Sciences in Health* **2**, 80-84.

Jordan S, Tunnicliffe C and Sykes A (2002) Minimising side effects: the clinical impact of nurse-administered 'side effect 'checklist. *Journal of Advanced Nursing* **37**, 155-165.

Kapborg I D (1994) Calculation and administration of drug dosage by Swedish nurses, student nurses and physicians. *International Journal of Quality in Health Care* **6**, 389-395.

Klein R (2006) *The Politics of the NHS: From Creation to Reinvention*, 5th edn. Oxford. Radcliffe Publishing.

Klein R (2007) Rationing in the NHS. *British Medical Journal* **334**, 1068.

Leininger M and McFarland M R (2002) *Transcultural Nursing: Concepts, Theories, Research and Practice*, 3rd edn. New York: McGraw Hill.

McGavock H (2000) My grave concern over nurse prescribing. *Prescriber* **11**, 45.

McKenna, H (2005) Commentary: dynamic effects of nursing roles with changing healthcare services. *Journal of Research in Nursing* **10**, 99-106.

Mead N and Bower P (2000) Patient-centredness: a conceptual framework and review of the empirical literature. *Social Science and Medicine* **51**, 1087-1110.

Moynihan R and Cassels A (2005) *Selling Sickness: How Drug Companies Are Turning Us All into Patients*. Crows Nest, Australia: Allen & Unwin.

Moynihan R, Heath I and Henry D (2002) Selling sickness: the pharmaceutical industry and disease mongering. *British Medical Journal* **324**, 886-891.

Mullally S (2002) Nurses of all levels can improve patients' experience of health care. *British Journal of Nursing* **11**, 424.

Murcott T (2005) *The Whole Story: alternative medicine on trial?* Basingstoke: Macmillan.

National Patient Safety Agency (NPSA) (2004) *Seven Steps to Patient Safety: An Overview Guide for NHS Staff.* **www.npsa.nhs.co.uk/patientsafety/improvingpatientsafety/7steps/**

National Patient Safety Agency (NPSA) (2007) *Safety in Doses: Improving the Use of Medicines in the NHS.* **www.npsa.nhs.uk/patientsafety/medication-zone/reviews-of-medication-incidents/**

NHS Confederation (2007) *From the Ground Up: How Autonomy Could Deliver a Better NHS*. London: NHS Confederation.

Nursing and Midwifery Council (2008) *Standards for Medicines Management*. London: Nursing and Midwifery Council. **www.nmc-uk.org/aFrameDisplay.aspx?DocumentID=4092**.

Nursing and Midwifery Council (NMC) (2006) *Standards of Proficiency for Nurse and Midwife Prescribers*. London: Nursing and Midwifery Council.

Payer L (1992) *Disease Mongers: How Doctors, Drug Companies and Insurers are Making You Feel Sick*. New York: John Wiley & Sons.

Pert C (1999) *The Molecules of Emotion*. London: Pocket Books.

Pierce J D, Fakhari M, Works K V and Pierce J T (2007) Understanding proteomics. *Nursing and Health Sciences* **9**, 54-60.

Playl J and Keeley P (1998) Non-compliance and professional power. *Journal of Advanced Nursing* **27**, 304-311.

Pollock A M (2005) *The NHS plc: the Privatisation of our Healthcare*. London: Verso Books.

Porter R (2002) *Blood and Guts: A Short History of Medicine*. London: Allen Lane.

Ramprogus V (2002) Eliciting nursing knowledge from practice: the dualism of nursing. *Nurse Researcher* **10**, 52-64.

Ranade W (1997) *A Future for the NHS? Healthcare for the Millennium*, 2nd edn. London: Longman.

Rang H P, Dale M M, Ritter J M and Moore P K (2003) *Pharmacology*, 5th edn. Edinburgh: Churchill Livingstone.

Rolfe G (1996) *Closing the Theory–Practice Gap: A New Paradigm for Nursing*. London: Butterworth Heinemann.

Sohn Y W and Doane S M (2003) Roles of working memory capacity and long-term working memory skill in complex task performance. *Memory and Cognition* **31**, 458-466.

Trefino J (1997) The courage to change: reshaping care delivery. *Nursing Management* **28**, 50-53.

Walsh M (1989) *Nursing Rituals, Research and Rational Actions*. Oxford: Butterworth Heinemann.

Wanless, D, Appleby J, Harrison A and Patel D (2007) *Our Future Health Service Secured? A Review of NHS Funding and Performance*. London: King's Fund.

Woodhead K (2000) Challenge a ritual or two. *British Journal of Perioperative Nursing* **10**, 2, 61.

Zaybak A, Güneş U Y, Tamsel L, Eşer I (2007) Does obesity prevent the needle from reaching muscle in intramuscular injections? *Journal of Advanced Nursing* **58**, 552-556.

Chapter 2

How to use information about medicines

This chapter introduces you to a different way of thinking about and using medicine information. Traditionally this information has been presented in a specific format. Most pharmacology books written for nurses introduce information related to body systems or conditions, for example 'medicines acting on the central nervous system/for neurological conditions' (Greenstein and Gould, 2004; Prosser *et al.*, 2000). A similar approach can also be seen in the *British National Formulary* (BNF) (**www.bnf.org**), a guide for prescribing and administering medicines. This can be a useful approach, particularly if the text offers some information about the body system to help you understand how the medicine works. There are also examples where a patient problem is identified, for example pain, so that **analgesics** (medicines used to relieve pain) can be discussed. However, we suggest that this kind of information gives only a limited perspective. As nurses administering medications, we might find a patient reluctant to take a medicine because of something they have read or because they are feeling nauseous. A knowledge only of what the drug or medicine 'does' may not prepare us adequately to assess the situation or provide meaningful information to patients. As Schwertz *et al.* (1997) note, traditional approaches have focused on drug action, but this does not necessarily prepare nurses to manage patients' medicines; rather, this demands knowledge and critical thinking skills.

Learning outcomes

By the end of this chapter you should be able to:

✔ Recognise the types of information nurses need in order to understand medicines

✔ Identify appropriate sources of information

✔ Interpret the information provided

✔ Begin to apply information to patient situations.

Chapter at a glance

The problem
Where will I find the information I need?
Do I understand what I am reading?
What kind of information do I need?
How can I use the information?
Quick reminder
References

THE PROBLEM

Although nurses need information about medicines for many reasons, for example to provide information to patients and to monitor the effect of medications, their main role is arguably related to the administration of medicines.

> **Medication administration is one of the fundamental tasks performed by nurses in everyday clinical practice.**
> (Grandell-Neimi *et al.*, 2005)

The Nursing and Midwifery Council (NMC) (2007) identifies the nurse's role in the administration of medicines in the following way:

> **You must exercise your professional judgment and apply your knowledge and skill.**

Although this suggests that nurses need both pharmacological knowledge and skills, many authors identify that nurses have insufficient pharmacological knowledge when they qualify and that students have difficulty in understanding the subject (Jordan *et al.*, 1999). Schwertz *et al.* (1997) suggest that students tend to be concerned with learning 'facts' and that they find the application of these facts to practice difficult. They go on to state that unless students can learn to apply pharmacological principles to their practice, they will not be able to keep up to date with new medicine developments. The NMC (2004) also states that nurses should acknowledge any limitations and, if necessary, improve their levels of knowledge and competence, because they are accountable for their practice.

One reason for this lack of knowledge might be that nursing has moved away from the 'medical' model of care (dominated by identifying and treating disease, signs and symptoms – that is, the physical manifestations of illness) and towards more holistic and individualistic care: the move from 'cure' to 'care'. This increased emphasis on 'softer' nursing skills, such as the interpersonal skills needed to establish therapeutic relationships with patients, has resulted in a loss of emphasis on, and a reduction of teaching related to, the biological sciences in nursing. This leaves many nurses feeling vulnerable about their knowledge of anatomy, physiology, pathology and pharmacology (Amos, 2001; King, 2004).

WHERE WILL I FIND THE INFORMATION I NEED?

For nurses today, there are countless sources of information available relating to medicines and drugs. These resources include not only pharmacology textbooks but also pharmacology journal articles, the BNF, *Martindale: The Complete Drug Reference* (a pharmacopoeia – an authorised handbook of drugs available around the world, including herbal and complementary products, nutritional products, vaccines and treatment reviews), Web pages and patient information leaflets.

We have used a range of sources to support the information provided in this book, including the BNF and several pharmacology textbooks written for nurses (Downie *et al.*, 2003; Greenstein and Gould, 2004; Prosser *et al.*, 2000). Full references can be found at the end of the chapter.

The BNF is probably the most frequently used and highly regarded of these resources. It is available to buy in both book and online format. The book is bought by almost all NHS trusts and given free of charge to their employees who supply or prescribe medicines to patients, to hospital wards and departments. It is also issued free to pharmacies and GPs. Most NHS trusts also have subscriptions to the online BNF (**www.bnf.org**) so that all healthcare professionals may access information through the trust's intranet. The online BNF is updated every six months, so it is a contemporary resource. Since 2005, there is also a BNF specifically for children's medicines. Updated annually, this provides information about the safe use of medicines for children, filling a previous gap in this area of practice (Novak, 2006).

The BNF is considered to be the definitive source of information about medicines, as it contains important information for prescribers. It is set out in a particular format to meet the needs of prescribers regarding the actions and uses of medicines. In addition, there are also many textbooks and journal articles that explain aspects of pharmacology in a variety of ways in order to appeal to different audiences. However, whatever information source is used, in order to find out whether the resource is useful we have to understand not only its format but also what it is saying.

Personal and professional development 2.1 Accessing information

Access a copy of the BNF and identify the format in which it presents information. Answers can be found at the back of the book.

Now consider:

- Is this information useful to you as a consumer?

- Is this information useful to you as someone who will be involved in patient education?

- Can you identify what further information about medicines you might need?

DO I UNDERSTAND WHAT I AM READING?

Getting to grips with any new subject discipline such as pharmacology (the study of drugs and their actions) can be daunting and difficult, besides being exciting and challenging. Often the process of studying a new discipline means having to learn a new language and this certainly applies to learning how to use information about medicines. Consider, for example, some of the terms used in this chapter. The language used comes from a variety of subject disciplines, including pharmacology, physiology and chemistry.

When a subject area has its own language, this is sometimes referred to as 'jargon' by those not familiar with the subject. Using the language immediately identifies those who understand the subject and therefore can be said to be 'inside the circle' and those who do not understand it and are therefore 'outside the circle'. A frequently used quote used to explain this is 'knowledge is power', attributed to Freire (1972), who was an influential thinker about education.

Personal and professional development 2.2
Using information

Take a moment to consider a recent patient encounter between a patient and a nurse or between a patient and a doctor. You might wish to reflect upon an example where you have consulted a nurse or doctor.

● What type of information was used? Did the discussion include a lot of medical terminology?

● Was there an attempt by the health professional to establish whether the patient understood?

● Was there an attempt to explain any of the jargon used?

● Was the health professional controlling the discussion, or was there an attempt to develop a partnership between the patient and the professional?

● Can we sum this up and identify who had the 'power' in this situation?

Related knowledge Sociology

An interesting and important sociological debate explores the power that is inherent in the use of such jargon, particularly that used by professional groups such as nurses and doctors. Although this debate will not be examined in this book, it is important that you understand how such power can influence relationships between patients/carers and healthcare professionals.

Qualified nurses need to be sensitive to the impact of jargon on patients and to develop communication skills with both service users and team members, in order to meet their needs in relation to the information that they require and the way in which they provide this information.

A contemporary issue for nurses is the wealth of information available on the Internet, not only for healthcare professionals but also for patients. Information can be posted on the Internet easily and we do not always know how reliable it is. Some information can be very biased, for example if a drug company disguises promotional material as independent advice. It is important that the resources we use, and recommend for patients, are both trustworthy and current (Aya, 2006).

Whichever source you use to access information about drugs and medicines, you will probably find a consistency of approach, such as the systems approach, which involves providing information mainly about how a medicine acts, although this is sometimes applied to patient care and patient education. Although this provides us with some useful information about medicines, it offers only a linear approach to learning and does not always prepare us for the complexities of patient care, for example when patients are taking complicated cocktails of medicines (polypharmacy). (We discuss this in relation to the older adult in Chapter 8.)

Greenstein and Gould (2004) suggest that one way to assist your learning about pharmacology is to develop a particular method of note-taking that involves recording:

- the name and class of the medicine,
- its source;
- what it is used for;
- its route of administration;
- its actions and effects;
- its adverse effects;
- any contraindications;
- its mechanism of action.

Consider how useful this method might be for you by using the following activity.

Personal and professional development 2.3
Identifying relevant information

A patient asks you what her tablets are for. She is concerned about whether they are safe to take. She is taking atenolol 50 mg.

▶ *(continued)*

What information would you need to know in order to answer her question? Are there any gaps in the range of information that Greenstein and Gould have identified above?

Greenstein and Gould (2004) state that atenolol is a selective beta-blocker, often given once a day to reduce blood pressure in patients with hypertension. The adverse effects include tiredness, lack of energy, depression, hallucinations, and cold hands and feet.

Essential terminology

Beta-blocker
A medicine that 'prevents stimulation of the beta-adrenergic receptors at the nerve endings of the sympathetic nervous system' (Martin, 2004).

Therapeutic effect
'The extent to which an intervention aids the well being of an individual' (Courtenay and Butler, 1999).

Side effect
An unwanted but predictable effect that is frequently experienced by patients.

Adverse effect
An unexpected and unpredictable reaction that occurs in some patients and that is not related to the usual effects of the drug when given in a normal dose.

Contraindication
A reason for not administering a medicine. Any factor in a patient's condition that makes it unwise to pursue a particular treatment, for example kidney disease (which limits the body's ability to metabolise and excrete some medicines) or pregnancy (there may be a risk that the medicine might pass through the placenta to the baby) (Audit Commission, 2001; Luker and Wolfson, 1999).

In the BNF, atenolol is identified as a beta-adrenoceptor blocker. The BNF states that this group of medicines 'block the beta-adrenoceptors in the heart, peripheral vasculature [peripheral means the outer parts of an organ or the body; vasculature refers to the blood vessels], bronchi, pancreas and liver' (www.bnf.org) and suggests that they can be used in the treatment of hypertension, angina and arrhythmia. They should be given with caution in patients with asthma.

Remembering what we have said about the impact of jargon on patients, if you have not come across this terminology before you may be feeling disempowered and 'outside' the circle. The next box explains these concepts.

Personal and professional development 2.4 Using this information

From the information above we can see that beta-blockers interfere with some activity. For example, they can be used to slow down heart activity in the patient with a fast and possibly irregular heart rate. This would constitute the therapeutic effect.

However, their blocking effect would be of concern in a patient with asthma because of their ability to block activity in the lungs. Thus, a history of asthma would be a contraindication for beta-blockers.

Slowing down of the heart's activity could result in a bradycardia; this would be a side effect.

> **Personal and professional development 2.5** Interpreting information
>
> Access a pharmacology book such as Downie *et al*. (2003) or Prosser *et al*. (2000) and try to identify why beta-blockers would be contraindicated in asthma. Answers can be found at the back of the book.

Using more than one source of information, such as consulting Greenstein and Gould (2004) and the BNF in the example above, can enhance our knowledge and understanding. Information sources often present knowledge in different ways and from a range of perspectives, depending on the purpose of the source. For example, a dictionary aims to give concise explanations, while a textbook is designed to provide more detailed information.

However, sometimes the information is confusing because of its presentation. In order to use this information effectively, we then need to consider other types and sources of information. In Chapter 1 we suggested that, in order to build up a sound knowledge base about medicines, we need to consider the nursing context as well as medicine information; we suggested that this involved additional knowledge, such as government initiatives, patient factors and your personal learning needs. If you think about the example above concerning the patient taking atenolol, we might need to consider the following:

- *Government initiatives*: Is this group of medicines identified within National Institute for Health and Clinical Excellence (NICE) documents? NICE provides information about medicines based on the most contemporary research and evidence available, including cost-effectiveness.

- *Patient factors*: What is this patient's diagnosis – that is, what is she taking the tablets for? Are there any other details you need to know about the patient? For example, is she forgetful or is she taking any other prescribed or over-the-counter medicines? Remember that atenolol can cause problems for patients with asthma, heart failure or diabetes mellitus.

- *Learning*: How would you best learn information such as this? What is your learning style? Do you learn by taking notes and memorising information? Most authors suggest that learning should be contextualised, that is related to practice (Lim and Honey, 2005; Schwertz *et al.*, 1997). Relating medicines to individual patient care, as in the example above, is a useful way of doing this. This is discussed further in Chapter 3, where we suggest that the knowledge we need should be generated from the individual patient.

It appears then that information relating to the medicine's actions and effects is only part of the information you need. You also need to be able to identify and/or categorise the information and apply it to specific situations.

Consider the following example.

> ## Personal and professional development 2.6
> ## Reviewing information
>
> Access any pharmacology textbook of your choice and identify the following information in relation to amitriptyline:
> - Drug group/classification
> - Action
> - Adverse effects

Amitriptyline

Greenstein and Gould (2004) provide the following information:

- Drug group/classification: Amitriptyline is classified as an antidepressant (a medicine used in the treatment of depression). It may also be described as a tricyclic antidepressant (named after the drug's molecular structure containing three rings of atoms).

- Action: Amitriptyline acts upon the central nervous system (CNS). It increases the production of a neurotransmitter amine (a substance produced by the body that enables the transfer of signals from one nerve cell to another, resulting in some action, e.g. movement or temperature regulation) such as serotonin or noradrenaline (also known as norepinephrine). Depression has been linked to a reduction of these substances.

  Amitripyline also has H2-receptor blocking activity (H2-receptors are part of the process of gastric acid production). Therefore, amitriptyline inhibits gastric acid secretion.

- Adverse effects: These include dry mouth, difficulty with micturition (passing urine) and constipation in older adults, postural hypotension (drop in blood pressure associated with a sudden change in position - usually moving from lying to standing), increased appetite and weight gain.

> ## Personal and professional development 2.7
> ## Reviewing information
>
> Having discovered the information about the actions of amitriptyline, could you have predicted any of the adverse effects?
> Read this section again and see how easy you found it to make links between the types of information offered.

Migraine

A migraine headache can be moderate or severe. It is often described as one-sided and pulsating and is usually associated with nausea, vomiting and visual disturbances. Migraine is a vascular headache; it is thought that the blood vessels of the brain initially constrict (narrow), causing visual disturbances, and then dilate (widen), raising the intracranial pressure and resulting in headache. Although there are specific medicines recommended for the relief of migraine attacks, such as sumatriptan, amitriptyline can be used when migraine headaches occur frequently; it is taken regularly in order to minimise the frequency of attacks.

If you read further, some texts acknowledge that amitriptyline can also be used in the treatment of diabetic neuropathy (damage to nerves and ultimately loss of nerve function, which is related to diabetes mellitus; see Chapter 14), the treatment of nocturnal enuresis (night-time bed-wetting in children) and the relief of migraine headaches (**www.bnf.org**). It is important to note that another of the tricyclic antidepressants, imipramine, is more commonly prescribed for nocturnal enuresis, but neither medicines would be the first choice of treatment because of their side effects, which include behavioural disturbances (**www.bnf.org**).

It might be difficult for you to understand why this medicine can be used in such a range of situations.

If we look at the use of amitriptyline in relation to nocturnal enuresis, this is based on the effect that the medicine has on the body (pharmacokinetics). As well as having an antidepressant effect, amitriptyline also blocks the parasympathetic nervous system (the parasympathetic nervous system is responsible for automatic body functions such as digestion and sleep), reducing the readiness of the detrusor muscle in the bladder (Figure 2.1) to respond to the impulses that initiate micturition ('detrusor' refers to a part of the body that 'pushes down').

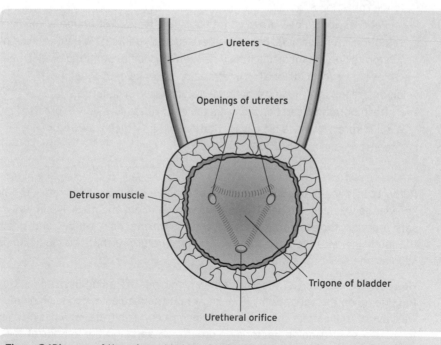

Figure 2.1 Diagram of the urinary bladder, showing the location of the detrusor muscle

If you check the information you found in relation to the activity above, you will note that retention of urine (the urine is retained in the bladder) is actually a side effect of this medicine (Courtenay and Butler, 1999). In the case of a child who wets the bed, we are using the side effect of this medicine as a therapeutic effect (the effect we are trying to achieve).

Pharmacological knowledge Contemporary approaches for the treatment of bed-wetting

Nocturnal enuresis occurs commonly in young children and so should be treated (e.g. using an alarm) only in children over 5 years of age. It may be treated using medicines in children over 7 years of age.

Desmopressin is described by the BNF as an analogue of vasopressin. Vasopressin (antidiuretic hormone; ADH) is produced by the pituitary gland (also known as the hypophysis); the pituitary gland has two lobes: the anterior pituitary (adenohypophysis) and the posterior pituitary (neurohypophysis). ADH is produced by the neurohypophysis and is responsible for increasing the reabsorption of water in the kidney, thus decreasing the amount of urine.

An analogue is a medicine that differs in minor ways from its parent substance. An analogue may be more effective or cause fewer side effects. Desmopressin is an analogue of vasopressin, which is more potent and has a longer duration of action.

Patients should be warned about the side effects of desmopression: fluid retention, stomach pain, headache, nausea and vomiting. Patients should be told to stop taking the medicine if they have an episode of vomiting or diarrhoea. Other side effects include hyponatraemia (a low level of sodium in the bloodstream), allergy and emotional disturbances in children.

Desmopression can be taken as a tablet or nasal spray for enuresis. If given as a nasal spray, it can cause nasal irritation and nosebleeds (www.bnf.org; Greenstein and Gould, 2004).

If you consider the information given above, we can start to identify the breadth of knowledge we need. We need to gain knowledge about the medicine in order to ensure safe practice, for example to understand the normal dose ranges and side effects of the medicine. Most sources will also identify the group that the medicine belongs to, such as analgesics or antibiotics.

However, we can understand why certain medicines are being used and start to predict the effects on the patient only if we know how the medicine works. A common example we can use to illustrate this is the medicine glyceryl trinitrate, which is often prescribed for patients with angina pectoris. In order to understand the actions of this medicine, we need to consider our current understanding of angina. Learning about the medication without learning about the normal physiology, disordered physiology (**pathophysiology**), disease processes and long-term conditions will not aid our understanding about the associated patient care and nursing interventions. We explain this approach in more detail in Chapter 3.

Related knowledge Patient conditions

Angina pectoris (chest pain) can be explained in simple terms as the consequence of an imbalance between supply and demand. In order for the body to work effectively, it needs a constant supply of nutrients, including oxygen. The heart muscle receives its nutrients and oxygen via the coronary arteries. If a patient has atheroma (a build-up of fatty deposits within the blood vessel wall; Figure 2.2), this will narrow the diameter of the blood vessel and therefore affect the volume of blood being pumped through the blood vessel, with a resulting lack of oxygen supply to the myocardium (heart muscle). Insufficient blood supply (ischaemia) causes tissues to become hypoxic or, if there is no oxygen at all, anoxic. A reduction or absence of oxygen can cause cell death – necrosis. There is some relationship between the pain experience and the degree of myocardial ischaemia. Angina is usually reversible, but it does cause decreased myocardial function. The heart is sensitive to lack of blood supply; however, ischaemia needs to be prolonged (3–4 hours) before it results in irreversible necrosis.

Usually the patient is aware of this only on exertion, for example when exercising or running for a bus, when there is a greater demand for nutrients and oxygen in order to sustain the increased activity. There is only a limited ability to supply nutrients and oxygen because of the narrowed blood vessel. The consequence of this is that the patient experiences pain (Alexander *et al.*, 2006).

This explanation refers to stable angina. In unstable angina, the onset and presentation of the pain are not predictable and achieving pain relief can be more difficult.

We have established that one of the features of angina is that the patient experiences pain on physical exertion. The medicines usually given to patients experiencing pain are called analgesics. However, when treating a patient's pain, the first step is always to establish the cause. If the cause can be eradicated, potentially then we can cure it, for example by removing a tooth or treating a gum infection if the patient has dental pain. If we cannot cure the cause, then we can try to relieve the pain and thus improve the situation for the patient – that is, we can relieve the symptom. There are a range of approaches to pain relief other than analgesics; these can be seen in Appendix 1.

Glyceryl trinitrate, a commonly used medicine for patients with angina, is identified in the BNF as a coronary **vasodilator**. This means that it **dilates** (widens or expands) the coronary arteries; it does this by relaxing the vascular smooth muscle of the artery wall.

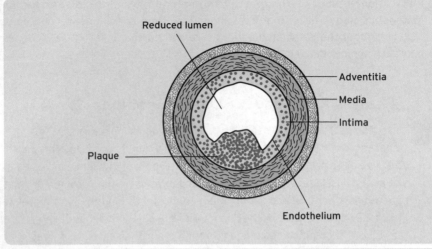

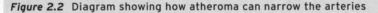

Figure 2.2 Diagram showing how atheroma can narrow the arteries

This information tells us where the medicine exerts its effect and what it does. By widening the diameter of the blood vessel in this way, more blood is delivered to the myocardium; the pain is relieved as a consequence of the increased delivery of oxygen to the tissue.

However, the BNF goes on to say that although glyceryl trinitrate is a potent coronary dilator, it also reduces venous return to the heart, which in turn reduces the work of the left ventricle; this is probably the most beneficial action of this medicine.

Related knowledge Anatomy and physiology

The amount of blood ejected from the left ventricle is dependent on a number of factors, one of which is venous return - that is, the amount and rate of blood returning to the heart. The main purpose of the venous circulation is to return blood to the heart so that it can exchange carbon dioxide for oxygen for recirculation. It might be useful to picture the circulation as a closed system and assume that the blood returning to the heart is the same as that leaving the heart via the left ventricle - that is, the ventricles pump as much blood as they receive from the venous system. The force of the ventricular contraction adjusts according to the volume of blood.

An adequate venous return needs to be maintained at all times, and so there are several mechanisms that manage the venous return.

The venous circulation may have to work against gravity, which will hinder venous return, for example if the person is standing. This is assisted by the use of valves within the veins and the action of the muscles surrounding the deep veins. If there is a loss of circulating blood volume, then the larger veins constrict in order to maintain blood pressure.

The venous circulation often functions as a large reservoir where blood can be 'stored' while still in the circulation in order to respond to changes in blood pressure that occur as a consequence of activity or emotion. This generally takes place in the larger veins by dilation of the veins. This decreases pressure and venous return, thus reducing the work of the left ventricle (Hinchliff *et al.*, 1996; Kindlen, 2003).

Reducing the work of the left ventricle will reduce the demand for oxygen, while dilating the artery will increase the supply of oxygen.

Related knowledge Anatomy and physiology

The heart consists of four chambers: two smaller chambers - atria - which essentially receive blood via the venous circulation, and two larger chambers - ventricles.

During the cardiac cycle the atria contract, forcing their contents (blood) into the ventricles. The ventricles then contract, forcing the blood out into the circulation, via the left ventricle into the systemic circulation and via the right ventricle into the pulmonary circulation (Figure 2.3).

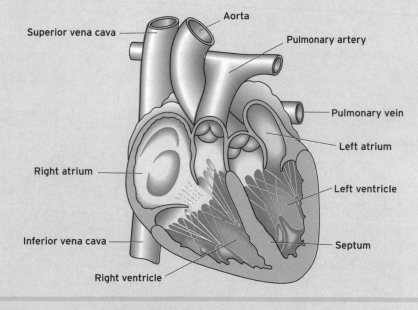

Figure 2.3 Diagram of the human heart

▶ *(box continued)*

Consider whether you need more information (and what type and from what source) in order to understand this medication and its actions.

As well as the two circulations described above, there is another important circulation to consider in relation to glyceryl trinitrate: the coronary circulation. This circulation services the heart itself. The myocardium receives its blood supply via the right and left coronary arteries (Figure 2.4), which branch from the aorta, immediately above the aortic valve.

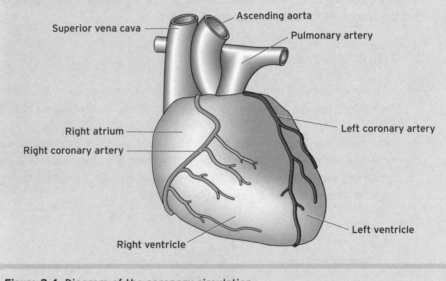

Figure 2.4 Diagram of the coronary circulation

Personal and professional development 2.8
Using information

In this situation, because of our knowledge about the patient's condition we can see that the choice of medicine would be related to the cause of the pain rather than being used simply to relieve the pain. Although we are improving the situation for the patient, we are not treating the source of the pain.

Because we are using this medicine to relieve pain, we need to consider the route of administration. Which route will deliver this medication quickly? For glyceryl trinitrate, the most usual route is the sublingual route via a spray. The rich blood supply under the tongue facilitates fast absorption. We could also consider whether we should continue to treat the pain only when it occurs or whether we should prevent the pain from occurring (**prophylaxis**) by using other nitrates in tablet form such as isosorbide mononitrate or by using skin (transdermal) patches. Transdermal patches deliver a small dose of the medicine over a prolonged period of time, with the intention of keeping the patient pain-free.

Routes of administration are discussed in Chapter 4.

Glyceryl trinitrate also exerts vasodilator (widening of the blood vessels) effects on the cerebral (referring to the cerebrum, part of the brain) arteries, so it is important to warn the patient that they might experience a throbbing headache as a consequence of the increased blood flow through the cerebral arteries. This medicine also has other side effects, such as flushing and headaches. A fuller list of side effects can be obtained by accessing a resource such as the BNF.

Related knowledge Pharmacological management of angina

So far we have discussed only approaches to pain relief. In the treatment of angina, we also need to consider the following:

- Preventing worsening of the patient's condition
- Improving the patient's quality of life

Therefore the following medicines may also be prescribed:

- *Aspirin*: Aspirin inhibits platelet aggregation – that is, it reduces the tendency of platelets (thrombocytes) to stick or clump together when blood flow is disrupted.
- *Atenolol or metoprolol (beta-blockers)*: Beta-blockers are discussed on page 28.
- *Verapimil or amlodipine (calcium channel blockers)*: The movement of calcium through channels into muscle cells is an essential part of the mechanism of muscle contraction. Using this group of medicines to prevent the movement of calcium encourages the muscles of the blood vessels to dilate, thus reducing blood pressure and reducing the work of the heart (Wiffen *et al.*, 2007).

Another example of pain that can be treated successfully with medicines from a group other than analgesics is the pain associated with shingles.

Related knowledge Disease processes

Shingles

Shingles (herpes zoster) is an infection caused by the varicella-zoster virus, which also causes chicken pox. After an attack of chicken pox, the virus lies dormant in the spinal cord. If the dormant virus is reactivated later, it travels down a specific sensory nerve to the skin, face or eye (ophthalmic zoster). This often results in a rash in the form of blisters, which can be seen to follow the pathway of the sensory nerve affected. Shingles can be an extremely painful condition; some patients are left with a chronic pain condition known as post-herpetic neuralgia, which is difficult to manage. Shingles can be treated with an antiviral such as aclicovir and analgesia, but another way of combating the pain is by using medicines that prevent the nerve transmission, such as anticonvulsants (**www.bnf.org**).

Medicines such as carbamazepine and phenytoin are classified as anticonvulsant medicines. They exert their effects by blocking sodium channels in nerve membranes; this reduces excitability of the nerve cells, thus preventing the spread of neuronal excitement. The transmission between one neuron and the next occurs via the mediation of neurotransmitters, which are released from nerve endings and diffuse across the synapse (the space between two neurons) to excite the next cell (Figure 2.5).

Carbamazepine and phenytoin are used in shingles where the severe pain experienced is a result of the virus being activated in a sensory dorsal nerve ganglion (a collection of nerve cells responsible for sensation). The pain follows the nerve fibre (Prosser *et al.*, 2000).

Think about the examples we have used so far of medicines that are described as belonging to a 'drug group', such as anticonvulsants, but are used in quite different situations. Unless we understand how the medication works, we cannot understand why medicines are used in such different situations. For example, if we have read about the use of carbamazepine only in the BNF, then it would be logical to assume that a patient taking the drug has epilepsy, but in the example above we can see that this is not necessarily the case.

Consider the following example: On 16 February 2007 it was reported on the BBC news website (**http://news.bbc.co.uk**) that doctors in a Newcastle hospital had used Viagra to 'save the life of a premature baby'. Viagra is the trade name for sildenafil, a medicine usually associated with its ability to treat erectile dysfunction. Erectile dysfunction can have many causes. It may be a side effect of certain medicines, such as methyldopa, a medicine used to reduce blood pressure. Sildenafil improves the blood flow to the penis. This effect was initially 'a lucrative side effect' discovered in the early testing of the drug (**http://news.bbc.co.uk**). A fuller discussion of this issue can be found in Shah and Ohlsson (2007).

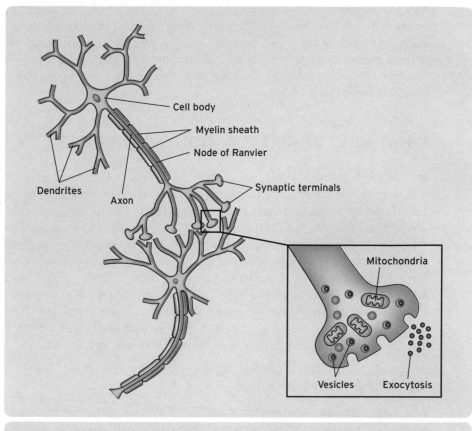

Figure 2.5 Diagram illustrating nerve cells (neurons)

Sildenafil was developed originally to lower blood pressure and treat angina. As we have seen in other examples in this chapter (e.g. amitriptyline), sometimes medicines are used for purposes other than that for which they were originally developed; thus, their therapeutic use changes.

Sildenafil works by blocking the enzyme phosphodiesterase. This enzyme is found in all body tissues (but with small differences in structure) and is responsible for the metabolism of a range of substances, including those responsible for maintaining dilation of blood vessels (Simonsen *et al.*, 2006).

Sildenafil is a specific phosphodiesterase inhibitor. It inhibits phosphodiesterase type 5, which is found predominantly in the arterioles of the penis. It acts as a potent vasodilator, widening the diameter of the blood vessels. The medicine was used to treat the premature baby because of its vasodilator effects: it enabled the transport of blood around the body (**http://news.bbc.co.uk**).

We can now start to understand why sildenafil should be avoided in patients with heart disease (it can cause systemic vascular dilation) receiving nitrates (medicines used in angina, e.g. glyceryl trinitrate). Sildenafil can greatly potentiate (increase) the effects of these medicines. Sildenafil is contraindicated in heart disease and in patients taking a range of other medicines because they can cause a drop in blood pressure (Greenstein and Gould, 2004).

WHAT KIND OF INFORMATION DO I NEED?

We can see from the examples above that the information we need about medicines includes not only the effects and dosages, so that we can administer medicines safely, but also details of how medicines exert their effects, so that we can assess and monitor the patient's response (Lim and Honey, 2005). We also need to know and understand the patient's disease/condition and how this affects the individual, their problems and symptoms. Lim and Honey (2005) suggest that, unless nurses understand how the medicine works and its 'related actions' on other body systems, they will be unable to anticipate the effects of the medication or transfer knowledge to new and complex patient situations. They go on to suggest that emphasis needs to be put on the 'principles, concepts and parameters' relating to how the drug exerts its effects, rather than just providing content about specific medicines (Lim and Honey, 2005).

Evidence-based practice

In recent years there has been great pressure on nurses and other healthcare professionals to base their practice on current, reliable and valid evidence. The NMC (2006) states clearly that registered nurses have a responsibility to deliver care 'based on current evidence, best practice, and where applicable, validated research'.

A number of international studies (Aiken *et al.*, 2002, 2003; Audit Commission, 2001; Tourangeau, 2005; Tourangeau *et al.*, 2006) have demonstrated clearly that the more highly educated the qualified nurse, the better the outcome, in terms of morbidity and mortality, for the patients that the nurse cares for. However, having the ability to use evidence in one's own practice also requires the skill to think critically in order to reach sound clinical judgements. We need to be able to judge the worth of the information we are presented with. It has been suggested that approaches to care have been based upon 'tradition, intuition, common sense and untested theories' rather than research (French, 1999).

Chapelhow *et al.* (2005) suggest that evidence-based practice is 'a way of working, which relies on retrieving and using information from a variety of sources ... to underpin practice'. They go on to state that this evidence base requires regular updating. However, a broader definition of evidence-based practice that might suit the purposes and philosophy of this book more effectively is that offered by Sigma Theta Tau International (STTI) (2006), which develops this into the following definition:

an integration of the best evidence available, nursing expertise, and the values and preferences of the individuals and communities who are served.

This definition encompasses the consideration of evidence, experience and patient choice.

Evidence-based nursing practice appears to have emerged from the concept of evidence-based medicine defined by Sackett *et al.* (1996) as 'the conscientious, explicit and judicious use of current evidence in making decisions about the care of individual patients'. The 'evidence' in this context is usually derived from systematic empirical (scientific) and/or quantitative research. Sackett *et al.* go on to state that neither alone is enough. This implies that healthcare practitioners need to have the skills to judge the information within the current context of care and in relation to a specific patient. Sackett *et al.* (2000) have recently recognised the need to acknowledge patient values.

French (1999) comments that there needs to be strong links between the evidence base and the nurse's understanding of the situation. NICE provides information relating to the efficacy and cost-effectiveness of new and existing treatments, while National Service Frameworks offer the evidence base for the interventions that they identify. These are two useful resources for healthcare professionals.

Personal and professional development 2.9

We have now provided several examples of situations where a range of knowledge is required. Think about some of the explanations offered about the identified medicines within this chapter. The information did not relate only to the medicine: it also identified information about normal body functioning.

Can you now start to identify the range of underpinning information, such as anatomy and physiology, that a nurse may need to access in order to understand the pharmacological information they are presented with?

Answers can be found at the back of the book.

HOW CAN I USE THE INFORMATION?

Although much literature (Latter *et al.*, 2000, 2001) identifies nurses' lack of knowledge, other authors would suggest that 'sometimes it is a lack of confidence in knowledge rather than a lack of knowledge' per se (King, 2004).

Clancy *et al.* (2000) and Latter *et al.* (2000) assert that pharmacological knowledge should be supported by skills such as autonomous learning, so that students can develop contemporary knowledge and a depth of understanding, in order to promote their confidence.

Personal and professional development 2.10

Aspirin is a medicine that is readily accessible and therefore a popular choice of pain relief. Consider what information you know about aspirin. You might have identified that asprin:

- is used for pain relief;
- forms part of some cold and flu remedies;
- can cause upset stomachs;
- can be taken by mouth, either as a tablet or dissolved in water;
- is used by patients who have had heart attacks in order to 'thin the blood';
- should not be used for young children.

If we have some knowledge about how medicines work and understand some of the language associated with pharmacology, we can organise the information we have regarding asprin, thus:

Classification	Pain relief (analgesic)	Also classified as a non-steroidal anti-inflammatory drug (NSAID)
	Antipyretic (often added to cold and flu remedies because it reduces temperature)	Anti-inflammatory action, which is related to its action on prostaglandins
	Antiplatelet and so used in secondary prevention of myocardial infarction and stroke in small doses for a long period	
Route	Oral	
Form/preparation	Tablets and soluble tablets	May be coated to render it gastro-resistant (this used to be referred to as 'enteric coated')
Side effects	Gastric irritation	Ulceration, bleeding, heartburn
Contraindications	Patients with asthma (potential for allergy), children under age 16 years (risk of Reye's syndrome)	Can cause brain damage

If we consult the BNF or another textbook, we can add the following information:

Chemical name	Acetylsalicylic acid	
Action	Inhibits production of prostaglandins (mainly local action), used for mild to moderate pain, e.g. headache, arthritis	Anti-inflammatory action, for pain associated with swelling/oedema
Patient education	Advise patient to take with milk or food to avoid stomach irritation Avoid alcohol	
Interactions	Anticoagulants Steroids Oral hypoglycaemics	Advise patient to inform doctor/dentist, as these medicines would be contraindicated

Source: Govoni and Hayes (1994)

Instead of trying to memorise information about medicines, for example potential adverse effects, understanding how a specific medicine works can enable us to predict its adverse effects (Schwertz *et al*., 1997).

If we take the example of furosemide, a diuretic (a medicine used to increase urine output and therefore fluid output), by looking at its site of action and how it exerts its effects we can predict its other potential effects. Furosemide is also further classified as a loop diuretic because of the part of the body it affects. Furosemide acts primarily on the ascending loop of Henle (part of the nephron, in the kidney; Figure 2.6), which is responsible for concentrating urine: 80% of the urine volume is reabsorbed here.

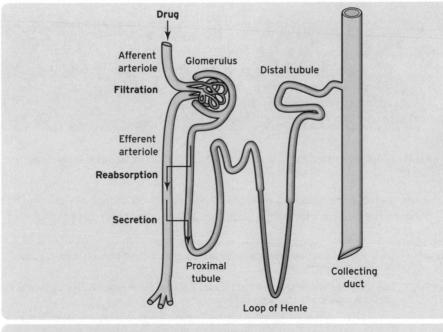

Figure 2.6 The nephron and urine production

Furosemide prevents reabsorption of sodium, chloride and water in the ascending loop of Henle, thus leading to an increase in the secretion of water, sodium, chloride and potassium. It is fast-acting and potent.

Knowing this limited information about furosemide enables us to predict two adverse (unwanted) effects:

● Loss of too much fluid

● Loss of too much sodium, chloride and potassium.

Personal and professional development 2.11
Using information

Identify the potential problems for a patient if too much potassium is lost:

● Mild muscle weakness

● Severe reduction of potassium (hypokalaemia) can result in cardiac arrhythmia (fast, irregular heart rate) (Kindlen, 2003).

Patients taking furosemide often need to go to the toilet frequently, and with some urgency. Therefore, they should be advised to take the furosemide early in the morning so that they do not have to get up repeatedly during the night to pass urine (Govoni and Hayes, 1994; Greenstein and Gould, 2004).

Personal and professional development 2.12

Can you think of a recommendation you should make to patients who are taking medicines to increase fluid output?
Answers can be found at the back of the book.

This is one way of applying pharmacological principles to patient care (Schwertz *et al.*, 1997).

Now consider the following example of digoxin. If you access any pharmacology text-book, it will provide information about digoxin in a similar format to this:

Source	Digoxin is a cardiac glycoside, a group of medicines derived from digitalis; it occurs naturally in some plants
Used for	Any condition that results in a fast, usually irregular heart rate, which if allowed to continue could cause the heart to fail

Action	Strengthens the contraction of the ventricles. Digoxin acts as a positive inotrope (an inotrope is an agent that increases or decreases the force of muscle contraction) by inhibiting sodium-potassium-ATPase (a transport molecule). This prevents sodium being pumped out of the cardiac muscle cells, which in turn increases the concentration of calcium in cells. This can result in a diuretic effect. Digoxin also acts upon the central nervous system to slow down the heart rate. It also increases the refractory period (the time when the heart is at rest). It depresses the conduction in the atrioventricular node and bundle of His (part of the electrical conduction system of the heart).

Personal and professional development 2.13
Using the information

We need to consider the implications of this information for nurses:

- Any medicine that reduces a patient's fast heart rate may result in the heart rate becoming too slow.

- The nursing observations required would involve recording the patient's pulse and heart rate (apical pulse) before administration. You would need to know normal heart rates related to age, and at what stage it would be appropriate to withhold the medicine and inform the medical staff of this decision.

- If digoxin is taken with medicines such as diuretics, then fluid balance should be monitored.

Route of administration	Orally by tablet or elixir, or by injection.
Dose	Determined in relation to the individual's age, renal function and body weight.
Fate of the medicine	The medicine is slowly absorbed; the half-life (in pharmacology, this term describes the time taken for the drug within the bloodstream to reach half the administered dose), regardless of the route, is 3-4 days.

Personal and professional development 2.14
Using the information

We need to consider the implications of this information for nurses. If we relate this to the adverse reactions noted below, we can conclude that the medicine will exert its effects for several days. The patient should be advised to take the medicine as prescribed and at the same time each day.

Adverse reactions	Digoxin toxicity: nausea, abdominal pain, vomiting, diarrhoea, fatigue, muscle weakness, headache, irritability, insomnia, arrhythmias.

Personal and professional development 2.15
Using the information

We need to consider the implications of this information for nurses:

● *Blood monitoring*: Digoxin is a medicine that needs to be monitored carefully; blood samples are taken on a regular basis in order to monitor plasma concentrations and assess for toxicity.

● *Assessment*: The patient's mood and sleeping patterns must be assessed.

● *Observation*: The patient's heart rate and fluid input and output should be measured and recorded.

Interactions   Many medicines can interact with digoxin, including antacids, beta-blockers and St John's wort.

Personal and professional development 2.16
Using the information

We need to consider the implications of this information for nurses. A careful medication history is required and the patient should be given advice about over the counter (OTC) medicines (Govoni and Hayes, 1994; Greenstein and Gould, 2004; Prosser *et al.*, 2000).

In order to be able to use information in this way, we need to link our knowledge and skills to our practice. Latter *et al.* (2001) suggest that 'the dynamic nature of pharmacology knowledge indicates that this will need to be complemented by self-directed and continuous learning in practice'. One approach that they recommend is experiential learning; this involves 'learning by doing' rather than listening and reading, and learning as a process of 'creating knowledge' (Kolb, 1984).

Within this chapter we have started this process of interpreting the medicine information available for use, based upon pharmacological principles that are introduced in more detail in Chapter 4.

Schwertz *et al.* (1997) suggest that any programme that incorporates pharmacological information should also include 'the process of pharmacological reasoning'. However, pharmacological reasoning is a complex skill that involves additional skills such as critical thinking and clinical judgement.

Complex skills

We need skills that allow us to use knowledge. Quinn (2000) identifies these skills as 'communication, problem-solving, evaluation, and critical thinking'. In this context the word 'critical' is used to imply that we 'examine and judge carefully' (McKeown and Summers, 2006). In other words, we should not take information at face value but instead think about the information and consider it. Quinn (2000) suggests that critical thinking involves drawing conclusions from the information, and then interpreting and speculating. In this case, it is about considering the information and knowledge we have gained, comparing it with previous experiences/situations and applying it to new situations and experiences. In order to develop the ability to engage in critical thinking, it is important to see it as a gradual process that involves trying out different learning strategies, constantly evaluating your progress, sharing ideas with others and considering how effective the approach is for enhancing your learning.

The NMC (2007) clearly identify the need for nurses to maintain their level of knowledge. Indeed, there is a requirement for qualified nurses to maintain a personal professional profile in order to support the learning undertaken in relation to their continuing professional development needs. This requires a commitment to continual learning. Think about this in relation to patients' medicines. Care is becoming increasingly complex, and so inevitably medicines are too. Patients are becoming more active in their care; we now seek patients' opinions and support their decision-making processes. Chapelhow *et al.* (2005) suggest that the nurse needs decision-making skills, risk-management skills, a sound evidence base and interpersonal and communication skills in order to enable the patient to make decisions. We therefore need to assess our knowledge and skills, identify whether we have the 'right' skills and then develop new skills.

Within nursing, we refer to this ongoing learning as 'lifelong learning'. This is defined by the NMC as 'more than simply keeping up to date. It requires an enquiring approach to the practice of nursing and midwifery as well as issues which impact on practice' (NMC, 2002).

Qualified nurses build up their knowledge over a period of time. Meerabeau (1992) describes this expert knowledge as 'tacit' knowledge and suggests it is refined each time the nurse meets a similar situation. However, inexperienced nurses need help to develop their knowledge and skills. This chapter has introduced a way of using information related to medicines that not only helps you develop your knowledge base but also equips you with skills to apply information to new situations.

Quick reminder

✔ There are many sources available for nurses to access information about medications, such as books, journals and Internet pages.

✔ Information about medicines is usually presented in specific formats, giving the effects of the medicine, its dose and route, etc.

✔ Medicines have both therapeutic and side effects. In certain circumstances, side effects may be considered a therapeutic effect.

✔ Patient medication regimes are often complex. In order to understand these, we need to understand how medicines work.

✔ If we understand the properties of a medicine, we can anticipate its effects upon the patient.

✔ Understanding medicines and the effects they have on patients requires sophisticated skills.

REFERENCES

Aiken L H, Clarke S P, Sloane D M, Sochalski J and Silder J H (2002) Hospital nurse staffing and patient mortality, nurses burnout, and job satisfaction. *Journal of the American Medical Association* **288**, 1987-1993.

Aiken L H, Clarke S P, Cheung R B, Sloane D M and Silber J H (2003) Educational levels of hospital nurse and surgical patient mortality. *Journal of the American Medical Association* **290**, 1617-1623.

Alexander M F, Fawcett J N and Runciman P J (2006) *Nursing Practice: Hospital and Home - the Adult,* 3rd edn. Edinburgh: Churchill Livingstone.

Amos D (2001) An evaluation of staff nurse role transition. *Nursing Standard* **16**, 36-41.

Audit Commission (2001) *A Spoonful of Sugar: Medicines Management in NHS Hospitals.* Wetherby: Audit Commission Publications.

Aya M (2006) Useful medicines information sources. *Practice Nurse* **32**, 32-38

Chapelhow C, Crouch S, Fisher M and Walsh A (2005) *Uncovering Skills for Practice.* Cheltenham: Nelson Thornes.

Clancy J, McVicar A and Bird D (2000) Getting it right? An exploration of issues relating to the bio-logical sciences in nurse education and nursing practice. *Journal of Advanced Nursing* **32**, 1522-1538.

Courtenay M and Butler M (1999) *Nurse Prescribing: Principles and Practice.* London: Greenwich Medical Media.

Downie G, Mackenzie J and Williams A (2003) *Pharmacology and Medicines Management for Nurses.* Edingburgh: Churchill Livingstone.

Freire P (1972) *Pedagogy of the Oppressed.* Harmondsworth: Penguin.

French P (1999) The development of evidence-based nursing. *Journal of Advanced Nursing* **29**, 72-78.

Govoni L E and Hayes J E (1994) *Drugs and Nursing Implications.* New York: Prentice Hall.

Grandell-Neimi H, Hupli M, Leino-Kilpi H and Puukka P (2005) Finnish nurses' and nursing students' pharmacological skills. *Issues in Clinical Nursing* **14**, 685-694.

Greenstein B and Gould D (2004) *Trounce's Clinical Pharmacology for Nurses.* Edinburgh: Churchill Livingstone.

Hinchliff S M, Montague S E and Watson R (1996) *Physiology for Nursing Practice*. London: Baillière Tindall.

Jordan S, Davies S and Green B (1999) The biosciences in the pre-registration nursing curriculum: staff and students' perceptions of difficulties and relevance. *Nurse Education Today* **19**, 215–226.

Kindlen S (2003) *Physiology for Health Care and Nursing*. Edinburgh: Churchill Livingstone.

King R L (2004) Nurses' perceptions of their pharmacology educational needs. *Issues and Innovations in Nursing Education* **45**, 392–400.

Kolb D (1984) *Experiential Learning: Experiences as a Source of Learning and Development*. London: Prentice Hall.

Latter S, Rycroft-Malone J, Yerrell P and Shaw D (2000) Evaluating educational preparation for a health education role in practice: the case of medication education. *Journal of Advanced Nursing* **32**, 1282–1298.

Latter S, Rycroft-Malone J, Yerrell P and Shaw D (2001) Nurses' educational preparation for a medication education role: findings from a national survey. *Nurse Education Today* **21**, 143–154.

Lim A G and Honey M (2005) Integrated undergraduate nursing curriculum for pharmacology. *Nurse Education in Practice* **6**, 163–168.

Luker K and Wolfson D (1999) *Medicines Management for Clinical Nurses*. Oxford: Blackwell Science.

Martin E A (2004) *Oxford Dictionary of Nursing*. Oxford: Oxford University Press.

McKeown C and Summers E (2006) *Collins English Dictionary*. Glasgow: HarperCollins Publishers.

Meerabeau L (1992) Tacit knowledge: an untapped resource or a methodological headache? *Journal of Advanced Nursing* **17**, 1108–1112.

Novak B (2006) The *British National Formulary for Children:* an important milestone. *Nurse Prescribing* **4**, 53.

Nursing and Midwifery Council (NMC) (2002) *Supporting Nurses and Midwives Through Life Long Learning*. London: Nursing and Midwifery Council.

Nursing and Midwifery Council (NMC) (2004) *Code of Professional Conduct*. London: Nursing and Midwifery Council.

Nursing and Midwifery Council (NMC) (2006) A-Z of Advice. **www.nmc-uk.org** (accessed 14 March 2007).

Nursing and Midwifery Council (NMC) (2007) *Standards for Medicines Management*. London: Nursing and Midwifery Council.

Prosser S, Worster B, MacGregor J, Dewar K, Runyard P and Fegan J (2000) *Applied Pharmacology. An Introduction to Pathophysiology and Drug Management for Nurses and Healthcare Professionals*. Edinburgh: Mosby.

Quinn F M (2000) *Principles and Practice of Nurse Education*, 4th edn. Cheltenham: Nelson Thornes.

Sackett D L, Rosenberg W M C, Gray J A M, Haynes R B and Richardson W S (1996) Evidence-based medicine: what it is and what it isn't. *British Medical Journal* **312**, 71–72.

Sackett D L, Richardson W S, Rosenberg W M C and Haynes R B (2000) *Evidence-based Medicine: How to Practice and Teach EBM*. Edinburgh: Churchill Livingstone.

Schwertz D W, Piano M R, Klienpell R and Johnson J (1997) Teaching pharmacology to advanced practice nursing students: issues and strategies. *AACN Clinical Issues* **8**, 132–146.

Shah P S and Ohlsson A (2007) Sildenafil for pulmonary hypertension in neonates. *Cochrane Database of Systematic Reviews* 3, CD005494.

Sigma Theta Tau International (2006) *Position Statement on Evidence-Based Nursing*. Indianapolis, IN: Sigma Theta Tau International.

Simonsen T, Aarbakke J, Kay I, Coleman I, Sinnott P and Lysaa R (2006) *Illustrated Pharmacology for Nurses*. London: Hodder Arnold.

Tourangeau A E (2005) A theoretical model for the determinants of mortality. *Advances in Nursing Science* **28**, 58–69.

Tourangeau A E, Doran D M, McGillis Hall L, O'Brien Pallas L, Pringle D, Tu J V and Cranley L A (2006) Impact of hospital nursing care on 30-day mortality for acute medical patients. *Journal of Advanced Nursing* **57**, 32–44.

Wiffen P, Mitchell M, Snelling M and Stoner N (2007) *Oxford Handbook of Clinical Pharmacy*. Oxford: Oxford University Press.

Chapter 3

Applying knowledge and skills: approaches to learning

The NHS Plan (DH, 2001b) states that 'patients need and deserve to have more say and greater choice'; in other words, patients need to be able to participate in decisions about their own care and about healthcare services in general. They also need reparation when things go wrong. It is also important to acknowledge that in some situations, such as the patient who has managed their chronic illness for some time, patients may know more about the management of their condition than nurses do (DH, 2001a).

Nurses are the largest group of healthcare professionals involved in care delivery. Nurses' roles are constantly developing, resulting in new ways of working, such as nurse prescribing and nurse-led services. This requires nurses to have experience and highly developed skills in giving information, communication and advocacy. Nurses need not only to participate in care but also to be able to influence care decisions at a range of levels. Mullally (2002) suggests that nurses are in a position to 're-shape care around the patient'.

Learning outcomes

By the end of this chapter you should be able to:

✔ Identify ways in which nursing roles are changing

✔ Justify the rationale for patient-focused care

✔ Consider different definitions of medicines management

✔ Identify the cognitive skills required by nurses to manage medicines effectively

✔ Identify sources for contemporary medicine information

✔ Describe enquiry-based learning

✔ Apply problem-solving strategies to practice situations in order to identify learning needs

✔ Describe a model of experiential learning

✔ Articulate the approach identified within this book to medicines management.

Chapter at a glance

Nursing roles
What information to use
Our approach
Conclusion
Quick reminder
References

NURSING ROLES

The traditional role of the nurse in relation to medicines has been to administer medicines that doctors have prescribed and pharmacists have dispensed. However, changes to nurses' roles have involved them in both dispensing and prescribing (NMC, 2007). It is important to note that the role of the other professionals is also broadening, for example pharmacists are becoming involved in prescribing (non-medical prescribing).

The Chief Nursing Officer (CNO) has identified ten key roles for nurses:

- To order diagnostic investigations such as pathology tests and X-rays
- To make and receive referrals, for example to a therapist or pain consultant
- To admit and discharge patients for specified conditions and within agreed protocols
- To manage patient caseloads, for example for patients with diabetes or rheumatological conditions
- To run clinics, such as for ophthalmology or dermatology
- **To prescribe medicines and treatments**
- To carry out a wide range of resuscitation procedures, including defibrillation
- To perform minor surgery and outpatient procedures
- To triage patients using the latest information technology to the most appropriate health professional
- To take a lead in the way local health services are organised and in the way that they are run (DH, 1999, 2001b, 2002).

The central focus of these new roles is the patient, making care more accessible and more related to their needs, including information and disease management. Wilson and DiVito-Thomas (2004) suggest that after the five 'rights' often cited in literature relating to the administration of medicines (right patient, right time, right route, right dose, right medicine), there is a sixth right that relates to the patient – 'the right response of the patient to the medication'. The patient therefore becomes the focus for the knowledge and skills required by nurses, but factors such as the context of, and influences on, care must always be considered.

The landmark Audit Commission (2001) report, *A Spoonful of Sugar*, calculated for the first time the amount of taxpayers' money that was wasted on medicines that were prescribed and dispensed but never taken, and also poor compliance (it is suggested that we should now use the term 'adherence' or 'concordance', rather than 'compliance'; reasons for this are discussed in Chapters 5, 9 and 10), leading to increased emergency hospital admissions and increased suffering through poor disease management. Using the patient experience as the focus of services, best practice was examined and a set of recommendations identified to enable NHS hospital and community trusts to modernise and develop the service delivery of all aspects of medicines supply to patients. As a result, the term 'medicines management' is used most commonly within the NHS to describe the processes that are involved to ensure the efficient prescribing and supplying of medicines to patients, both in hospitals and in the community.

The Medicines and Healthcare Products Regulatory Agency (MHRA) (**www.mhra. gov.uk**) defines medicines management as follows:

> **The clinical, cost effective and safe use of medicines to ensure patients get the maximum benefit from the medicines they need, while at the same time minimising potential harm.**

Both pharmacists and prescribers are encouraged to use systems that:

- regularly scrutinise medication use;
- regularly review prescriptions;
- promote efficient administration of any repeat prescription service;
- provide patient education about medication use;
- improve the primary care–secondary care interface;
- provide an agreed local formulary (list of approved medications);
- encourage the use of patient self-administration;
- promote the use of patients' own medicines when admitted to hospital (Audit Commission, 2001).

These processes ensure both clinical governance and financial probity. However, for nurses, the term 'medicines management' encompasses the wider aspect of a nurse's role in relation to medicines. Traditionally this role was primarily rooted in the administration of medicines, partly because knowledge of many medicines was limited. Our knowledge and understanding has now grown in relation to medicines, and there has also been development in our understanding of psychology, sociology and interpersonal and communication skills. Allied with this are improvements in nutrition, living conditions, public health and medicine that have led to many more people living longer with long-term conditions, such as chronic chest conditions (DH, 2001a). As a result, not only are many nurses now involved in something more than the task of medicine administration but also there are greater expectations of nurses regarding their role in medicines management.

Therefore we would argue that nurses should also use the term 'medicines management'. In this context, we feel that it best describes the process that

> facilitates the engagement of patients, so enabling them to make what they see as best use of their prescribed medicines.

In order that the nurse can facilitate this process, they must not only have some understanding of certain aspects of pharmacology, along with a variety of other understandings, but they should also have developed their emotional intelligence (their ability to know and understand themselves in order to work more effectively with others) and their communication skills.

Skills

Not all nurses are comfortable with taking on new nursing roles. There has been some concern about taking on the traditional roles of junior doctors and potentially 'mopping up' after initiatives such as Junior Doctors: The New Deal (NHS Management Executive, 1991), which was introduced to improve the working conditions of junior doctors and bring them in line with EU directives on working hours. There also appears to be an assumption that career development for nurses was associated with the adoption of medical tasks. Walsh (1999) queries whether the nurse practitioner (the nurse who works in an advanced role) is a 'mini doctor or maxi nurse'. In other words, nurses' career development and therefore status previously were often linked to adopting 'technological' tasks such as prescribing and cannulation. However, more recently there has been development of 'separate but equal' roles for nurses (Rafferty et al., 1996).

Any role development requires nursing as it currently exists to be examined in order to create a considered view of professional nursing. Allen (2004) suggests it can be challenging for members of a profession to analyse their own roles. However, Hughes (1984), a social scientist, suggests that if any professional group is to 'define proper conduct with respect to their work activities, for themselves and society at large' and then to claim a mandate, the group must explore the culture and ideals of the profession. Mandates encourage professionals to strive towards ideals and generate status, thus broadening their roles as opposed to a licence; providing certain activities for payment. However, this can be at odds with employers, who usually want the best deal for their money, which is often achieved based upon industrial task-centred models of working. Arguably, nurses' roles should broaden as a response to patient care needs and care delivery. Inherent within the medicines management initiative are the aims of promoting health, improving patient care and patient satisfaction, developing professional skills, improving quality (clinical governance), improving resources and reducing waste.

Allen (2004) sought to identify nursing activities and identified several complex 'interrelated bundles of activity':

- Managing multiple agendas
- Circulating patients
- Bringing the individual into the organisation

- Managing the work of others
- Mediating occupational boundaries
- Obtaining, generating, interpreting and communicating information
- Maintaining records
- Prioritising care and rationing resources.

Allen suggests that nurses resolve tensions between the needs of patients and the needs of healthcare organisations, managing resources and different sources of information. In doing so, Allen highlights the difference between the popular image and the realities of nursing.

Nurses' role in relation to medicines management

Nurses involved in administering medicines interpret, assess, administer, communicate, provide information and support, anticipate, monitor, review, record and report. They may also diagnose, solve problems, prioritise and analyse in order to make decisions. Leathard (2001) suggests that nurses also use clinical observation and history-taking.

Manias and Bullock (2002) suggest that nurses' thinking in relation to administration is based on recognition and intuition – hypotheticodeductive reasoning. However, Eisenhauer *et al.* (2007) belive that not enough studies have been carried out on the cognitive (thinking) skills used by experienced nurses. Their study concludes that nurses' thinking skills are sophisticated. Eisenhauer *et al.* (2007) recorded examples of the following:

- *Monitoring of medication*: This involved assessment skills, for example considering the dose and route of medication in the context of the patient's condition. Pain relief was an example of this, where the nurse felt the patient needed more medication.
- *Communication with other health professionals*: Communication with doctors and pharmacists was based on an analysis of the situation, as in the example above, and on patient advocacy. Nurses routinely judged the patient's response to medication based upon interpretation, using their knowledge and experience of the patient.
- *Evaluation of the treatment*: This was related to the patient's response, for example blood pressure monitoring, the effectiveness of pain relief, relief of nausea or agitation. This also involved a consideration of whether there was a 'better' choice of medication.
- *Teaching*: This was individualised for the patient based upon an interpretation of the patient's needs and capacity to understand.
- *Anticipating*: The anticipation and prevention of adverse effects was based on using information such as patients' laboratory reports.
- *Risk-taking*: In order that patients received medicines when they needed them, risks were sometimes taken, for example using verbal prescriptions.
- *Anticipatory problem-solving*: For example, giving pain relief before procedures.

Eisenhauer *et al.* (2001) suggest that this evidence refutes the concept that administration of medicines is simply a task but demonstrates complex thinking and application of theory to practice. They go on to suggest that administration is only one aspect of the nurse's role in relation to medicines management. Figure 3.1 offers a visual overview of the elements of the nurse's role in relation to medicines management.

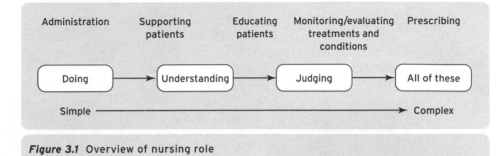

Figure 3.1 Overview of nursing role

Other authors have sought to explain the complexity of administering medicines to a single patient. Chapelhow *et al.* (2005) apply their model (Meaningful Assimilation of Skills for Care, MASC) to help uncover the intricacy of this nursing skill, which is often invisible and difficult even for experienced and skilled nurses to articulate. They identify a range of knowledge and skills required, including five categories of 'underpinning concepts and theories' that support the nurse's thinking, relating to the:

- patient, e.g. condition, beliefs, religion;
- personal, e.g. the nurse's philosophy, learning style, social skills;
- professional, e.g. legislation, ethics, emotional labour (personal cost);
- context, e.g. trust policies, resources;
- evidence, e.g. physiology, medicines, nursing interventions (Chapelhow *et al.*, 2005).

They stress the importance of skills to use these theories in a specific situation. Such skills are known as 'enablers'. Chapelhow *et al.* (2005) offer some examples of how they can be interpreted:

- Assessment: working with the patient
- Communication: language, body language, advocacy, patience
- Risk management: relating to medication effects
- Professional judgement and decision-making: considering alternatives
- Record-keeping and documentation
- Managing uncertainty: supporting patients' decisions.

Figure 3.2 shows the various factors that need to be considered in medicines management.

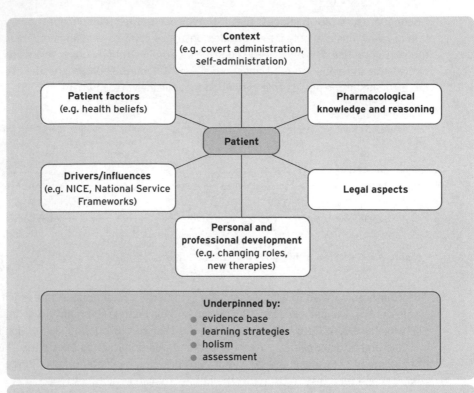

Figure 3.2 Visual representation of factors to consider in medicines management

Vigilance

The Eisenhauer *et al.* (2007) study into the complex thinking required highlighted some very clear examples of how and where these skills were used by nurses to 'prevent harm and promote good patient care outcomes'. For example, they suggest that nurses assessed patients' needs for medication, monitored adverse effects, and made judgements about the timing of medications and information needs of patients. The authors also note that the act of administering medication was a small part in the whole process. They go on to identify the need for nurses to use 'professional vigilance', which they sum up as the thinking processes identified above, which are particularly pertinent for nurses in helping patients to manage their medication regimes safely and effectively. They refer to the work of Meyer and Lavin (2005), who offer the following definition of professional vigilance:

> ... a state of scientifically, intellectually, and experientially grounded attention to and identification of clinically significant observations/signals/cues; calculation of risk inherent in nursing practice situations and readiness to act appropriately and efficiently to minimise risks and respond to them.

One of the nurses in the Eisenhauer *et al.* study (2007) sums this up quite effectively: 'The sixth R is the registered nurse who makes sure the previous five Rs are correct.'

Meyer and Lavin (2005) suggest that 'it has not always been as easy for nurses to attach a label to what they think and to communicate the judgements that result from the mental work of professional vigilance', but such thinking and communication involves:

- assessment of observations and cues;
- assessment of risk;
- prevention of risk.

This involves thinking about what they are doing, in order to make decisions about care.

Much of the nurse education literature identifies the difficulty for students in relating classroom teaching to their clinical experience – the theory–practice gap. This is said to exist when 'the knowing that' of theory is divorced form 'the knowing how' (applying theory to practice) of clinical practice (Jordan, 1994). Two strategies have been suggested to close this gap: the adoption of heuristic learning strategies such as problem-solving, and drawing theory from practice (exploring the clinical problem). Problem-solving is an approach to learning that has been adopted in both nursing and medical education, where it is often called problem-based learning.

Within nurse education, we have tended to move towards enquiry-based learning, placing the emphasis on patient needs rather than problems, and promoting the importance of the student identifying what they need to know and so directing their own learning. Like any strategy, this needs practice and some initial direction.

This and many other books and articles are written to help both student nurses and qualified nurses to develop a greater understanding of pharmacology. There is no doubt that qualified nurses who are involved in administering medication and/or educating patients about their medication need to have a sound knowledge and understanding of the medicines that they are commonly administering, but such understanding strictly speaking is not pharmacology. Pharmacology is the science of how drugs act on the body. However, there is no widely accepted term to describe the aspects of pharmacology that are needed by nurses. Along with skills related to medicine administration, patient education and patient assessment, it involves emotional intelligence, knowing the patient/carer, recognising and interpreting body language, user/carer involvement, interpersonal skills, record-keeping, documentation and evaluation of the effects of the medicine.

WHAT INFORMATION TO USE

There are thousands of medicines available for use, and it is impossible to memorise all the information related to them all (Lim and Honey, 2005). Choosing which medicines to include in a book such as this can be difficult. Schwertz et al. (1997) suggest that all nursing students should have some knowledge about all of the 'major medicine groups'. This is not the purpose of this book; we aim to provide a means of learning about medicines in any situation; a framework or model. Schwertz *et al.* (1997) comment that it is often necessary when teaching pharmacology to recommend two or three texts, as no one book will provide the breadth and depth of information required. Leathard (2001), on the other hand, suggests that nurses should have an understanding of the medicines that are commonly administered within their area of practice rather than have detailed knowledge about a lot of medicines, as the latter is not realistic. She goes on to suggest that nurses should have the skills to be able to research other medicines that they meet.

Miller (1992) suggests that, unless theory is related to practice and specifically to the individual patients, students may see it as irrelevant. Latter *et al.* (2001) support this idea, suggesting that pharmacological knowledge is valued when it has clear importance for practice. Latter *et al.* suggest that 'the dynamic nature of pharmacology knowledge indicates that this will need to be complemented by self-directed and continuous learning in practice'. They identify the need to provide students with the means to develop this aspect of their learning. Their study identified that currently there is a lack of opportunity for students to integrate knowledge and skills in practice, and that this should be supported by the use of experiential and problem-based learning.

Manias and Bullock (2002) undertook a study that identified that students felt inadequately prepared for issues related to medication in practice. Reasons for this, suggested by Gerrish (2000), include the lack of opportunity to get involved in medication administration because of 'workload pressures' and shorter clinical practice. Gerrish also recommends 'active' learning strategies.

Within this chapter, we provide some information and a rationale for why we have adopted an approach to learning about medicines related to patient care situations (contextualised learning). This involves taking a situation and teasing out the information we need in order to understand a patient's prescribed care. The process of using patient groups begins in Chapters 7 and 8, and then we move on to look at individual patient scenarios in Chapter 9 onwards.

We have deliberately avoided using a systems approach – for example, looking at medicines related to the respiratory or cardiovascular systems – in this book. Equally, we have avoided looking at themes such as infection. We feel these approaches are reductionist because they do not acknowledge that patients may have problems with more than one body system. Instead, as nurses, we need to understand how systems, conditions and treatments interrelate. An important aspect of any patient's care is their reaction to treatment, including not only the physical response but also their feelings and ability to manage their treatment.

We have also avoided trying to relate treatments to branch-specific scenarios, which we feel can perpetuate the barriers between the separate disciplines of nursing and does not reflect the true nature of the patient's experience. Consider the reality of a patient accessing an A&E department with mental health problems, for example. This approach would also be at odds with the current government drive towards enhanced multiprofessional/interprofessional working. The Audit Commission (2001) stresses the importance of a multiprofessional approach to medicines management, and so nurses need to develop skills of collaborative working as well as gaining pharmacological knowledge.

Explaining our choice of information

The scenarios within the book have been chosen to reflect situations that student nurses are likely to meet regularly in practice. We have accessed a range of information sources to validate the situations we have chosen, including National Service Frameworks (NSFs), which reflect areas that the government has highlighted as priorities, and the National Institute for Health and Clinical Excellence (NICE) guidelines in order to make sure that the medicines discussed are contemporary.

We have considered the recommendations from the British Pharmacological Society (BPS, 2002), which has outlined a core curriculum for pre-registration nurses, identifying topics such as drug development, pharmacokinetics, pharmacodynamics, specific drug groups (e.g. anticonvulsants and analgesics) and certain skills (e.g. interpretation and reflection).

Another resource we have used is the Prescription Analysis and Cost (PACT) tool, which analyses data from the Prescription Pricing Division (PPD). This provides up-to-date information about the patterns of prescribing and enables us to identify the most commonly prescribed medicines. The PPD processes prescriptions on a monthly basis (**www.ppa.org.uk**). For example, information up to March 2007 informs us that the number of prescriptions is increasing and in which areas. These prescriptions are identified as being for medicines used in cardiovascular and endocrine diseases. The PPD suggests that one key influence on this in general practice has been the NSFs for coronary heart disease, diabetes and older people.

We have considered these recommendations and identified the core group of medicines that seem to be reflected in all these resources. We have also tried to provide a wide-ranging source of information about medications. We compared the information above, which, apart from that of the BPS, focuses upon groups of medicines or patient groups, with recommendations within nursing literature about the extent of knowledge required by nurses for safe practice in relation to medicines. These are effectively summed up by Leathard (2001) as classifications, pharmacodynamics, pharmacokinetics, drug interactions and drug development. These are introduced as concepts in Chapter 4, but they emerge in a more realistic and valid way from the patient scenarios in this book. Bullock and Manias (2002) add clinical decision-making and patient education to this list.

We begin in Chapters 7 and 8 by looking at two groups identified within the NSFs: older adults and cancer care. This will allow us to explore commonalities of treatments and patient needs. It also enables us to start applying information to patient groups before we start the more complex process of exploring the information we need in order to understand medicines from an individual patient perspective. We have decided to use cancer care and the older person, as both are such vast topic areas. Care of the older person highlights issues pertinent to this age group, such as the altered physiology related to the ageing process and the vulnerability of older people, using examples such as polypharmacy and compliance. However, being as this NSF focuses on a group of patients rather than on a disorder, we also offer a scenario in Chapter 13 in which an older person has a diagnosed disease process.

In each situation, whether patient group (older person) or individual scenario, as in Part 4, the information is presented using a standardised framework that always includes:

- the evidence base for the underpinning knowledge required to understand the situation;
- pharmacological knowledge;
- nursing knowledge regarding interventions and implications;
- related knowledge, such as explanations of disordered physiology;
- personal and professional development activities to engage you in the learning process;
- essential terminology.

Using patient scenarios

The use of patient scenarios to develop knowledge and understanding is not a new approach. Schwertz *et al.* (1997) describe this approach as 'excellent' for developing pharmacological reasoning as it provides examples of realistic pharmacological interventions in patients with complex health problems. Thus, it is a popular technique because it enables the integration of theory and practice. However, Schwertz *et al.* comment that, when applied to promoting the understanding of pharmacology information, there is a 'potential loss of emphasis on pharmacologic principles'. The focus of this book on understanding patient situations generated from practice means that the patient scenario drives the choice of information. Some issues may be revisited in more than one situation, enabling the transfer of knowledge into new situations in order to generate new understandings in the context of that patient. However, this does mean that some aspects of pharmacology may not be addressed. Our priority in writing a book such as this is to provide an approach to understanding patients and their medications – a learning strategy – rather than covering every aspect of pharmacology.

Using scenarios in this way, we tease out the important information that we need to know in order to make sense of the situation. To do this, we highlight what we believe are the key components of the scenario to be explored. This is an approach that any of us might use in order to try to make sense of a situation. This is a technique employed by teachers who are trying to encourage students to both direct and be active in their own learning, and is described as being either problem-based or enquiry-based learning. The key feature is that the student identifies within the scenario or situation those issues that they need to investigate in order to enhance their understanding.

Problem-/enquiry-based learning

Problem-based learning uses situations or scenarios that are context-related – that is, they are examples generated from practice. Price (2001) suggests that this method confirms the pledge to 'how to' learning in nursing rather than simply 'doing'.

King (2003) maintains that students do not effectively learn abstract concepts. Rather, ideas become much more meaningful when they are clearly related to the student's own world of work. Another strength of this approach is that the student identifies their own individual learning needs. Bath and Blais (1993) suggest that problem-based learning is an approach used in, for example, medical education because it generates problems to understand and solve from real situations. The problem-based learning approach is advocated by Beers and Bowden (2005) as a strategy that 'facilitates effective learning and promotes long-term knowledge retention' due to its focus on the application of knowledge, which is one of the aims of this book.

Many nursing curricula have adopted this approach but have dropped the term 'problem' because nursing activities are related to patients' needs as well as problems; they then refer to the approach as 'enquiry-based learning'. The student gets involved in their own learning by identifying what they do not know and then finding out the relevant information. This involves learning from experience: students investigate the experience and develop a critical stance to understanding practice. This then equips them with skills to adapt to changing healthcare delivery. Price (2001) argues that this approach also reinforces the 'need to work effectively with others'. Healthcare professionals from different disciplines will see the patient from different perspectives, which will enhance students' understanding and develop shared appreciations of the situation.

One of the strengths of this approach is that it helps you visualise the whole picture, for example in the patient with more than one condition and taking more than one medicine. In such a situation, it is important to find out whether the medications are prescribed or over the counter (OTC), whether the medicines interact with each other, whether the patient is able to manage a potentially complicated medication regime, and whether the patient believes that taking prescribed medication is the best way of managing their condition.

Wilkes and Batt (1998) remind us that 'nurses bring their world to the classroom' and that this involves shared understanding, images and language learned within clinical areas. We feel it is important to use this world to understand medicines and how they are used in practice. This enables students to understand that there are reasons for care interventions and that using a 'reasoning approach' is a useful way to understand care (Wilkes and Batt, 1998).

Latter *et al.* (2000) suggest that 'the dynamic nature of pharmacology knowledge indicates that this will need to be complemented by self-directed and continuous learning in practice'. They identify the need to provide students with the means to develop this aspect of their learning. Their study identified that currently there is a lack of opportunity for students to integrate knowledge and skills in practice, and that this should be supported by the use of experiential and problem-based learning. Price (2001) suggests that enquiry-based learning can provide 'an exciting and relevant way to learn' that will improve your practice and help you make decisions.

Skills development

Enquiry-based learning involves comparing the practice situation with the student's existing knowledge and understanding in order to identify areas for development. This encourages students to develop problem-solving skills, to review the value of the information obtained and to transfer knowledge into new situations. If managed successfully, this process of learning can develop 'skilled, knowledgeable and reflective practitioners' (Frost, 1996).

Problem-solving involves information-processing, the aim of which is to assist the decision-making process. This is a useful process when choosing appropriate patient outcomes and nursing interventions; we can also transfer this process to learning. This process is based on the assumption that we bring to the problem some previous knowledge, such as our experience of similar problems (Price, 2003). The first step in the process is identifying the problem. In enquiry-based learning, we start by identifying what we don't know.

Personal and professional development 3.1

You could now skip to any of the patient chapters and read the patient scenarios. The first step is to identify what information within the scenario you need to research in order to understand the situation.

If you read the scenario about Katie, a young girl with epilepsy, in Chapter 12, you could start by asking yourself the following questions:

- What do you know about epilepsy?
- What do you know about treatments for epilepsy?
- What would be the effects of alcohol and anticonvulsant drugs?
- Why has Katie had a convulsion after being well-controlled on her treatment?
- What are the consequences of unprotected sex?
- Would this treatment have any potential action on a developing foetus?
- What are the implications for the nurse?

However, this is just the first stage. We also need to know how we find this information, how we can judge its worth, and how we decide what information we need.

Learning tools

Maule (2001) suggests that in order to 'judge' we need to integrate different aspects of information. When faced in a care environment with a patient who is receiving medication, we need to be able to identify the type of information that we need, for example information about the medication, information about the patient and information about legislation. We need to identify appropriate sources of information, such as a pharmacology book that presents information in a format that is easy to access and understand, professional sources (e.g. DH and NMC websites), and books providing information on disease processes, disordered physiology and nursing care/interventions. Another useful strategy is to identify people who can help, such as mentors, lecturers, doctors, pharmacists, dieticians, patients and carers.

This is a lot of information, and so we need to be focused and discerning. We need to follow the process of identifying some initial information, reviewing it and then identifying further information needs. This needs to be compared with the patient's situation: Does the information provide an adequate overview of the topic? Are there any gaps? Does it raise more questions? Does it direct us to other useful sources that we had not considered initially?

This process involves ongoing review of our understanding and how we are managing it – that is, what are we learning, what is it that enhances our learning, and what is it that inhibits our learning? Inhibitors to learning are usually lack of appropriate language (see Chapter 2) and/or lack of specialist knowledge. As learners, it is also easy to compare our knowledge with that of experienced practitioners, the result being another inhibitor – lack of confidence.

Models are available that guide you through a process for learning, such as experiential learning described by Kolb (1984). This starts with the 'problem/experience' and involves identification of learning needs, carrying out some action and evaluating our progress in order to identify 'where next'. Jasper (2003) identifies this as a useful approach to 'understanding practice'. Practice reinforces learning, but only if this practice is 'scrutinised' and subject to discussion and critical appraisal with colleagues and/or clients (Leathard, 2001). Figure 3.3 shows the stages of Kolb's model.

Jasper (2003) describes practice as meaningful learning; by working with 'real people in real settings', you develop knowledge and skills. Engaging with experiences in this way is consistent with 'deep' approaches to learning (Entwistle and Tait, 1994). Deep learning involves understanding information, relating it to our own experience and then evaluating the value of what we are reading. Surface learning, on the other hand, is concerned with memorising information (Quinn, 2000). Deep learning is more appropriate for practitioners working in challenging and dynamic care environments, as it

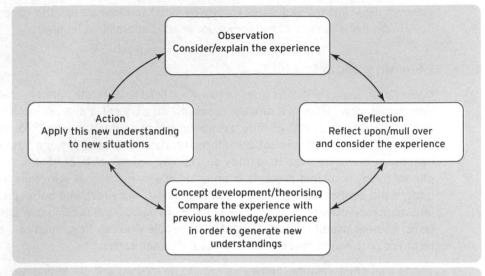

Figure 3.3 Adaptation of Kolb's (1984) experiential learning cycle (Kolb, 1984)

fosters understanding, transferability of knowledge and autonomous learning, bases learning around patients and practice, encourages the application of theory to practice, and generates an understanding of theory from practice.

Most qualified nurses over the past two or three decades have recognised how useful the problem-solving cycle is. However, McAllister (2003) has established that using such a cycle can be restrictive. She argues that this is mainly because there are two ways of thinking (confirmation bias and fixation) that seem to get in the way when, as nurses, we use the problem-solving cycle. McAllister suggests that this is compounded in times of stress, when 'thinking becomes rigid'. Although she does not explain fully the reason for this, there is evidence that the complexity of the work that some people do has a major impact on their thinking processes. As they work through multiple problems at the same time, their thought processes start to fill their working memory to such an extent that there is little 'space' left (Hecht, 2002; Sohn and Doane, 2003).

It may be that there simply is not sufficient power left to enable us to easily take a different view of a situation, and so we stick with our familiar patterns of activities and ideas. Instead of using the problem-oriented approach, McAllister (2003) supports the idea that clinical reasoning benefits from solution-orientation as it brings 'creative, non-rational thinking processes'. She argues strongly that instead of 'aiming to do work on a client', nurses should aim 'to work with and for' a patient.

Essential terminology

Confirmation bias and fixation

These terms are used in psychology to describe a particular set of cognitive (thinking) processes. The former describes how we much more readily seek data that corroborate our ideas rather than data that disprove them. The latter term is used to explain the difficulty that we all have in taking a completely different view of something.

> ## Personal and professional development 3.2
>
> As a student working in a healthcare environment with a medicine unfamiliar to you, what would be the first information source that you would use to find out more about that particular medicine?
>
> Consider how this fits with the previous discussion. Do you choose information that is familiar, or do you choose to use a range of sources, some of which challenge conventional wisdom?
>
> Consider the discussions in previous chapters regarding the various uses of a single medication, according to the patient's condition.

It is important to keep up-to-date with new medicines (e.g. genetic therapy, which has the potential to challenge our previous understandings of causes of disease) and to appreciate why in some situations (e.g. relating to the patient's genetic profile) medicines do not act in the way in which we expect them to or do not exert any effect. Consequently, we need to acquire a broad understanding and a flexible approach to working effectively with patients. 'Learning how to learn' enables us to be safe and competent and to cope with new roles and new medicine developments – the 'changing dimension of health care' (Lim and Honey, 2005).

OUR APPROACH

Using the term 'medicines management' in the way that we do in this book can be seen as somewhat controversial. We use the term in a very different way from that used since it was first introduced into the NHS by the Audit Commission (2001). Medicines management for nurses is more than administration of medicines. Nurses also monitor the effectiveness of treatments, advise patients about treatments (e.g. the diabetic nurse specialist who helps the patient manage **hyperglycaemia**), educate patients, recommend changes to treatments, and now, increasingly, prescribe medicines. Inevitably, this requires knowledge about how medicines affect the patient, information about the patient so that we can make judgements, and understanding of the context in which we work (policies, administration systems, ordering and the wider context of nursing), professional advice and new roles. Much of the literature on role transition (Amos, 2001) identifies that students feel that their pharmacology knowledge is inadequate and worry about this aspect of their role after qualifying, particularly as their responsibilities change in relation to medicines management. Therefore, it is important to have the skills in order to maintain a contemporary evidence base for our actions and interventions.

CONCLUSION

The approach taken in this book is not purely an overview of how medicines act. Within this book, we look at the wider issues associated with treatment-related interventions for patients. It is important to know how medicines work, but we also need to know how to deal with patients' responses to treatment, for example a sudden drop in blood pressure after medication, and how to deal with issues that might arise, such as responding to a verbal prescription. These responses, although based on certain similar principles, vary in relation to the individual patient and individual care environment.

Leathard (2001) suggests that the development of nurse prescribing provides us with a 'timely prompt' for considering the 'understanding of medicines' that is needed by nurses. The amount of knowledge and understanding that we need about medicines will vary in relation to practice responsibilities, but expanding roles demand 'expanding understanding'. Meyer and Lavin (2005) suggest that unless we acknowledge this and try to raise awareness of the sophisticated skills that nurses use in patient interactions, we 'risk having this unique aspect of our work be invisible to others'.

Quick reminder

✔ Pharmacology information is readily available.

✔ Pharmacology knowledge needs to be linked to patient care in order to be meaningful.

✔ Students perceive pharmacological knowledge as being difficult to learn.

✔ There are contemporary approaches to learning that encourage the application of theory to practice.

✔ To be meaningful, learning involves the development of skills, identifying the problem, retrieving information, reviewing information, making judgements about the values of information and applying this theory to practice.

REFERENCES

Allen D (2004) Re-reading nursing and re-writing practice: towards an empirically based reformulation of the nursing mandate. *Nursing Inquiry* **11**, 271-283.

Amos D (2001) An evaluation of staff nurse role transition. *Nursing Standard* **16**, 36-41.

Audit Commission (2001) *A Spoonful of Sugar: Medicines Management in NHS Hospitals.* Wetherby: Audit Commission Publications.

Bath J B and Blais K (1993) Learning style as a predictor of drug dosage ability. *Nurse Educator* **18**, 33-36.

Beers G W and Bowden S (2005) The effect of teaching method on long-term knowledge retention. *Journal of Nursing Education* **44**, 511–515.

British Pharmacolgical Society (2002) at **http://www.bps.ac.uk**.

Bullock S and Manias E (2002) The educational preparation of undergraduate nursing students in pharmacology: a survey of lecturers' perceptions and experiences. *Journal of Advanced Nursing* **40**, 7-16.

Chapelhow C, Crouch S, Fisher M and Walsh A (2005) *Uncovering Skills for Practice*. Cheltenham: Nelson Thornes.

Department of Health (DH) (1999) *Making a Difference: Strengthening the Nursing, Midwifery and Health Contribution to Health and Healthcare*. London: The Stationery Office.

Department of Health (DH) (2001a) *The Expert Patient: A New Approach to Chronic Disease Management for the 21st Century*. London: The Stationery Office.

Department of Health (DH) (2001b) *The NHS Plan: A Plan for Investment, A Plan for Reform*. London: The Stationery Office.

Department of Health (2002) *Liberating the Talents: Helping Primary Care Trusts and Nurses to Deliver the NHS Plan*. London: The Stationery Office.

Eisenhauer L A , Hurley A C and Dolan N (2007) Nurses' reported thinking during medication administration. *Journal of Nursing Scholarship* **39**, 82-87.

Entwistle N J and Tait H (1994) *The Revised Approaches to Studying Inventory: Centre for Research into Learning and Instruction*. Edinburgh: University of Edinburgh.

Frost M (1996) An analysis of the scope and value of problem-based learning in the education of healthcare professionals. *Journal of Advanced Nursing* **24**, 1047-1053.

Gerrish K (2000) Still fumbling along? A comparative study of the newly qualified nurse's perception of the transition from student to qualified nurse. *Journal of Advanced Nursing* **32**, 473-489.

Hecht S A (2002) Counting on working memory in simple arithmetic when counting is used for problem solving. *Memory and Cognition* **30**, 447-455.

Hughes E C (1984) *The Sociological Eye*. London: Transaction Books.

Jasper M (2003) *Beginning Reflective Practice*. Cheltenham: Nelson Thornes.

Jordan S (1994) Should nurses be studying bioscience? A discussion paper. *Nurse Education Today* **14**, 417-426.

King R L (2003) Nurses' perceptions of their pharmacology educational needs. *Journal of Advanced Nursing* **45**, 392-400.

Kolb D (1984) *Experiential Learning: Experiences as a Source of Learning and Development*. Englewood Cliffs, NJ: Prentice-Hall.

Latter S, Rycroft-Malone J, Yerrell P and Shaw D (2000) Evaluating educational preparation for a health education role in practice: the case of medication education. *Journal of Advanced Nursing* **32**, 1282-1298.

Latter S, Rycroft-Malone J, Yerrell P and Shaw D (2001) Nurses' educational preparation for a medication education role: findings from a national survey. *Nurse Education Today* **21**, 143-154.

Leathard H L (2001) Understanding medicines: extending pharmacology education for dependent and independent prescribing (part II). *Nurse Education Today* **21**, 272-277.

Lim A G and Honey M (2005) Integrated undergraduate nursing curriculum for pharmacology. *Nurse Education in Practice* **6**, 163-168.

Manias E and Bullock S (2002) The educational preparation of undergraduate nursing students in pharmacology: clinical nurses' perceptions and experiences of graduate nurses' medication knowledge. *International Journal of Nursing Studies* **39**, 773-784.

Maule A J (2001) Studying judgments: some comments and suggestions for future research. *Thinking and Reasoning* **7**, 91-102.

McAllister M (2003) Doing practice differently: solution-focused nursing. *Journal of Advanced Nursing* **41**, 528-535.

Meyer G and Lavin M A (2005) Vigilance: the essence of nursing. *Online Journal of Issues in Nursing* **10**, 8.

Miller A (1992) From theory to practice. *Journal of Clinical Nursing* **1**, 295-296.

Mullally S (2002) Nurses of all levels can improve patient's experience of health care. *British Journal of Nursing* **11**, 424.

NHS Management Executive (1991) *Junior Doctors: The New Deal*. London: NHS Management Executive.

Nursing and Midwifery Council (NMC) (2007) *Standards for Medicines Management*. London: Nursing and Midwifery Council.

Price B (2001) Enquiry-based learning: an introductory guide. *Nursing Standard* **15**, 45–52.

Price B (2003) Understanding the origins of practice problems. *Nursing Standard* **17**, 47–53.

Quinn F M (2000) *Principles and Practice of Nurse Education*. Cheltenham: Nelson Thornes.

Rafferty A M, Allcock N and Lathlean J (1996) The theory/practice 'gap': taking issue with the issue. *Journal of Advanced Nursing* **23**, 685–691.

Schwertz D W, Piano M R, Klienpell R and Johnson J (1997) Teaching pharmacology to advanced practice nursing students: issues and strategies. *AACN Clinical Issues* **8**, 132–146.

Sohn Y W and Doane S M (2003) Roles of working memory capacity and long-term working memory skill in complex task performance. *Memory and Cognition* **31**, 458–466.

Walsh M (1999) Nurses and nurse practitioners: priorities in care. *Nursing Standard* **13**, 38–42.

Wilkes L M and Batt J E (1998) Nurses' understanding of physical science in nursing practice. *Nurse Education Today* **18**, 125–132.

Wilson D and DeVito-Thomas P (2004) The sixth right of medication administration. *Nurse Educator* **29**, 131–132.

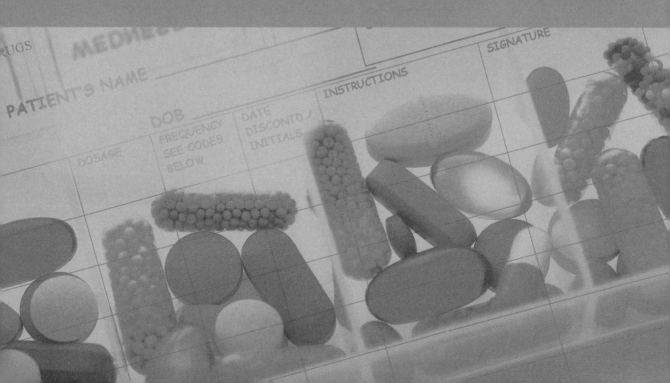

Part 2

Important concepts and principles

Chapter 4

Underpinning pharmacological principles: pharmacodynamics and pharmacokinetics

There are a bewildering number of drugs on the market. Understanding how drugs and medicines work is crucial for the qualified nurse. Nurses can contribute to treatment decisions only if they understand how medicines exert their effects, can recognise side effects and know about interactions. This knowledge equips the nurse to monitor and evaluate the effectiveness of a medicine for the patient and to provide the patient with the information they need to manage their treatment regimes effectively. It would be impossible for most people to have an in-depth knowledge of all available medicines, but the Nursing and Midwifery Council (NMC) (2007) suggest that:

> ... you must know the therapeutic uses of the medicines to be administered, its normal dosage, side effects, precautions and contra-indications.

Essential terminology

Professional knowledge

The Nursing and Midwifery Council (NMC) is the regulatory body for nursing and midwifery and is responsible for public safety. The NMC offers professional advice to qualified nurses and produces minimum standards to which qualified nurses should adhere. The NMC (2007) has recently produced a set of standards in relation to medicines management.

This implies a breadth of knowledge about the medicines that nurses administer regularly. Before you move on to read the chapters containing information about the medicines administered for specific patients and their conditions, consider your current understanding of how medicines work and how they can affect the patient. You also need to consider your responsibilities in relation to these drugs (this is explored in the next chapter).

Ensuring that medicines are administered safely is one of the most important roles of the nurse. The NMC (2007) states:

> The administration of medicines ... is not solely a mechanistic task ... it requires thought and the exercise of professional judgment.

This implies an underpinning knowledge and skills base related to medicines. In order to understand the effect (or lack of) that a drug or medicine is having on a particular patient, we need to understand how the medicine exerts its effects. We cannot know all information about all medicines in use today, but we should have knowledge about the commonly used medicines and the core medicines given to patients within the patient care context in which we are working, whether hospital-based, in patients' homes or in residential care.

Learning outcomes

By the end of this chapter you should be able to:

✔ Describe the process of drug development
✔ Identify and explain some of the terminology used when discussing drugs and medicines
✔ Explain how drugs exert their effects on the body
✔ Outline how drugs reach their target sites
✔ List the routes by which medicines are administered
✔ Identify some formulations of medicines in common usage.

Chapter at a glance

This chapter will introduce some of the essential underpinning information:

Sources of information
Terminology
Understanding pharmacology
Drug development
Aims of drug treatment
Pharmacodynamics
Pharmacokinetics
Adverse drug reactions and drug interactions
Routes of administration
Preparations
Quick reminder
References

SOURCES OF INFORMATION

If we do not know about an individual medicine, then we need to know where to find the relevant information and how to find it.

There are many textbooks that provide information about drugs and medicines for nurses and other health professionals. One useful resource is the British National Formulary (BNF), which is produced twice a year and sent free of charge to health professionals involved in administration and/or prescribing of medicines. The BNF is also available online at **www.bnf.org**. The BNF claims to provide 'UK healthcare professionals with authoritative and practical information on the selection and clinical use of medicines in a clear, concise and accessible manner… Its guidance is continually refined to reflect the latest evidence' (**www.bnf.org**).

Whatever resource you choose to use, you need to be able to find what you are looking for. This is not always as straightforward as it sounds: as with any new undertaking, we need to learn the specialist language in order to make sense of the situation (see Chapter 2).

TERMINOLOGY

You may wish to start the process of understanding the language used in relation to medicine administration and the underpinning knowledge required to understand how medicines work (e.g. physiological principles) by considering what is meant by the term 'drug'. If we look up this term in a dictionary or encyclopaedia, we might find a definition that reflects that a drug is a substance that produces a beneficial effect on the body, relieves problems, prevents the development of disease or restores health. Wikipedia (**http://en.wikipedia.org**), for example, defines a drug as 'any biological substance, synthetic or non-synthetic, that is taken for non-dietary needs … it will produce some effects or alter some bodily functions'. This is a standard definition, but Wikipedia offers an interesting differentiation between naturally occurring substances and synthetically produced substances. Consider the example of the **hormone** insulin: when produced naturally by the body, would be referred to as a hormone; but when given to a patient with insulin-dependent diabetes mellitus, as part of the patient's treatment, it is considered a drug. We need to become familiar with the technical language that we use to describe and explain drugs and drug actions, as the language used in conversations does not always adequately describe the way in which drugs are used in a clinical context. The example of insulin reminds us that some drugs and medicines are given to replace substances that the body is unable to produce; other examples are dopamine (given to patients with Parkinson's disease) and levothyroxine (given to patients with an underactive thyroid gland) – that is, replacement therapy.

In reality

One concern when accessing information is the accuracy and therefore validity of the information. Websites are useful, but peer-reviewed sources, which may be Web-based, are the most reliable. One of the benefits of using a Web-based resource is that it is easily accessible and therefore may be used widely by patients. It is often useful for healthcare professionals to access the same source as the patient so that we have some insight into the patient's level of knowledge. One useful Web-based resource for health professionals is the BNF online.

We explore this 'familiar' language within this chapter and introduce some language and terminology that you might not be as familiar with.

Personal and professional development 4.1
Underpinning knowledge

You may wish to do some further reading or remind yourself about the following terms and processes before moving on to read the rest of this chapter.

Cell: The basic unit of all living organisms. Cells can replicate exactly.

Diffusion: The process involved when gases and liquids of different concentrations combine until they become of equal concentration.

Diuresis: Increased production of urine by the kidneys.

Electrolyte: In clinical contexts, this term refers to ions such as sodium ions.

Enzyme: A protein that in small amounts can increase the rate of a biological reaction, thus acting as a catalyst.

Hormone: A substance that is produced by the body (by an endocrine gland) and then transported via the bloodstream to an organ or tissue in order to exert a modifying action on that organ's or tissue's structure or function.

Metabolism: The chemical and physical processes that take place within the body in order to maintain its functioning and development.

Molecule: A particle that consists of two or more atoms held together by chemical bonds.

Receptor: A particular area of the cell membrane that binds with a specific hormone.

Drug names

Some drug names are indicative of their chemical constituents – the chemical name. Pharmaceutical companies also market their drugs under trade (brand) names. An analogy is Hoover and vacuum cleaner: Hoover is the brand name, but vacuum cleaner describes the product; however, many people use the terms interchangeably.

The brand name may or may not reflect the drug's chemical constituents. The brand name is often short or easy to remember; for example, Detrusitol™ (tolterodine tartrate) indicates its effect of relaxing the detrusor muscle in the bladder (this drug is classified as an antimuscarinic; it reduces detrusor contractions and increases bladder capacity and is used when incontinence occurs as a result of detrusor instability (**www.bnf.org**).

Different pharmaceutical companies may produce different versions of the same drug, and so the same drug may have several brand names. It is important to use the generic name (the approved or official medical name; also referred to as the international non-proprietary name; and often derived from the chemical name) in order to minimise errors in care situations.

It is recommended that when writing the generic name, the name has a lower-case initial letter; brand names, on the other hand, have capital initial letters. For example, tramadol (generic name), a synthetic analgesic based on opioids, has several trade names, including Zydol, Dromadol and Zamadol (Dewar, 2000; **www.bnf.org**).

Name changes

Until 2003 the UK used a drug-naming system of British approved names (BANs), despite European and UK legislation (European directive 92/27/EEC) that recommended the use of international non-proprietary names (rINNS). There was a reluctance to change because of the potential for mistakes when moving from one system to another. However, the use of two systems across Europe and the UK added to the risk of error; following wide consultation, the Medicines Commission advised that rINNS be adopted by 30 June 2004 (**www.mhra.gov.uk**; Simonsen *et al.*, 2006).

The words 'drug' and 'medicine' are often used interchangeably. For example, we frequently hear nurses referring to drug administration. However, many authors suggest that we should use the term 'medicines' when referring to drugs used in clinical situations. This is reinforced by the NMC (2007), which goes even further and suggests the term 'medicinal product' to describe:

> … any substance or combination of substances presented for treating or preventing disease … administered … with a view to … restoring, correcting or modifying physiological functions.

There are some important distinctions to be made between drugs and medicines.

A drug:

- is a chemical substance;
- can be any chemical taken for its physiological effect;
- is the active ingredient of a medicine.

A medicine:

- contains the drug and inactive materials (**excipients**), depending on the form, e.g. tablet, capsule. Excipients include flavourings, diluents to add bulk, binders to enable the ingredients to be formed into a tablet, and lubricants to ensure a smooth surface. Sometimes substances are added to slow down the absorption of the drug; this sustained-release format produces a prolonged effect, therefore limiting the number of doses required per day;
- is a substance that cures/arrests disease or relieves symptoms.

In a clinical context, we need to have a broader perspective of what constitutes a 'medicine' – for example, medical gases such as oxygen and intravenous fluids – and is therefore subject to legislation in relation to storage, availability and administration.

To complicate things further, drugs and medicines are classified according to the action they exert or the body system they affect and are described as belonging to drug groups such as analgesics, antibiotics, laxatives, antihistamines, anti-emetics, anxiolytics, antidepressants, corticosteroids and anticonvulsants.

A full list of these can be obtained from the BNF or a pharmacology textbook for nurses.

It is interesting to note how many of the drug groups we can identify begin with 'anti'. In other words, they prevent something occurring. Many drugs routinely prescribed are for the management of symptoms and/or conditions such as pain, nausea, depression and raised blood pressure. In fact, we have very few actual 'cures'. The most familiar example of a cure is the **antibiotic**, which can eliminate infections by destroying bacteria.

Although knowledge of drug groups is a useful way to begin to learn about medicines, it does not help us understand why, for example, we use some anticonvulsants for pain relief in certain situations, such as neuralgia (see Chapter 2) . It is therefore important to understand how the medicine exerts its effect.

So far within this book we have used the terms 'drug' and 'medicine' interchangeably. For the rest of the book we use the term 'drug' to describe the chemical used to produce an effect on the body and use the term 'medicine' to refer to the use of the chemical therapeutically – that is, its actions and uses. For example, the medicine co-codamol contains two drugs – paracetamol and codeine phosphate. However, paracetamol and codeine phosphate individually can also be described as medicines.

UNDERSTANDING PHARMACOLOGY

For nurses, we might assume that the key knowledge required is related to the pharmacology of medicinal drugs – that is, those prescribed as treatments. It is important to note that there are several non-prescription social drugs that have an impact upon treatments, such as caffeine, alcohol and nicotine. Also, patients may be using illegal recreational drugs. The nurse's knowledge base therefore should reflect not only the effects of medicines but also the impact of social drugs, poisons, pharmacologically active foods and pollutants (Comerford *et al.*, 2005). The nurse therefore needs an understanding of psychology, social customs, religious practices and legislation. The potential for drug development using genetic material and the current issues relating to drug costs and availability also pose difficult moral and ethical problems.

> **Personal and professional development 4.4 Thinking about treatments**
>
> Can you identify some of the wide range of uses of drug therapies that are available today?
>
> Answers can be found at the back of the book.

Rang *et al.* (2003) define pharmacology as 'the study of the effects of chemical substances on the function of living systems'. Pharmacology is a relatively new subject and was 'born in the mid-19th century' (Rang *et al.*, 2003). The development of clinical pharmacology is usually attributed to a physician, William Withering, who conducted early studies into the use of digitalis. We can trace the origins of clinical pharmacology – that is, the effects of drugs on humans (Rawlins, 2001) – to early therapeutics (treatment of disease) related to magic potions and herbal remedies. This reflects early beliefs that illnesses were the result of witchcraft, magic or misfortune, which had very little scientific basis. We also have evidence that some pharmacologically active substances such as opium, derived from the poppy, were used for pain relief.

According to Rawlins (2001), the progress in pharmacology since Withering's work has been informed by chemistry, pathology and human biology. The developments in these subjects have provided us with a basis for understanding the effects of chemicals on humans.

Although now produced in laboratories, drugs were originally derived from many sources, such as plants, minerals, microbial cultures and animal tissues. Many natural sources are still used: for example, digoxin and vincristine are produced from plants and insulin is produced from genetically modified bacteria.

Some drugs in regular use have been available for a considerable period of time. The longer we have used a drug, the more information we can gather about how it behaves. As our knowledge about illness and its causes develops, we can develop new and improved versions of traditional drugs. For example, we know that aspirin can be used to treat mild to moderate pain, but we also understand that it has an anti-inflammatory action (and thus it is known as a non-steroidal anti-inflammatory drug or NSAID) and an antiplatelet action. Aspirin and other NSAIDs interrupt the synthesis of prostaglandins from arachidonic acid by inhibiting the enzyme cyclo-oxygenase (COX). COX-1 is an isoenzyme of COX found in tissues and responsible for tissue homeostasis; it regulates platelet aggregation and exerts a protective effect on the lining of the stomach. COX-2 is the isoenzyme whose action results in the production of prostaglandins, chemicals produced by the body in response to injury. Prostaglandins cause inflammation. NSAIDs are believed to reduce inflammation by inhibiting COX-2 and thus the production of prostaglandins.

Another example is angiotensin-converting enzyme (ACE) inhibitors, which were developed to reduce blood pressure by interfering with the renin–angiotensin–aldosterone system, the body's normal physiological mechanism for maintaining blood pressure. The first ACE inhibitors had problematic consequences; for example, a patient's blood pressure could fall more quickly than desired, and hence careful observation of the patient was important. This is still important, but companies developing the newer, second-generation ACE inhibitors have fine-tuned their effect so that this is not such an alarming effect.

DRUG DEVELOPMENT

Drugs are produced by pharmaceutical companies both to address gaps in therapeutics – that is, to provide treatments for diseases or improve current treatments – and to be profitable.

Having identified that clinical pharmacology is concerned with the effects of chemicals on humans and that there is the potential for any drug or medicine to be used incorrectly (either deliberately or inadvertently), it is important that we consider the safety of drugs. We need to balance this safety against the efficacy of drugs; for example, some important groups of drugs can cause serious and distressing side effects, such as chemotherapy drugs used in the treatment of cancer. Some textbooks refer to this as the 'risk-to-benefit ratio' (Rawlins, 2001).

It is very important, therefore, that before new drug treatments are available for use by the general public, we are confident about the drug's expected therapeutic and unwanted effects. Drugs need to be tested appropriately before licences can be granted for their use.

Essential terminology

Licence

All medicines for use in the UK must be granted a product licence, which outlines the conditions under which the medicine can be used (Downie *et al.*, 2003).

The NMC (2004, 2007) suggests that, in most cases, crushing tablets renders them unlicensed. This is particularly true of medicines formulated to be administered once daily, when crushing would change their properties, such that they would be used outside the manufacturer's recommendations, e.g. nifedipine LA, a longer-acting medicine used in the treatment of angina and hypertension. In this situation, the person crushing the tablet takes responsibility for administering the medicine out of licence; for example, they are responsible for any unwanted effects that occur. If the prescription identifies the medicine to be given in this way, the prescriber takes responsibility.

If a patient is being fed by enteral feeding tubes (e.g. percutaneous endoscopic gastrostomy, PEG), this can cause problems with administration of medicines, which have to be delivered via the tube. If the nurse crushes tablets in order to administer

In reality

There is widespread use of unlicensed medicines in children's nursing. Permanan *et al.* (2007) suggest that this is because 'the development and testing of drugs for children is far from satisfactory'. Using children in clinical trials raises ethical issues, which are not easily resolved. In other words, because medicines are not routinely tested on children, medicines used for children are often those licensed for use in adults, therefore, the format may be unsuitable for children; doses are based upon adult doses but reduced in relation to the weight or age of the child. This may put the child at risk as specific recommended doses for children have not been established as part of the drug development process.

Medicines licensed for use in adults but used for children (informed use) are described as being 'off label' (**www.bnf.org**).

In response to this issue, new legislation for children's medicines came into effect on 26 January 2007 (Commission of the European Communities: Regulation (EC) No. 1901/2006). This sets out changes in relation to the development and accessibility of children's medicines, including ethical research.

Drug trials are undertaken over a considerable period of time to establish the mode of drug actions and to eliminate harmful effects. Thus, when a drug becomes available to the public, we know as much as we can about the drug, such as its effects on the body and the duration of those effects so that we can establish the route and frequency of doses (Greenstein and Gould, 2004).

The first stage of drug testing takes place in the laboratory to determine the drug's properties and identify potential short-term toxic effects. It is then tested to establish its effects and actions. This process begins with tests on cell and tissue samples; many drugs are rejected at this stage.

Once the pharmaceutical firm can predict with some confidence the effect of the drug, it is tested on animals. The effects on animals cannot be assumed to be the same as those on humans, however, and therefore inevitably the next stage involves testing the drug on humans. There are several carefully controlled phases in the process of testing on humans. Drug trials in healthy volunteers (phase 1 trials – see below) require authorisation from the the Medicines and Healthcare Products Regulatory Agency (MHRA), the government agency responsible for ensuring that medicines are 'acceptably safe'.

Human testing

Phase 1

This involves giving the drug for the first time to humans. Healthy volunteers are used to see whether the effects in animals can be replicated in humans. This usually involves a small number of volunteers; for example, in the high-profile drug trial in which six young men suffered serious adverse effects after taking an anti-inflammatory drug (TGN1412), there were only eight volunteers. The drug is tested for safety and side effects. The drug is administered initially in a small dose, which is increased gradually to assess for the maximum tolerated dose (Wiffen *et al.*, 2007).

Phase 2

This involves testing the drug on a small sample of people with the relevant illness or disease, under close supervision. This phase is concerned with effectiveness, side effects and the relationships between dose, therapeutic effects and side effects.

Phase 3

This involves testing on large numbers (300–3000) of people with the relevant illness or disease, over a longer period of time, and across a range of test centres. This phase is concerned with confirming the results of the previous phases and testing for full information about the drug (Wiffen *et al.*, 2007).

Testing involves the use of randomised controlled trials (RCTs), which involves the comparison of groups of patients. One group receives the experimental drug, while the other receives a 'treatment' that has no therapeutic effect (**placebo**). The patients are allocated randomly so that neither the patient nor the researchers know which group of patients is receiving the experimental drug. This double-blind testing is considered to produce very strong evidence and is often described as the 'gold standard' for evidence-based care (Walsh and Wigens, 2003).

> **Essential terminology**
>
> **Placebos**
> 'Substances with no known pharmacological effects' (Simonsen *et al.*, 2006)

In randomised controlled trials, blind testing can take two forms:

- *Single-blind study*: the researcher does not know which drug has been administered.
- *Double-blind study*: neither the subject nor the researcher knows which drug has been administered (Wiffen *et al.*, 2007).

If the Committee for the Safety of Medicines (CSM) is satisfied that the drug is safe and effective, then the drug is licensed.

Phase 4

Having successfully reached this stage and generated a lot of data, the drug is used to treat patients. This allows for wider testing against other drugs and testing for further side effects and long-term risks and benefits, involving scrutiny of the **yellow card scheme** reports (Downie *et al.*, 2003; Simonsen *et al.*, 2006).

Further information about drug testing can be found on the MHRA website (**www.mhra.gov.uk**).

AIMS OF DRUG TREATMENT

The aim of drug treatment is to achieve a concentration of drug in the blood or tissue that lies somewhere between the minimum effective level and the maximum safe concentration. Drugs are identified as having a **therapeutic range** (index) - that is, the range between toxicity and safety (Figure 4.1). The wider the therapeutic index or range, the safer the drug.

Digoxin, a medicine given to slow down a fast heart rate, has a low therapeutic index; that is, the therapeutic and toxic doses are close, and the patient taking digoxin must be monitored carefully. With most drugs, we can monitor the patient by blood sampling

Not everyone responds in the same way to a medicine, and in many cases the dose has to be adjusted to allow for such factors as the age, weight or general health of the patient.

The dose of any medicine should be sufficient to produce a beneficial response but not so great that it will cause excessive adverse effects. If the dose is too low, the medicine may not have any effect, either beneficial or adverse; if it is too high, it will not produce any additional benefits and may produce adverse effects.

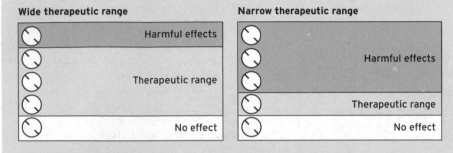

Wide therapeutic range

Harmful effects

Therapeutic range

No effect

Narrow therapeutic range

Harmful effects

Therapeutic range

No effect

Dosage of medicines with a wide therapeutic range can vary considerably without altering the drug's effects.

Dosage of medicines with a narrow therapeutic range has to be carefully calculated to achieve the desired effect.

Figure 4.1 Therapeutic range (after BMA, 2002)

- that is, taking a specimen of blood and measuring the amount of drug in the bloodstream. With digoxin, we can also record the patient's pulse and heart rate; if this becomes too slow, then it is an indication that the dose needs to be reviewed.

In reality

Blood monitoring can not only identify the amount of drug in the bloodstream but also identify an improvement or deterioration in the patient's condition. In the patient with an underactive thyroid gland, for example, treatment should reflect an improvement in thyroid function, determined by checking the levels of circulating thyroid hormones. A patient taking a diuretic, on the other hand, may have regular blood tests for electrolytes in order to determine whether the patient is losing too much potassium.

Blood monitoring is an invasive and potentially distressing procedure and therefore used only when necessary. Other tests, such as urine samples, may be used to establish the amount of the drug eliminated and therefore an estimate of the drug in the bloodstream, or the patient's condition and behaviour may be observed and assessed.

Dose response

Drugs are identified as having a therapeutic index or margin of safety, which is interpreted in texts such as the BNF as recommended normal dose ranges. This therapeutic index is determined by extensive drug trials (Dewar, 2000). For example the dose for paracetamol given in the BNF is 0.5-1g every 4-6 hours, to a maximum of 4g daily (**www.bnf.org**). This dose is for an adult taking the drug orally. The range gives some flexibility for individual patients, as not all patients achieve pain relief with the same dose. Factors taken into account when determining the dose of a medicine include the patient's age and condition, and the route of administration (Dewar, 2000). These factors are discussed later in this chapter.

PHARMACODYNAMICS

Pharmacodynamics is the effect of drugs on the body and the mode of drug action – that is, the study of how drugs interact with the body in order to produce a response. Despite a great deal of research that allows us to predict how drugs will act, we do not always know why drugs work in a particular way. We can, however, put forward some theories as to how drugs work. An underpinning principle is that the drug interacts with cells and tissues in order to exert its effects, and therefore the drug must be delivered to the tissues in an appropriate dose if it is to bind to the tissues. Drugs cannot change the function of cells, but they can affect how well the cell functions or the rate at which it functions by interacting at a cellular or molecular level, usually with proteins (Simonsen *et al.*, 2006).

The purpose of administering drugs is 'to achieve a certain, predicted effect within the body' (Dewar, 2000).

All body functions are controlled by substances such as enzymes, receptors on cell surfaces, carrier molecules and specific receptors/macromolecules (proteins that are integral parts of cell membranes). Most drugs act by interfering with these control systems at a molecular level. This chemical interaction between the drug and the cell brings about some change to the cell's function, because the 'attached drug and cell' function differently; this constitutes the drug's effect (Dewar, 2000).

Most drugs produce their effects by binding to protein molecules (targets), such as enzymes, carrier molecules/transport mechanisms, ion channels and receptors (Rang *et al.*, 2003). Groups of drugs bind to specific targets, which recognise the drug group. This combination of drug and target is reversible. Figure 4.2 shows the interaction between drugs and target sites.

Essential terminology

The physiological response that is produced by a drug binding to a protein is referred to in most pharmacology textbooks as a 'target protein-ligand interaction'.

Target protein

A protein molecule that allows another molecule to bind to it.

Ligand

Ligand is a broad term for a substance that binds to a target protein to produce a response. The response can be agonist or antagonist (producing or preventing responses). Ligands can be hormones, neurotransmitters (produced within the body and therefore described as endogenous) or drugs (produced outside the body and so described as exogenous).

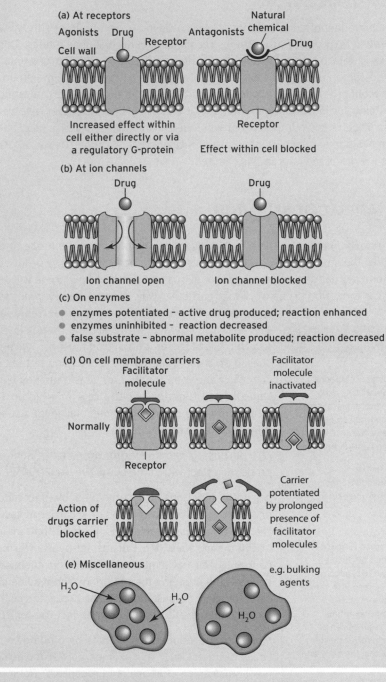

Figure 4.2 Mechanisms of drug action (after Prosser *et al.* 2000)

Enzymes

Enzymes are proteins that are biological catalysts. They speed up a wide variety of chemical processes within the body. Enzymes may be extracellular or intracellular (Simonsen *et al.*, 2006). Drugs may enhance/increase or, more commonly, inhibit/decrease the action of enzymes and thus interfere with a variety of chemical processes; examples include aspirin, some diuretic drugs (transport-inhibiting diuretics, such as furosemide) and ACE inhibitors.

Carrier molecules

Although some drugs move freely within the fluid compartments of the body, many drugs need a carrier to assist them across the cell membrane, because the drug molecules are insufficiently lipid-soluble to be able to pass through the lipid membranes unaided. The carrier is usually a protein and which may be specific (Dewar, 2000), such that the carrier recognises the molecule it transports. Rang *et al.* (2003) describe the carriers as having 'a recognition site', and this makes them specific.

Ion channels

Ion channels are selective pores in the cell membrane that allow the movement of ions such as sodium, potassium and calcium in and out of the cell. Some drugs, such as lidocaine and calcium channel blockers (e.g. verapamil), block these ion channels, which interferes with ion transport and causes an altered physiological response. Calcium channel blockers are vasodilators and are used in the management of angina. Calcium is necessary for muscle contraction: low calcium levels reduce both the force and the rate of muscle contraction, in this case in the heart muscle (Simonsen *et al.*, 2006). Other drugs, such as nifedipine, bind with proteins in the ion channel wall.

Other, newer drugs, such as nicorandil, open ion channels; in this case potassium channels. In angina, chest pain occurs because narrowed coronary arteries restrict the amount of oxygen able to be delivered to heart muscle (myocardium). Giving a drug to open the potassium channels in the membrane of the muscle allows an influx of potassium; this prevents the calcium channels from opening and prevents calcium from becoming available. The result is a relaxation of the muscle walls of the coronary arteries, which causes arterial vasodilation (Conway and Fuat, 2007; Galbraith *et al.*, 2007).

Receptors

It is thought that most drugs exert their effects by binding with a receptor (target molecule) on the cell surface or in the cell cytoplasm, forming a drug–receptor complex. A drug may have an affinity for a certain receptor; receptors bind only with drugs that have compatible structures, rather like a key fits in a lock. Once the drug has bound to a receptor, a specific response occurs. If this activates the receptor, it is said to potentiate (stimulate) the action of the cell; this is known as the agonist effect. Examples of drugs that cause an agonist response are nicotine, insulin and corticosteroids. The opposite response is the antagonist effect, in which the action of the cell is blocked. In this case, the receptor is 'occupied' but no effect is produced. Figure 4.3 shows how agonists and antagonists affect the cell.

Morphine, an opioid analgesic, produces its action by binding to opioid receptors. It is a full agonist, which means it produces a maximum response. The result is a diminished sensation of pain for the patient (see Chapters 7, 9, and 10 for more detailed explanations of opioids). Naloxone is an antagonist; it occupies the opioid receptor without producing an effect. It can therefore be considered as an antidote to morphine. Naloxone stops the unwanted effects of respiratory depression that occur following large doses of morphine by occupying the opioid receptor (Dewar, 2000; Downie *et al.*, 2003; Simonsen *et al.*, 2006).

However, drugs rarely exert a maximum response; instead, they produce a limited response related to the drug's ability to occupy the receptor. They are then known as **partial antagonists** (Rang *et al.*, 2003). Greenstein and Gould (2004) define partial antagonists as drugs able to either potentiate or block an action, depending on the dose or length of action; often, the higher the dose, the more effective the drug.

Many medicines are thought to produce their effects by their action on special sites called *receptors* on the surface of body cells. Natural body chemicals such as neurotransmitters bind to these sites, initiating a response in the cell. Cells may have many types of receptor, each of which has an affinity for a different chemical in the body. Drugs may also bind to receptors, either adding to the effect of the body's natural chemicals and enhancing cell response (agonist drugs) or preventing such a chemical from binding to its receptor, and thereby blocking a particular cell response (antagonist drugs).

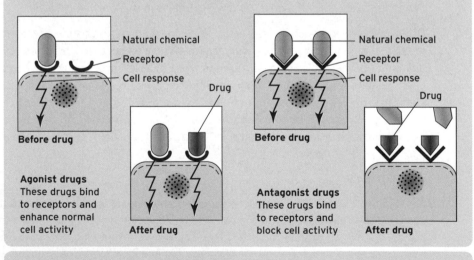

Figure 4.3 Agonists and antagonists (after BMA, 2002)

Sometimes drugs compete with the naturally occurring agonist to prevent a response. An example of this is beta-blockers, a group of medicines that compete with the body's naturally occurring stimulants to block a response, for example to slow down a fast heart (see also Chapter 10).

Receptor subtypes

It has become apparent that there are variations – subtypes – of receptors. Receptors may be very similar but possess subtle differences that help to explain the effectiveness (or ineffectiveness) of some drugs. In theory, it should be possible to produce a drug that will bind only to a specific subtype of a receptor and therefore be more effective. Figure 4.4 helps to clarify this.

There are some drugs whose actions cannot be explained by the mechanisms described above. For example, laxatives and antacids act on the contents of the gastrointestinal tract rather than at a cellular level (Dewar, 2000).

PHARMACOKINETICS

If you consider some experiences you have had with patients or discussions you have had with your friends and family, you will probably recognise that some people favour one medicine over another. One patient's condition, such as hypertension (high blood pressure), might be controlled adequately by their treatment, but another patient with hypertension may not be able to achieve effective blood pressure control. Rusnak *et al.* (2001) suggest that only 27% of patients with hypertension achieve blood pressure

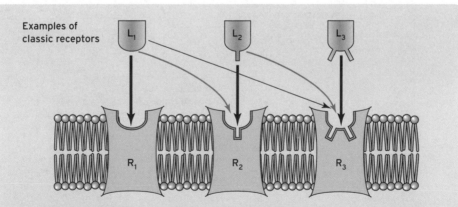

Formation of complexes. The same ligand can bind to different targets (in this example, classic receptors), but not all the complexes that are formed lead to the same effect. Ligand L_1 fits all receptors but produces the best response by binding to R_1. L_2 fits R_2 and R_3 but provides the best response in R_2. L_3 fits only R_3.

Figure 4.4 Receptor subtypes (after Simonsen *et al.*; 2006. Reproduced by permission of Roy Lysaa and Edward Arnold (Publishers) Ltd)

control. This difference in response is thought to relate to our individual genetic makeup and thus how our body deals with drugs (Read, 2002).

Thus, there are several factors to consider when assessing and monitoring a patient's medication needs. Pharmacokinetics is the study of drug action within the body. *Kinetics* refers to movement, and therefore pharmacokinetics can be defined as 'the study of the "movement" or fate of drugs in the body' (Simonsen *et al.*, 2006). In other words, pharmacokinetics is about how the body deals with the drug. It refers to all the processes involved from the moment the drug or medicine enters the body to the time it leaves the body. These processes are known as absorption, distribution, metabolism and elimination (ADME; Figure 4.5):

● *Absorption*: The process by which a drug enters the bloodstream. Some injections, such as via the intravenous route, bypass this by depositing the drug directly into the bloodstream. When drugs are given orally, they first travel through the gastrointestinal tract before entering the bloodstream.

● *Distribution*: The process by which the drug passes from the bloodstream into the target tissues.

● *Metabolism*: The process of transforming a drug so that it attracts water or becomes more water-soluble, ready for excretion.

● *Elimination*: The removal of the products of metabolism from the body. Drugs are excreted mainly by the kidneys, but also by the liver via the biliary system and in smaller quantities via the skin and lungs.

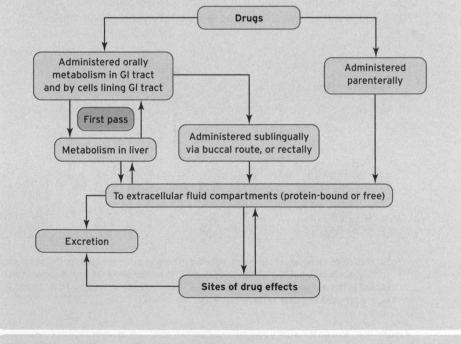

Figure 4.5 ADME (after Prosser *et al.*, 2000)

Absorption

Absorption refers to the journey of the drug from the site of administration (in the case of oral medications, this is through the intestinal wall) and into the plasma, ready to be delivered to its point of action. If a drug is absorbed through the intestinal wall, it is first transported to the liver, via the hepatic portal vein, before being circulated to body tissues. One function of the liver is to detoxify substances it recognises as toxic, which may include drugs. This is called the **first pass effect**. Some drugs manage to pass through the liver without being metabolised, while others are converted to an active metabolite that then exerts the therapeutic effect (e.g. atenolol, a beta-blocker).

It is the amount of the drug that survives its journey through the liver that is available for use by the body. This is one consideration when deciding upon the route of administration, because giving the drug by a different route – for example, by injection – can avoid the first pass effect.

With certain drugs, if given repeatedly, the breakdown process becomes more effective. Therefore, larger doses are then required in order to produce the same effect – this is known as **drug tolerance**. Tolerance can be seen when opioid analgesics are used for pain relief. Another familiar example is the tolerance that develops to alcohol: as our body gains 'more experience' of alcohol, we are able to drink more before we notice the symptoms of intoxication; alcoholics can drink very large quantities of alcohol without becoming inebriated or sick. The explanation for this is that the liver increases its production of enzymes such as alcohol dehydrogenase, which hastens the metabolism of alcohol and so there is less alcohol available to reach the receptors. Explanations for tolerance to other drugs include a reduction in the mechanism of action, a decrease in the number of receptors (downregulation) and receptor desensitisation (this might explain the tolerance that develops to morphine) (Simonsen *et al.*, 2006; Wickens, 2005).

Some drugs, such as glyceryl trinitrate, are not usually administered orally because they are metabolised almost completely and therefore largely inactivated by the first pass effect. However, the main reason for not administering glyceryl trinitrate orally is that it needs to be available rapidly to relieve the pain (see Chapter 2).

Absorption is enabled by specific transport systems:

- *Passive diffusion* via a concentration gradient, that is, from an area of high concentration (in the gastrointestinal tract) to an area of lower concentration (in the bloodstream). This is the most common and the most significant transport system. The drug molecules diffuse across the cell membranes (Figure 4.6), which requires no cellular energy. The process stops when the concentrations become equal.

- *Active transport* requires cellular energy as the drug moves from an area of low concentration to one of high concentration, therefore working against the concentration gradient. These drugs make use of the physiological mechanisms that exist to transport some substances across cell membranes. Usually these transport

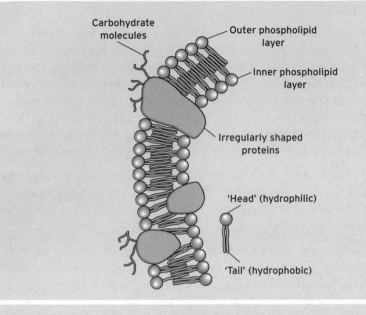

Figure 4.6 The cell membrane (after Hinchliff, Montague and Watson, 1996)

systems involve a carrier molecule such as a transmembrane protein. Examples include drugs that resemble natural body substances, such as levodopa, which resembles dopamine, a neurotransmitter that is missing in Parkinson's disease (Downie *et al.*, 2003; Rang *et al.*, 2003).

● *Filtration* through a pressure gradient via pores between cells. Filtration applies only to small molecules, and therefore the number of drugs absorbed in this way is limited.

● *Facilitated diffusion* allows drugs that are not lipid-soluble, such as glucose, to be transported across the cell membrane by a carrier, usually a protein (Figure 4.7). This uses a concentration gradient but requires no energy.

Distribution

Distribution is the delivery of the drug to the various body tissues and fluids via the bloodstream. Distribution is dependent upon the following:

● *Blood flow*: The high vascularity (presence of blood vessels) of some organs, such as the heart, liver and kidneys, means that drugs are distributed to them rapidly, whereas distribution to skin and fat, which have fewer blood vessels, is slower. The patient's activity levels and body temperature also affect blood flow.

● *Solubility of the drug*: The ability of the drug to cross a cell membrane depends upon whether the drug is soluble in water or fat (lipid). Lipid-soluble drugs easily cross cell membranes, but water-soluble drugs do not. Lipid-soluble drugs can therefore cross the

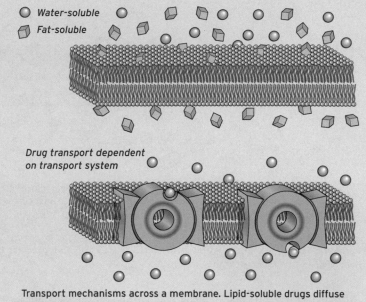

Transport mechanisms across a membrane. Lipid-soluble drugs diffuse through he membrane by passive diffusion, while other drugs need the help of specialised transport systems.

Figure 4.7 Transport systems (after Simonsen *et al.*, 2006. Reproduced by permission of Roy Lysaa and Edward Arnold (Publishers) Ltd)

Essential terminology

Blood–brain barrier

The mechanism that regulates which molecules can enter the cerebrospinal fluid and tissue spaces surrounding the cells of the brain. The barrier prevents potentially harmful substances such as drugs passing into the brain. The cells that make up the walls of the capillaries surrounding the brain are closer together than in other capillaries in the body, which enables them to block the passage of some substances but allow other substances through.

blood–brain barrier and enter the brain, but water-soluble drugs are not successful here because the capillaries of the central nervous system (CNS) lack channels between cells, therefore blocking their means of access. We also need to consider storage sites; for example, fat acts as a storage site for lipid-soluble drugs such as anticoagulants (drugs that delay or prevent blood clotting). This means that the drug accumulates within fat and may remain there for some time, being released slowly.

- *Plasma protein binding*: Most drugs attach to a carrier (plasma protein) within the bloodstream. When the drug and protein are bound, the drug is not available for use; only the unbound portion of the drug is active. A drug is said to be highly protein-bound if more than 80% of the drug is bound. If a patient is taking more than one drug that binds to a plasma protein, the drugs may compete for the protein (Figure 4.8). This process explains some drug interactions; for example, warfarin can dislodge other drugs from plasma proteins, with the result that the dislodged drug is more active, with potentially toxic effects.

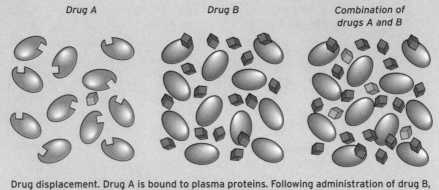

Drug displacement. Drug A is bound to plasma proteins. Following administration of drug B, some of drug A may be displaced from binding sites, resulting in an increase in the free drug concentration of drug A.

Figure 4.8 Drug displacement (after Simonsen *et al.*, 2006. Reproduced by permission of Roy Lysaa and Edward Arnold (Publishers) Ltd)

- *Diffusion*: Drugs diffuse out of the bloodstream into tissue spaces and cells, entering the fluid compartments of the body. The more widely a drug diffuses, the lower the concentration of the drug. If the patient has **dehydration**, there is less fluid for the drug to diffuse into and therefore the drug is present in a greater concentration (Downie *et al.*, 2003). As an example, consider the difference in concentration between a mug of coffee that contains a spoonful of sugar and a smaller espresso cup that contains a spoonful of sugar.

Metabolism

Metabolism is the transformation of a drug in preparation for excretion from the body (biotransformation). The pharmacological activity of the drug is usually removed over time, making the drug less active. This occurs mainly in the liver, by hepatic enzymes, but also in the kidneys, intestinal mucosa, lungs, plasma and placenta. Changes to the liver, for example due to age or disease, can affect liver function: hepatic enzymes can be increased (enzyme induction) or can be inhibited (enzyme inhibition), and thus the drug dose needs to be reviewed (Simonsen *et al.*, 2006).

The products of metabolism are called metabolites. Inactive metabolites are excreted, while active metabolites have their own pharmacological properties. Some drugs are administered as prodrugs and are not active until they are metabolised; for example, desloratidine is converted to loratidine (an antihistamine used to relieve the symptoms of allergy) in the body.

Metabolism is an ongoing process that occurs in two stages:

- *Phase I metabolism*: This includes chemical reactions such as hydrolysis (the reaction between a compound and water to produce another compound), oxidation (a reaction in which a molecule or atom loses electrons, e.g. glucose is oxidised during cellular respiration) and reduction (a reaction in which a molecule or atom gains electrons). The reactions change the chemical properties of the drug, producing metabolites. These reactions are produced by enzymes such as cytochrome P459, found in liver cells. The metabolites are still active at this stage (Dewar, 2000).

- *Phase II metabolism*: The drug/phase I metabolite is now conjugated (fused with another compound) with water-soluble substances to render the drug soluble and largely inactive, ready for excretion via all body fluids. Drugs that remain in a lipophilic (lipid-soluble) state are mostly reabsorbed in the intestine; they then reach the liver again and are reconjugated. They are said to circulate in the enterohepatic circulation, staying longer within the body; an example is digoxin (see Chapter 2). Some drugs compete for enzyme metabolism, which can cause an accumulation of drugs when they are administered together, increasing the risk of adverse reactions and toxicity.

Elimination

Elimination is the removal of a drug from the body. Drugs are eliminated in two main ways:

- *Metabolism*: As outlined above, drugs may be broken down or combined with some other chemical so that they are no longer pharmacologically active and can be excreted more easily. This usually happens in the liver and is brought about by enzymes.

- *Excretion via the kidneys*: This is via a combination of processes within the kidneys, including glomerular filtration (filtration of plasma by the kidneys), tubular secretion (transfer of substances from the blood vessels of the tubule into the lumen of the tubule) and tubular reabsorption (removal of water and other substances from the fluid in the tubule and transportation into the blood). The kidneys' regulatory and excretory processes are responsible for urine production. Figure 4.9 shows the location of these processes within the nephron.

    Renal function is therefore important in the excretion of drugs from the body. One test that we use to measure kidney function is the creatinine clearance test, which compares the level of creatinine (a waste product of protein and nucleic acid metabolism) in the urine aagainst the level in the bloodstream. This usually involves collection of the patient's urine for 24 hours and collection of a blood sample at the end of this period. This establishes the effectiveness of glomerular fitration and therefore provides us with an assessment of renal function.

Drug elimination is mainly via the kidneys (in urine) or via the liver and biliary system (elimination in faeces). Elimination also occurs in much smaller quantities through the skin (in sweat, e.g. elimination of vitamin B) and the lungs (in expired air, e.g. anaesthetic gases, small amounts of alcohol). Drugs may also be eliminated in other body fluids, such as saliva.

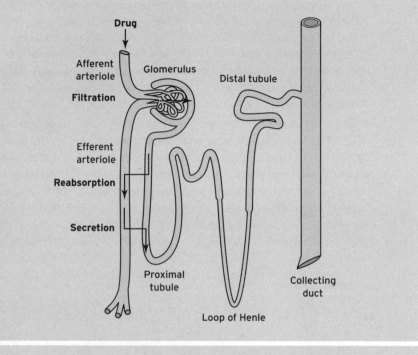

Figure 4.9 The nephron and urine production

Half-life

The half-life is 'the rate at which the active drug is removed from the body' (Prosser *et al.*, 2000); that is, the time taken for the drug to fall to half its initial dose. Knowledge of the half-life is used to establish the dose and frequency of dose required to maintain circulating blood levels of the drug at a therapeutic level. This requires an understanding of the metabolism of the medicine, as metabolites can also be active and therefore exert a similar therapeutic effect to that of the administered drug.

The half-life is affected by absorption, metabolism and elimination. Knowledge of the drug's half-life, and therefore how long it remains in the body, influences how often the drug needs to be administered – that is, the dosing intervals (Figure 4.10). The aim of dosing is to produce a stable concentration of the drug in the bloodstream. A drug that is administered regularly is said to reach a **steady state** (concentration); that is, the drug levels within the body stay at a 'therapeutically effective concentration' below toxic levels and above the minimum effective level (Greenstein and Gould, 2004).

There are two easily recognisable examples that help to demonstrate this: pain relief and alcohol. If you have had experience of taking analgesics to relieve pain, you may have found yourself watching the clock for the next dose because the dose you are taking is not effective and you are not maintaining an adequate therapeutic level within

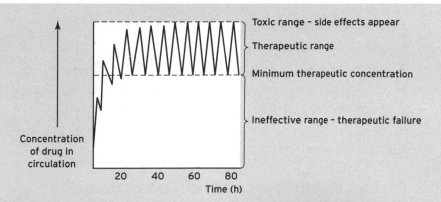

In the example illustrated above, the drug is scheduled to be administered four times per day, or every six hours. If this is done strictly, for example at 6am, 12 noon, 6pm and midnight, the concentrations fluctuate but they remain within the therapeutic range.

However, if the ward is busy, the dosing may be rescheduled to accommodate other tasks, with the result that the drug is administered at 10am, 2pm, 6pm and 10pm. Therefore, the concentrations fluctuate wildly. At times the drug is below the minimum therapeutic concentration and ineffective, but at other times it causes toxicity, as illustrated below:

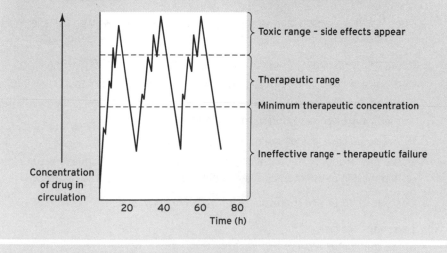

Figure 4.10 Dosing intervals (after Jordan, 2002)

the bloodstream. Studies have shown that when people self-medicate, they tend to be cautious about the dose they take and the frequency of doses (Bird and Hassall, 1993).

Conversely, you may have witnessed the effects when people take several 'doses' or units of alcohol close together. Alcohol remains in the bloodstream until it is metabolised by the liver. Allen (1996) suggests that the effects of alcohol can be seen approximately ten minutes after drinking; if someone consumes several units of alcohol in a short time, then the blood alcohol level will rise, as the person is consuming alcohol at a faster rate than the body metabolises it.

To take this a little further, several factors affect how a drug is 'used' by the body. These factors can be related to:

- specific groups within the population, such as children;
- general situations, such as the presence of food in the stomach;
- the individual, such as the presence of liver disease, which will impact upon the body's ability to metabolise and eliminate drugs.

These factors should be taken into consideration when drugs are prescribed for, and administered to, patients.

Factors that influence the effects of drugs

Factors relating to potentially vulnerable groups of patients

Older patients

The effects of ageing may reduce the first pass effect and affect excretory processes, thus increasing the amount of drug available to the body, with potentially toxic effects for the older person (Chapter 8 discusses the effects of drugs on the older person).

Children

Neonates have more water and less fat than older children. Organs and organ systems in children are immature. Maturity is related to age. As a consequence:

- gastric emptying is reduced in children under the age of 6 months;
- drugs are absorbed more readily through the skin of neonates;
- the higher proportion of water in neonates enables an increased distribution of medicine, often resulting in the need for higher doses;
- neonates have less plasma proteins;
- the immaturity of neonatal organs such as the liver and kidneys results in reduced elimination of the medicine and a delay in achieving a steady state.

Doses in children are therefore usually age-related (Simonsen *et al.*, 2006).

Pregnant women

Some medicines are contraindicated in pregnant women because of the potential of the drugs to harm the baby. As a general principle, medicines should be avoided during pregnancy. Simonsen *et al.* (2006) suggest that three risks need to be considered when making decisions about treatment of pregnant women:

- The risk to the mother if the medicine is not used
- The risk to the baby if treatment for the mother's illness is not given or continued
- The risk to the baby if the medicine is used.

The following points regarding treatment of pregnant women should be considered:

- Some lipid-soluble drugs cross the placenta and therefore put the foetus at risk of injury. The term 'teratogenesis' describes the potential of drugs to cause development abnormalities in the foetus; e.g. warfarin is an anticoagulant, but may also cause death or miscarriage.

- Some groups of drugs, e.g. **barbiturates** (sedatives), may cause drug **dependence** (which used to be referred to as addiction) in the foetus.

- In the pregnant user of narcotics (opioids), at birth the baby may exhibit narcotic withdrawal unless weaned off the narcotic by using decreasing doses of methadone.

- A drug can cause fetal abnormalities because of its mode of action rather than crossing the placenta; e.g. a **vasoconstrictor** may cause vasoconstriction of the blood vessels within the placenta.

- The effect of the drug upon the fetus depends upon the foetal stage of development and the potential sensitivity to drugs.

- Some drugs, given just before or during labour, may cause maternal or neonatal complications; e.g. drugs such as opioids used for pain relief in labour may sedate the baby.

- Pregnancy can affect the body's ability to distribute, metabolise and excrete drugs; e.g. in pregnancy, there is a reduction in plasma proteins, an increase in enzyme activity in the liver, an increase in the percentage of water in the body and a doubling of renal blood flow.

Nursing implications Using information about medicines

Using the information provided earlier in the section on absorption, distribution, metabolism and excretion, can you identify the potential effects and nursing implications of the following:

- Reduction in plasma proteins
- Increased liver enzyme activity
- Increased renal blood flow.

Answers can be found at the back of the book.

Breastfeeding mothers

It is possible for medications that the breastfeeding mother takes to affect the baby. Generally medicines are in a lower concentration in breast milk compared with in the bloodstream, and so the potential dose the baby may receive will be small. As a general principle, the mother should be encouraged to breastfeed even if she is taking medications. However, there are some important points to consider:

- Medicines can be excreted in breast milk.
- The effect upon the infant depends upon the stage of development and therefore its sensitivity to drugs; e.g. elimination may be slower.

- Some drugs can affect or even stop the production of breast milk, e.g. the combined oral contraceptive pill. High doses of oestrogen may inhibit the production of breast milk (Downie *et al.*, 2003; Simonsen *et al.*, 2006; Wiffen *et al.*, 2007).

General factors affecting the absorption of medicines and distribution from the gastrointestinal tract

- *Gut motility*: An increase in the motility of the gut means that medicines and other substances move through the gut quickly and there will be less time for medicines to be absorbed. Some antibiotics modify the gut flora (the bacteria that exist within the body without causing ill-effects), such that the gastrointestinal contents move through the gut faster; this leads to ineffective absorption of some drugs, such as oral contraceptives. It is also necessary to consider factors such as intestinal infection and the presence of disease processes such as irritable bowel syndrome (IBS).

- *Gastric emptying*: If this is fast, medicines will be absorbed quickly; if emptying is slow, medicines will be absorbed slowly. The rate of gastric emptying can be affected by the presence of food.

- *Surface area*: The potential for absorption is greater in the small intestine because of its large surface area.

- *Gut pH*: The stomach has an acidic medium, but this changes progressively to an alkaline medium lower down the gastrointestinal tract; the greatest variability is between the stomach and the duodenum. For drugs to be absorbed effectively, they need to be lipophilic (fat-loving) in order to pass through cell membranes. Many drugs are weak acids or weak base. Weak acidic drugs are lipophilic in acidic mediums, whereas weak base drugs are lipophilic in base or alkaline mediums. Aspirin is an example of a medicine that is lipophilic in an acidic medium and therefore absorbed more effectively in the stomach; pethidine is a weak base (Galbraith *et al.*, 2007; Rang *et al.*, 2003).

  Taking antacids or a glass of milk with tablets in order to prevent the gastro-irritant effect of the medicine can change the pH of the stomach to a more alkaline one. Some medicines are designed specifically to be absorbed in the lower gastrointestinal tract within an alkaline medium; for example, medicines may be provided with a special coating to render them gastro-resistant, which means that they do not become active until dissolved in the alkaline medium in the small intestine. It can take up to 4 hours for a drug to reach the small intestine. This information is important for nurses. Diclofenac, an analgesic, is gastro-irritant and is available in a gastro-resistant preparation. Because of the length of time it takes for the drug to be absorbed in this form, it cannot be used for acute pain.

- *Blood flow*: The small intestine has a good blood supply and so absorption is fast in this part of the body.

- *Presence of food and fluid*: Food in the stomach can hasten, slow or impair the absorption of medicines. It is therefore important that the patient follows any specific instructions relating to taking the medicine with food or on an empty stomach. Some antibiotics should be given before food to enable the achievement of a high plasma level. As a general principle, for fast absorption, medicines should be taken on an empty stomach (Mason, 2002).

- *Medicine composition*: The formulation (preparation) of the drug affects the ability of the drug to be absorbed and reach peak blood concentration levels. For example, liquids are absorbed more rapidly than solids.

Individual patient factors

- *Age*: Older adults and very young children can be particularly vulnerable when receiving medicine therapies.

- *Body weight*: The larger the individual, the larger the area for medicine distribution. Lipid-soluble drugs may be stored initially; therefore, to begin with they are unavailable but then they remain active within the body for longer, for example diazepam. Some doses of medicines are weight-related, particularly in young people.

- *Nutritional status*: Patients who are malnourished usually have less body protein, resulting in fewer proteins to act as carriers and enzymes and fewer storage sites for lipid-soluble drugs.

- *Food-medicine interactions*: The presence of food in the stomach can enhance or inhibit the absorption of a medicine. Grapefruit juice can reduce drug metabolism and therefore interfere with or inhibit the action of certain medicines, such as simvastatin. (More information about grapefruit and grapefruit juice can be found in Chapter 6.)

- *Disease processes*: As most absorption of oral medicines occurs in the small intestine, factors that affect the small intestine also affect the medicine; for example, surgery reduces the absorption of a drug, but intestinal irritation such as that due to IBS can mean that a drug passes through the small intestine quickly and has limited ability to be absorbed.

    Disease of the liver has the potential to inhibit metabolism and slow excretion, and so it is important to understand how a patient's specific medicines are detoxified and then take this into consideration when prescribing decisions are made.

    The condition of the patient can also affect absorption. If a patient experiences postoperative shock (a situation in which the circulation is maintained to vital organs such as the heart and brain but the peripheral circulation is reduced), this can result in a potential reduction in drug delivery, even to vital organs, particularly if the shock persists (Collins, 2000).

- *Mental and emotional factors*: Pain, anxiety and stress can decrease the amount of drug absorbed because of a change in blood flow or reduced movement through the gastrointestinal tract or gastric retention caused by the effect of pain on the autonomic nervous system. Patients who are confused or depressed may also take too much or too little of their medication.

- *Genetic and ethnic factors*: The enzyme systems that control the metabolism of drugs are genetically determined. For example, the level of rosuvastatin in the bloodstream in Asian people can be twice as high as that in non-Asian people following the same dose; that is, 5 mg in Asian people may produce the same effect as 10 mg in non-Asian people. Therefore, it is important to start the treatment with a small dose and monitor blood levels. Chinese people metabolise beta-blockers such as propranalol faster compared to white people. The pharmacological effects of the drug are altered and so Chinese people may experience increased cardiovascular effects (Rang *et al.*, 2003).

Bioavailability

One key influencing factor is bioavailability. Before a drug can be effective, it must reach the receptor site in an adequate quantity to produce a response. Drugs given intravenously have a high bioavailability because they are delivered directly into the bloodstream. Administration via other routes involves processes that reduce the amount of drug available.

Bioavailability is affected by:

- dose;
- duration of action (plasma half-life);
- route of administration;
- patient factors, e.g. disease processes.

In reality

Bioavailability can vary between different brands of the same drug, and so sometimes it is important to ensure that a patient always receives the same brand.

It is important to recognise that all medicines have the capacity to cause the following types of unwanted effect:

- *Side effect*: An unwanted medicine response that we know about. Side effects are predictable and we can warn patients about them in advance.
- *Adverse effect*: An unwanted and unexpected medicine response.

Contraindications are factors related to the individual, such as their condition or age, that mean the treatment is inappropriate and should not be given. Think about the previous examples of medicines that cross the placenta.

In reality

We use the term 'side effect' to describe the unwanted effects of a medicine that we know about. The term 'adverse effect' traditionally was used to describe unexpected effects but in many textbooks was used interchangeably with 'side effect'. More recently, 'adverse effect' has become more of an umbrella term to describe any unwanted effect of the medicine for the patient.

The term 'adverse effect' will now be used throughout this book.

Personal and professional development 4.5

Access a copy of the BNF and identify the side effects of and contraindications for aspirin.

ADVERSE DRUG REACTIONS AND DRUG INTERACTIONS

The unwanted and inadvertent effects of medicines that appear even when the medicine is taken as directed or prescribed are described as adverse drug reactions (ADRs). The World Health Organization (WHO, 1975) defines an ADR as 'a response to a drug which is noxious and unintended'; the MHRA (2002) takes this further, stating:

> ... an adverse drug reaction is an unwanted or harmful reaction experienced following the administration of a drug or combination of drugs under normal conditions of use and is suspected to be related to the drug.

Unfortunately, most medicines have the potential to cause ADRs, and this is often compounded by individual patient factors such as age, disease and genetic makeup. ADRs can impact upon patient adherence, resulting in the patient's loss of confidence in the treatment, subsequently delaying recovery and adversely affecting quality of life (Luker and Wolfson, 1999). ADRs can be classified into two groups:

● *Type A reactions*: These are exaggerated and therefore predictable responses. If we administer a medicine to slow down a patient's heart rate, we can predict that there is the potential for the heart rate to be too slow, and therefore we would monitor the patient carefully as the treatment was commenced (Shepherd, 2002).

- *Type B reactions*: These are less predictable, unexpected and often idiosyncratic (related to a particular patient) responses. This is often as a result of the individual genetic profile of the patient. Unfortunately, such reactions often mean that the treatment has to be discontinued or have serious consequences for the patient.

One important aspect of drug development is to minimise ADRs as much as possible. As healthcare professionals, we can help to minimise ADRs by reporting them, so that the collected knowledge about a medicine is as up-to-date as it can be. In the UK we use the yellow card system. Any prescribed or OTC medicine, including blood products, vaccines, herbal products and radiographic contrast media, has the potential to cause adverse reactions. Resources such as the BNF are updated regularly so that they contain the most up-to-date information about medicines. The yellow card scheme was introduced to facilitate the prompt reporting of serious adverse reactions, such as anaphylaxis, blood disorders, endocrine disturbances, haemorrhage and renal impairment (**www.bnf.org**). Until recently, only doctors, dentists, coroners, pharmacists and nurses were asked to report adverse reactions; now, however, patients and carers have also been included in this list. This information is reported to the MHRA by post or via the website (**www.yellowcard.gov.uk**). Information about the scheme and the yellow cards themselves are available within the BNF and from the MRHA (**www.mhra.gov.uk**). Unfortunately, adverse reactions are not always reported (Luker and Wolfson, 1999), because the system remains voluntary. However, the NMC (2007) states that the registered nurse must notify an adverse reaction via the yellow card scheme immediately.

We need to balance the beneficial effects of medicines, such as pain relief and management of mental illness, against our knowledge of the unwanted effects such as ADRs.

Iatrogenesis

Secondary disease induced by medicines and treatments is referred to as 'iatrogenic disease'. Common examples include the cumulative effects of cocktails of medicines given to older people (polypharmacy), hair loss as a consequence of chemotherapy, and antibiotic resistance due to the overuse of antibiotics. Iatrogenesis can have short- or long-lasting effects or even permanent effects.

It is estimated that 5–17% of admissions of older patients to hospital are related to adverse reactions to medicines (DH, 2001).

Iatrogenesis is not related solely to conventional medicine. Patients may also experience ill-health as a result of complementary therapy. Iatrogenesis has been described as 'doctor-induced', as traditionally doctors were the main prescribers. However, some authors suggest that iatrogenesis can occur as a result of nursing treatment, such as pressure ulcer development, healthcare-associated infections (HAIs) and patient dependency.

> **Essential terminology**
>
> **Iatrogenesis**
>
> 'Iatro' comes from the Greek *iatros*, meaning 'healer', and *genesis*, meaning origin. Thus, 'iatrogenesis' means ill-health or ill-effects relating to treatment.

Where iatrogenesis occurs due to complicated therapeutic regimes – for example, if the patient is taking many medicines – then the iatrogenic effects may be as a consequence of drug interactions where the action of one drug is potentiated or decreased by the presence of another drug.

Drug interactions

When two or more medicines are given together, they have the potential to interact. The effects of the individual medicines may then be enhanced, diminished or otherwise altered. The greater the number of medicines given, the higher the potential for interaction (Simonsen *et al.*, 2006).

Receptors

- Drugs may compete to occupy the same receptor, e.g. morphine and naloxone.
- Drugs that act on different receptors but within the same body system, such as the CNS, can cause cumulative effects. For example, the suppression of the CNS caused by sedatives can be enhanced by alcohol: the drugs produce their effects by different mechanisms, but the result is the same (Simonsen *et al.*, 2006).
- Drugs that act on different receptors within different organs can also have cumulative effects. For example, warfarin and aspirin interact by producing an exaggerated effect on coagulation (blood clotting; the process by which blood is converted from a liquid to a solid state, involving the interaction of coagulation factors – see Chapter 5), despite the two drugs having different actions.

Absorption

Medicines that slow down the activity of the gastrointestinal tract will slow down the absorption of other medicines taken; for example, some treatments for migraine slow down absorption. Activated charcoal is an example of a substance given because we know it blocks absorption of drugs by making them insoluble; it is commonly used in the treatment of overdose of drugs taken orally.

Distribution

Drugs compete to bind with plasma proteins. Only the unbound portion of the drug is pharmacologically active, and so competition can alter the effects of some drugs. If a patient is receiving two medicines with a high degree of binding to the same plasma proteins, then there is the potential for one medicine to displace the other medicine, leading to an altered effect. This is usually only a problem for medicines that are highly protein-bound and with a narrow therapeutic index, such as warfarin. An increased concentration of free drug usually results in increased elimination (Downie *et al.*, 2003; Simonsen *et al.*, 2006).

Drugs can have an effect on enzyme activity in the liver, either increasing or reducing enzyme activity and thus reducing or increasing the impact of the drug. The presence of alcohol, for example, can depress liver enzyme activity and therefore reduce the metabolism of some drugs. However, if a patient with chronic alcoholism has a period free from alcohol intake, there may be a rebound effect, causing enzyme activity and therefore metabolism to increase in the short term.

Excretion

Some drugs affect the kidneys, usually by inhibiting processes such as secretion and reabsorption and thus reducing the ability of the kidneys to excrete certain drugs (Simonsen *et al.*, 2006).

Enhanced effects

Giving two medicines together can have positive benefits for the patient. Consider the patient coping with pain caused by cancer, which can be very difficult to treat. If we give two medicines together, the overall effect may be cumulative; that is, the combined action may be greater than the action of the individual medicines. The medicines do not have to belong to the same group, and often a combination of medicines from different drug groups is the most beneficial. For example, amitriptyline has been found to increase the effectiveness of analgesics for certain types of pain (see Chapter 7). We use the word 'adjuvant' to describe the 'other drug' in this situation.

> **Essential terminology**
>
> **Adjuvant**
> A substance (in this case, a drug) that aids the action of another, increasing the efficacy or potency of the other when administered at the same time.

In reality

Warfarin and aspirin are now prescribed in combination. Although the two medicines have the same outcome, their mode of action is different: warfarin is an anticoagulant, while aspirin is an antiplatelet. A patient prescribed warfarin is advised not to take certain OTC medicines, such as aspirin, because of its potential for enhancing the actions of warfarin. However, if a healthcare professional is managing the patient who requires anticoagulant therapy such as warfarin, it is recommended that warfarin and aspirin are used together. This produces a more beneficial effect and also is easier to manage than using warfarin alone.

ROUTES OF ADMINISTRATION

As adults we are usually familiar with taking medicines to relieve the symptoms of illnesses. Even if you had a relatively illness-free childhood, you may have been vaccinated, taken antibiotics or pain relief. This provides us with some experience from which to generate examples of routes of administration; for example, vaccines are usually given by injection, and antibiotics are often given by mouth. There are many other routes that can be used for administration in care settings.

We use the term **'enteral'** when discussing medicines administered by mouth/orally (by far the most common route used in the British healthcare system) and the term **'parenteral'** to describe medicines administered by methods other than the oral route, for example by injection.

Personal and professional development 4.6

Can you speculate as to why the oral route of administration is the most common?
Answers can be found at the back of the book.

It is possible to introduce medicines by a variety of different means, to reach specific areas of the body, depending on the availability of access. Some of the main routes to consider are as follows:

- *Oral*: given by mouth.
- *Sublingual*: given under the tongue.
- *Buccal*: placed between the top lip and the gum.
- *Inhaled*: breathed in via the respiratory tract.
- *Injected*: into the soft tissues by a number of means:
  - *Intravenous*: injected into a vein.
  - *Intramuscular*: injected into the muscle.
  - *Intra-articular*: injected into a joint cavity.

- *Intraspinal*: injected into the spinal column.
- *Subcutaneous*: injected under the skin.
- *Topical*: applied to the skin or mucous membranes.
- *Transdermal patch*: applied to be absorbed through the skin.
- *Optical*: applied into the eye.
- *Aural*: applied into the ear.
- *Vaginal*: inserted into the vagina.
- *Rectal*: inserted into the rectum.

Personal and professional development 4.7

Can you suggest some reasons for choosing one route rather than another?

If the patient is in pain, then they will probably want to take some pain relief that will act quickly. Some routes allow the drug faster access to the bloodstream and therefore the target site. So, for example, if we can deposit the medicine directly in the bloodstream by injection, then its action will be faster.

Some routes are more acceptable than others; for example, most patients prefer to take a medicine by mouth than have an injection. However, there might be several reasons why the injection route is more desirable. Consider the ability of the patient to swallow a tablet: the patient might have a dry mouth or be 'nil by mouth' following surgery on the gastrointestinal tract.

We consider the routes of administration in more detail below.

Oral route

The oral route is most common route used in the UK. The medicine is swallowed and so passes through the gastrointestinal tract; it is then absorbed mainly in the small intestine. The gastrointestinal tract has a huge surface area, which readily allows for absorption. The oral route is convenient because it does not usually require the intervention of a health professional; that is, the patient can self-administer. Because we use the mouth to eat food and drink, we find the oral route easy to access. This is usually the cheapest route.

Essential terminology

Local
The medicine effect is limited to a specific area.

Systemic
The medicine exerts effects on the body as a whole.

The patient has to be conscious and able to swallow if the oral route is used.

Medicines given by the oral route are used systemically; that is, they produce a generalised effect throughout the body. Antibiotics taken in this way target bacteria in a number of different locations, while medication given to treat cancers affects normal cells as well as cancer cells. However, treatments can often be produced so that they are more selective or targeted.

Sometimes, however, we give medicines for their localised effects, for example lozenges taken to soothe a sore throat.

Personal and professional development 4.8

Another example of medicines used for their local effects within the gastrointestinal tract are antacids given to relieve dyspepsia.
Can you identify some other examples of medicines given via this route for local effect?
Answers can be found at the back of the book.

Medicines that are given orally for systemic effect have to travel via the gastrointestinal tract before they can be absorbed and transported to their target. This inevitably means that the oral route can be slow. This is an important consideration when considering pain relief. Also, absorption of medicines via the oral route can be variable and therefore difficult to predict. We have previously identified that the presence of food in the stomach can slow down absorption (Greenstein and Gould, 2004). The co-administration of other medicines and the presence of disease can increase or slow absorption.

There are other disadvantages to the oral route, including poor patient adherence for many reasons, such as the medicine irritating the stomach and the first pass effect, which can result in a reduced amount of the active drug reaching the target site.

Personal and professional development 4.9

It is important to consider nursing interventions that enable the patient to take oral medication appropriately. Identify some appropriate strategies.
Answers can be found at the back of the book.

Sublingual route

This involves placing the medicine under the tongue so it can be absorbed directly into the bloodstream via the blood vessels under the tongue. This enables the medication to take effect quickly (Downie *et al.*, 2003). A familiar example of medication taken this way is glyceryl trinitrate, a vasodilator used to dilate (open) coronary arteries in order to allow increased blood flow and reduce preload (see Chapter 2), thus reducing the pain associated with ischaemia and the workload of the heart in angina. Glyceryl trinitrate can be administered sublingually in the form of tablets or an aerosol spray. This is a straightforward way of administering medication quickly for the patient experiencing the pain of angina; the route avoids the first pass effect and there is a low risk of overdose. However, the patient does need to understand how to take the medicine correctly, and there is a risk of side effects.

More recently, 'wafers' have been developed that dissolve quickly under the tongue. An example is rizatriptan used to treat migraine, where nausea can be a problem (**www.nursingtimes.net**).

Buccal route

With the buccal route, the medicine is held in the mouth between the top lip and the gum for absorption through the mucous membrane. Prochlorperazine to prevent nausea is given in this way if there is a risk that oral tablets may be vomited. The buccal rate avoids the first pass effect. If the patient is receiving medication on a regular basis using the buccal route, the tablet site should be varied in order to reduce the risk of dental problems (Downie *et al.*, 2003).

Inhaled route

Medicines may be administered via the respiratory tract by breathing in via the mouth or nose. This can be for a local effect on the mucous membrane of the nose or lungs or to introduce anaesthetic gases. Entonox, a mixture of nitrous oxide and oxygen often associated with pain relief in labour, is administered this way; this drug is used in the maintenance of anaesthesia and, in smaller concentrations (not enough to induce anaesthesia), for analgesia. Medicines given via the inhalation route are well absorbed because the lungs have a large surface area and good blood flow (Rang *et al.*, 2003).

Some medicines are available as gases, such as oxygen, while others driven by a gas become droplets for inhalation and are delivered by a mask, such as in the use of a nebuliser for patients with acute respiratory distress.

The medicine may be administered via an inhaler, using a device to deliver the drug in a metered dose aerosol or as a fine dry powder. Inhalers can be self-administered, but this needs special considerations, such as the patient's adherence to technique. The inhaler may be enhanced by the attachment of a *spacer* device such as a volumatic spacer (discussed in detail in Chapter 15).

In reality

Some authors make a distinction between medicines inhaled and given intranasally (Galbraith *et al.*, 2007).

> ### Intranasal administration
>
> This route is used mainly for treatment of conditions such as nasal congestion – that is, for local use – but a small number of medicines can be given via this route for systemic effect. An example of this is vasopressin (see Chapter 2). Vasopressin is absorbed through the nasal epithelium. Medicines administered via this route are usually delivered by sprays and drops.

Personal and professional development 4.10

Identify the correct inhaler technique for a metered dose such as salbutamol.

A benefit of the inhalation route is that medicines used to target the pulmonary system can be administered directly into the lungs, which achieves high concentrations at the desired site of action. Very little drug is absorbed into the general circulation and so there are limited systemic adverse effects. This is considered a safe route for medicines such as inhaled corticosteroids. Medicines can also be given via an endo-tracheal tube in emergencies.

Injection routes

These routes are also described as parenteral administration (medicines given by any route other than via the gastrointestinal tract). Medicines are deposited by injection into the soft tissues by a number of means. This usually involves a trained member of staff or in some circumstances a trained carer. Problems related to patient adherence are therefore usually avoided (**www.nursingtimes.net**).

Types of injection include the following:

- *Intramuscular*: The medicine is injected into a muscle. There is no first pass effect and so the medicine acts quickly. This route is convenient for administering medicines that could cause vomiting or gastric irritation. Injections require special equipment and an aseptic technique. They can be painful for the patient and there are some associated risks, such as nerve damage, infection and local irritation. Side effects happen quickly. Absorption depends on the muscle being used and the patient's condition (e.g. hypovolaemic shock (a consequence of blood loss) results in a reduction of the peripheral circulation). Only small volumes of a medicine can be administered in this way.

- *Subcutaneous*: This involves depositing small amounts of medicine into the subcutaneous tissue, the fatty (adipose) tissue just below the skin. It is a commonly used route. Absorption is slower than with the intramuscular route as the medicine is absorbed via capillaries, but it is faster than the oral route (Downie *et al.*, 2003; Greenstein and Gould 2004; Simonsen *et al.*, 2006).

- *Intradermal*: The medicine is placed just under the surface of the skin; this raises a 'bleb' (blister). This route is used for some vaccinations, local anaesthetics and investigations e.g. tuberculosis, allergy.

- *Intravenous*: The medicine is injected directly into the bloodstream via a vein. This route can be used for medicines, replacement fluids such as saline and blood, and contrast agents, which can be seen on x-ray and therefore used for diagnostic purposes. Doses can be given as a bolus or as a continuous infusion. Medicines given via this route take effect quickly; the whole dose is available since it bypasses the gastrointestinal tract, and so often a lower dose can be given. Intravenous injection requires a qualified healthcare professional and special equipment. There is a risk of accidental overdose and ill-effects. Intravenous injection is potentially the most dangerous route, because after the drug is given it is very difficult to 'retrieve' it (although antidotes may be available) (Downie *et al.*, 2003; Simonsen *et al.*, 2006). When administering some medicines such as benzylpenicillin with a potential to cause anaphylaxis (an abnormal and immediate allergic response), it is advisable to have adrenaline (epinephrine) at hand.

- *Intra-articular*: The medicine is injected into a joint cavity. A familiar example is that of corticosteroids injected into an inflamed and painful joint to relieve stiffness and inflammation and thus improve mobility. Medicines given via this route are long-acting, as absorption from the synovial fluid is slow. This route involves special precautions to prevent infection and requires an appropriately qualified practitioner.

- *Intraspinal*: The medicine is injected into the spinal column, where it mixes with spinal fluid. The route is commonly used for medicines that exert an effect on the nervous system (Simonsen *et al.*, 2006). This means of injection should be undertaken only by a qualified practitioner with training in the technique.

  - *Intrathecal*: The medicine is injected between the meninges, the membranes that surround the brain and spinal column, into the subarachnoid space and thus the cerebro-spinal fluid via a spinal needle. This route bypasses the blood–brain barrier and is a route for administering antibiotics (some of which are insufficiently lipid-soluble to penetrate the blood–brain barrier) in meningitis (inflammation of the three membranes that line the skull and vertebral canal and enclose the brain and spinal cord) (Rang *et al.*, 2003).

  - *Epidural*: This route is usually used for the administration of a local anaesthetic into the epidural space (outside the dura) in the lumbar region of the spinal cord. One use is to relieve the pain of childbirth. It requires an appropriately qualified healthcare professional and can be uncomfortable for the patient. Figure 4.11 shows the sites of spinal injection.

- *Intra-arterial*: Not commonly used, this involves the injection of opaque substances into the circulation. It is used mainly for diagnostic purposes. It may also be used to administer some cytotoxic (anticancer) medications in order to introduce the drug directly into a tumour (Downie *et al.*, 2003; Simonsen *et al.*, 2006).

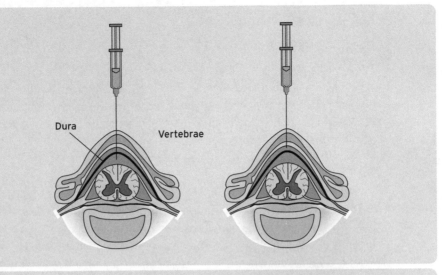

Figure 4.11 Sites of spinal injection: (a) spinal, (b) epidural (after Simonsen *et al.*, 2006. Reproduced by permission of Roy Lysaa and Edward Arnold (Publishers) Ltd)

The parenteral route is used for a number of reasons, for example, if the medication cannot be taken orally, if the medication is destroyed in the stomach and if careful control over the medication is required. However, there are some risks that we need to be aware of when administering injections.

Nursing implications Factors to consider when giving injections

There are some general considerations when giving injections:

- Follow the correct procedure for medicine administration (see Chapter 5).
- Consider the comfort, dignity and information needs of the patient.
- Eliminate infection and prevent cross-infection:
  - Wash hands to prevent cross-infection.
  - Choose a suitable work surface if preparation of the injection is required.
  - Use gloves to protect yourself.
  - Check the local policy for use of alcohol swabs to clean the skin.
- Preparation of the injection:
  - Consider the choice of equipment, needle size, etc.
  - Use the correct diluent, e.g. water, for injection.

▶

▶ *(continued)*

Specific safety issues

The appropriate choice of medicine preparation related to the route is essential. You may remember the case of Wayne Jowett who died following an injection of vincristine (a cytotoxic medicine) indicated for intravenous use into his spine. The report into his death suggested that only expert staff should be allowed to administer spinal injections.

The DH has issued national guidance on 'the safe administration of intrathecal chemotherapy' (**www.dh.gov.uk**).

Nurses on pre-registration nursing programmes are taught to give injections via the subcutaneous and intramuscular routes. On qualifying, and after receiving further training, nurses may be involved in administering intravenous medications. Injections via the other routes described in this section are usually administered by doctors and often require extra training, e.g. in relation to spinal injections (Jamieson *et al.*, 2002; Parish, 2001).

Personal and professional development 4.11
Identifying risks

Identify at least three risks to the nurse when administering medicines via injection.

Answers can be found at the back of the book.

Topical routes

Greenstein and Gould (2004) suggest that the correct use of the term 'topical' indicates 'application of the drug directly to the surface where its action is wanted'. Examples of this therefore include application of a medicine to the skin or mucous membranes, inhalation of medicines directly into the respiratory tract, application of medicines to the eye and insertion of medicines into the rectum or vagina for local treatment.

Most commonly in clinical areas, however, we tend to link the topical route to the application of creams, ointments, lotions and paints to the skin. These are usually used for the treatment of skin conditions such as psoriasis. This route is also used in children when a local anaesthetic cream (Emla™, a combination of two local anaesthetics, lidocaine and prilocaine) is applied before some painful procedures. It is important to remember the timing of the application of this anaesthetic: in order to be effective, it needs to be applied 30 minutes before the procedure.

Because topical medicines are poorly absorbed, they are considered to be reasonably safe; however, they still need to be used with caution. If a cream is applied to treat the skin, we can assume that it will treat whatever skin it comes into contact with; therefore, nurses need to protect their own skin by using gloves or applicators. Some skin treatments, such as corticosteroid creams, carry more risk. These are prescribed in small doses and the prescriber's instructions for use should always be followed. Absorption of medicines delivered topically can be enhanced by applying a dressing. An occlusive dressing raises the surface skin temperature and dilates the blood vessels, which increases the absorption rate.

Transdermal route

This route involves the use of an adhesive patch. The medicine is placed within the patch and applied to the skin for absorption through the skin and into the tissues. This absorption is slow, and so this route is used for replacement therapy such as nicotine or hormone replacement therapy (HRT) where a slow but steady release of the medicine is required. The route may also be used for medicines such as glyceryl trinitrate and the analgesic fentanyl, used for prophylaxis, where the intention is that the patient should not experience pain. One advantage of giving medicines in this way is that they are absorbed through the skin into the bloodstream, thereby avoiding the first pass effect (Greenstein and Gould, 2004; Simonsen et al., 2006).

Personal and professional development 4.12

We need to be careful where we apply the transdermal patch. Identify some general rules we should follow when using transdermal patches.
Answers can be found at the back of the book.

Optical route

This route delivers medicines to treat the eye, such as eye drops and ointments. Drops are placed in the lower eyelid fold. It is thought that the medicine is absorbed through the cornea, although there is also some unpredictable systemic absorption. This route is used to relieve irritation and infection, and to lubricate dry eyes with artificial tears. Eye drops are also used for diagnostic purposes, such as to dilate pupils or to introduce a dye in order to aid examination of the cornea. It is important to warn the patient beforehand that they might experience blurred vision (Fegan, 2000; Simonsen et al., 2006).

Aural route

This route is used for the delivery of medicines into the ear for local effect to treat infections or soften ear wax. The medicine is usually in the form of a spray or drops (Fegan, 2000).

Vaginal route

This involves insertion of medicines into the vagina for the treatment of local dryness, irritation or infection, such as thrush, using creams or pessaries.

Rectal route

This route involves the insertion of the medicines into the rectum, for retention or evacuation purposes.

Retention

Suppositories or enemas can be given to treat local irritation or infection, or for systemic use. Because of the blood supply in the rectum, medicines are readily absorbed from this route and can be used to treat a variety of conditions. The rectal route can also be used for local effects, such as the use of local corticosteroids in patients with ulcerative colitis or treatments for haemorrhoids.

However, the patient may not find the rectal route acceptable, and the dose may be expelled in the faeces before it has all been absorbed.

Evacuation

Evacuants in the form of enemas or suppositories are used to empty the rectum.

Advantages of this route include the avoidance of the first pass effect and gastro-irritation seen with some medicines given orally.

Other routes

There are some other routes of administration that are not classified very easily. Medicines can be deposited wherever we can access a site. For example, medicines can be deposited into the pleural cavity if the patient is undergoing a pleural tap (withdrawal of fluid from the lungs), into the peritoneal cavity or intra-osseous (into the vascular network of a long bone, used in emergency situations where intravenous access might be difficult, e.g. in burns and in children under 6 years of age).

The choice of route depends upon many factors, including the part of the body we wish to treat, how quickly we require the medicine to have an effect, the length of time the medicine stays in the body, and the medicine's unwanted effects. Some of these factors are concerned with the medicine and how it works, but we also need to consider patient factors:

- How easy is the treatment for the patient to manage?
- If the medicine produces side effects such as weight gain (e.g. associated with administration of corticosteroids), will the patient continue with the treatment?
- Complex treatments may be difficult for the patient to adhere to, and so treatments involving one dose per day may be more successful.

For patients who are 'needle-phobic', a 'needle-less' injector is available. This involves a gas-drug formulation; the release of the compressed gas drives the medicament into the tissues. This can be used for subcutaneous and intramuscular injection. The rationale for use is to improve adherence (Dewar, 2000).

PREPARATIONS

Medicines are available in a number of different preparations (formulations), such as tablets, caplets, capsules and suppositories.

Personal and professional development 4.13

What other preparations can you identify?
Answers can be found at the back of the book.

Quick reminder

✔ The terminology related to drugs and medicines can be complex and confusing. It covers what a medicine should be called and is related to the medicine's effects and the type of medicine.

✔ Clinical pharmacology, the study of drugs and their effects on humans, is a relatively new discipline, informed by chemistry, pathology and human biology, and involved with synthetically producing drugs and medicines from plants, minerals and animal sources.

✔ The process of drug production is lengthy and thorough and is aimed at establishing efficacy and safety.

✔ Drugs are developed to produce a predictable effect on the body in terms of toxicity and efficacy at a determined dose and dose frequency.

✔ Pharmacodynamics is the study of how drugs exert their effects on the body, usually by interacting with target proteins.

✔ Pharmacokinetics refers to the fate of drugs in the body. Four processes are involved: absorption, distribution, metabolism and excretion.

✔ There are general and specific factors relating to individual patients and patient groups that influence pharmacokinetics.

✔ Medicines exert therapeutic effects and adverse effects. Some of these result from drug interactions. Some medicines can cause secondary disease.

▶

continued

✔ Medicines can be administered by a variety of routes depending upon the speed of action required, the accessibility of the target site and the acceptability of the route to the patient.

✔ Medicines are available in a variety of forms, such as capsules, which can be further modified depending upon the response required, for example slow absorption.

REFERENCES

Allen K M (1996) *Nursing Care of the Addicted Client*. Philadelphia, PA: Lippincott.

Bird C and Hassall J (1993) *Self Administration of Drugs: A Guide to Implementation*. London: Scutari Press.

British Medical Association (BMA) (2002) *British Medical Association Guide to Drugs and Medicines*. London: Dorling Kindersley.

Collins T (2000) Understanding shock. *Nursing Standard* **14**, 35–43.

Comerford K, Haworth K and Weinstock D (2005) *Clinical Pharmacology Made Incredibly Easy*, 2nd edn. Philadelphia, PA: Lippincott, Williams & Wilkins.

Conway B and Fuat A (2007) Recent advances in angina mangement: implications for nurses. *Nursing Standard* **21**, 49–58.

Department of Health (DH) (2001) *National Service Framework for Older People*. London: The Stationery Office.

Dewar K (2000) Introduction to pharmacology. In Prosser S, Worster B, MacGregor J, Dewar K, Runyard P and Fegan J *Applied Pharmacology: An Introduction to Pathophysiology and Drug Management for Nurses and Healthcare Professionals*. London: Mosby.

Downie G, Mackenzie J and Williams A (2003) *Pharmacology and Medicines Management for Nurses*. Edinburgh: Churchill Livingstone.

Fegan J (2000) Drugs and head and neck disorders. In Prosser S, Worster B, MacGregor J, Dewar K, Runyard P and Fegan J *Applied Pharmacology: An Introduction to Pathophysiology and Drug Management for Nurses and Healthcare Professionals*. London: Mosby.

Galbraith A, Bullock S, Manias E, Hunt B and Richards A (2007) *Fundamentals of Pharmacology: An Applied Approach for Nursing and Health Care*, 2nd edn. Harlow: Pearson Education.

Greenstein B and Gould D (2004) *Trounce's Clinical Pharmacology for Nurses*. Edinburgh: Churchill Livingstone.

Hinchliff S M, Montague S E and Watson R (1996) *Physiology for Nursing Practice*. Oxford: Balliére Tindall.

Illich I (1976) *Medical Nemesis: The Expropriation of Health*. New York: Pantheon.

Jamieson E M, McCall J M and Whyte L A (2002) *Clinical Nursing Practices*. Edinburgh: Churchill Livingstone.

Jordan S (2002) *Pharmacology for Midwives*. Basingstoke: Palgrave.

Jordan S, Griffiths H and Griffiths R (2003) Administration of medicines. Part 2: pharmacology. *Nursing Standard* **18**, 345.

Luker K and Wolfson D (1999) *Medicines Management for Clinical Nurses*. Oxford: Blackwell Science.

Mason P (2002) Food and medicines. *Pharmaceutical Journal* **269**, 571–573.

Medicines and Healthcare Products Regulatory Agency (MHRA) (2002) *Adverse Drug Reactions: A Potential Role for Liaison Officers*. London: Medicines and Healthcare Products Regulatory Agency.

Nursing and Midwifery Council (NMC) (2004) *A-Z Advice Sheet: Medicines Management*. London: Nursing and Midwifery Council.

Nursing and Midwifery Council (NMC) (2007) *Standards for Medicines Management*. London: Nursing and Midwifery Council.

Parish C (2001) Agency launched to help reduce NHS mistakes. *Nursing Standard* **15**, 8.

Permanant G, Mossialos E and McKee M (2007) The EU's new paediatric medicines legislation: serving children's needs? *Archives of Disease in Childhood* **92**, 808-811.

Prosser S, Worster B, MacGregor J, Dewar K, Runyard P and Fegan J (2000) *Applied Pharmacology: An Introduction to Pathophysiology and Drug Management for Nurses and Healthcare Professionals*. London: Mosby.

Rang H P, Dale M M, Ritter J M and Moore P K (2003) *Pharmacology*, 5th edn. Edinburgh: Churchill Livingstone.

Rawlins M D (2001) *Pharmacology. The Oxford Companion to Medicine*. Oxford: Oxford University Press.

Read C Y (2002) Pharmacogenomics: an evolving paradigm for drug therapy. *Medsurg Nursing* **11**, 122-125.

Rusnak J M, Kisabeth R M, Herbert D P and McNeill D B (2001) Pharmacogenomics: a clinician's primer on emerging technologies for improved patient care. *Mayo Clinic Proceedings* **76**, 299-309.

Shepherd M (2002) Medicines. *Nursing Times* **98**, 43.

Simonsen T, Aarbakke I K, Coleman I and Sinnott R L (2006) *Illustrated Pharmacology for Nurses*. London: Hodder Arnold.

Walsh M and Wigens L (2003) *Introduction to Research*. Cheltenham: Nelson Thornes.

Wickens A (2005) *Foundations of Biopsychology*. Harlow: Pearson Education.

Wiffen P, Mitchell M, Snelling M and Stoner N (2007) *Oxford Handbook of Clinical Pharmacy*. Oxford: Oxford University Press.

World Health Organization (WHO) (1975) *Safety, Efficacy and Utilization*. **www.who.int/medicines/areas/quality_safety/safety_efficacy**

Chapter 5

Nursing implications and responsibilities

Those of us with some experience of care, whether as a nurse, patient or relative, can readily identify the importance placed upon administering prescribed medicines to patients in order to improve their condition. We may also be able to identify some problems, such as availability of medicines, the reluctance of some patients to take medicines and instructions in relation to specific medicines. One important and time-consuming aspect of the nurse's role, therefore, is the administration of medicines.

In an attempt to improve the service to patients in relation to medicines, the Audit Commission (2001) undertook a review of how this medicines service was managed in the NHS. The report identified what it described as the 'central component' of medicines in healthcare; this included the development of new medicines and the increase in chronic illness that has resulted in large numbers of medicines being administered. The Audit Commission also highlighted that medicines use 'was not being optimised'. For example, it identified that not all patients given a prescription actually have the prescription dispensed, and that sometimes patients make mistakes when taking medicines. This comprehensive report examined a wide range of issues in relation to medicines, hence the development of the term 'medicines management'. The Audit Commission defines medicines management as the process that 'encompasses the entire way in which medicines are selected, procured, delivered, prescribed, administered and reviewed'.

A wide range of issues related to medicines management as it applies to the nurse's role will be introduced and explored within this chapter.

Learning outcomes

By the end of this chapter you should be able to:

✔ Identify the key aspects of medicines management for nurses

✔ Identify nursing responsibilities related to the administration of medicines

✔ Outline the implications of current drug legislation for nurses

✔ Identify other sources of information related to medicines management that nurses need to be aware of

✔ Discuss the advantages of self-administration

✔ Suggest appropriate strategies in response to issues arising from practice, such as 'remote' prescriptions.

Chapter at a glance

Introduction
Drug legislation
Ordering and storage
Administration of medicines
Self-administration
Patient compliance
Patient education
Issues relating to the administration of medicines
Professional requirements
Quick reminder
References

INTRODUCTION

Griffith *et al*. (2003) state that administration of medicines is a 'key element of nursing care', and the Audit Commission (2001) suggests that up to 40% of nurses' time is spent in medicine administration. Added to this, many authors identify the complexity of this nursing activity; Chapelhow *et al*. (2005) offer some reasons for this:

● Administration of medicines is a skill that is performed frequently, but evidence suggests that despite our efforts to do this safely the error rate is increasing (Audit Commission, 2001).

- Medicines administration is a skill made up of many other skills, such as cognitive skills; maintaining an appropriate knowledge base, assessment and interpretation, interpersonal skills; communication, and professional skills; making judgements and decision-making.

This is supported by Eisenhauer *et al.* (2007), who describe medicine administration as 'complex and many-faceted' and requiring thought to prevent errors, prevent harm and promote therapeutic responses. Nearly all patients are given medicines as a result of a visit to hospital (Audit Commission, 2001), and administration of medicines is therefore one of the most important responsibilities of the nurse. Administration of medicines is also one of the required competencies for entry to the professional register (NMC, 2007); competency requires ability, experience and confidence.

DRUG LEGISLATION

There are two key pieces of legislation relating to the administration of medicines: the Medicines Act (1968) and the Misuse of Drugs Act (1971).

Medicines Act (1968)

The Medicines Act is the principal statutory framework. It is a very comprehensive piece of legislation that identifies administration systems, licensing systems, sale and supply of medicines to the public, packaging and labelling. It is important to note that this legislation applies to all healthcare workers, and not only nurses, and so the Act also covers retail pharmacies and the British Pharmacopoeia.

The availability of medicines direct to the public is regulated by the Medicines Act (1968), which classifies medicines into three categories, with another category relating to medicines available by prescription:

- *General Sales List*: These are medicines that are available in pharmacies and retail outlets and are considered relatively safe if taken as directed. The range of medicines and their availability (i.e. package size, doses) are regulated by Section 53 of the Medicines Act.

- *Pharmacy-only (P) medicines*: These medicines can be sold only in registered pharmacies by or under the supervision of a registered pharmacist. This list may include medicines available in retail outlets but supplied in larger doses or quantities.

- *Prescription-only medicines (POMs)*: These medicines must be prescribed by a licensed practitioner (a doctor, dentist or, more recently, non-medical prescriber such as a nurse, pharmacist or optometrist). With the introduction of supplementary prescribing, some allied health professionals such as physiotherapists, radiographers and podiatrists may also be involved in prescribing. Hospitals are exempt from these prescription-only provisions (Dimond, 2005). Prescription medicines may be sold or supplied by a hospital providing they are in accordance with the written instructions of a doctor, although these instructions need not be contained in a formal prescription (Nursing and Midwifery Council (NMC), 2007).

Since 2002, all new medicines are POM for their first 5 years on the market (**www.pjonline.com**).

The Medicines Act (1968) is intended to be followed by all healthcare professionals. Some of the key implications of the legislation for nurses working in clinical areas are:

- All medicines should be kept in a suitable locked container.
- Keys should be carried on the person of the nurse in charge.
- Preparations for external and internal use should be stored separately.
- Only a pharmacist, medical officer or dentist may label or change the label on any pharmaceutical product.

Misuse of Drugs Act (1971)

This act controls those drugs that have the potential for addiction. The Misuse of Drugs Act and further legislation in the Misuse of Drugs Regulations (2001) regulate the import, export, supply and use of these drugs, classifying them according to their potential to cause harm if abused as follows:

- *Class A*, e.g. morphine, methadone.
- *Class B*, e.g. barbiturates, codeine.
- *Class C*, e.g. cannabis, most benzodiazepines.

Cannabis is a contemporary example of a drug that has been moved from one category (class B) to another (class C) because of a reconsideration of its toxicity and comparison with other drugs in its class. Although it is still illegal to possess cannabis, trials are currently being undertaken into its therapeutic benefits. The Home Office currently states that there is insufficient evidence to classify cannabis for therapeutic use, but it will consider this in the future (DH, 2002). The current government is now considering whether to reclassify cannabis as Class B.

The Misuse of Drugs Act (1971):

- lists and classifies controlled drugs;
- creates criminal offences in relation to the manufacture, supply and possession of controlled drugs;
- gives the Secretary of State power to make regulations and directions to prevent the misuse of controlled drugs;
- creates advisory council in the misuse of drugs;
- gives powers of search, arrest and forfeiture.

Drugs within this group can have enormous therapeutic value, for example in pain management.

Personal and professional development 5.1

Can you identify other uses for controlled drugs that are used in patient care environments?
Answers can be found at the back of the book.

The Misuse of Drugs Regulations (2001) further classify controlled drugs into categories that reflect their potential for misuse. The categories are referred to as schedules, of which there are five. The schedule denotes the requirement for import, export, production, supply, possession, prescribing and record-keeping:

- *Schedule 1* covers drugs such as lysergic acid diethylamide (LSD) that are used recreationally rather than therapeutically. Their possession and supply is prohibited, unless the Home Office stipulates otherwise.
- *Schedule 2* covers drugs subject to full controlled drug requirements (see below). Examples include morphine and pethidine.
- *Schedule 3* includes drugs such as barbiturates.
- *Schedule 4* includes benzodiazepines, prescription-only drugs.
- *Schedule 5* drugs have only limited potential for abuse, such as kaolin and morphine, but invoices must be kept for two years.

Controlled drugs

Although all medicines in clinical areas are subject to regulations regarding storage and administration, controlled drugs, because of the potential for misuse, have specific regulations. In patient care areas, controlled drugs are categorised as Schedule 2 and, more recently, Schedule 3. The principles in relation to this category of drugs involve maintaining checks in relation to stock balance (keeping registers for ordering and administration) and secure ordering, administration and destruction of drugs. Controlled drugs are ordered using a specific order book, delivered to the ward in a locked container and stored 'in a locked cupboard within a locked cupboard', which should be identified clearly (Prosser, 2000). It is usually accepted that administration of controlled drugs should involve two practitioners, one of whom should be a registered nurse.

Personal and professional development 5.2
Implications for nurses

The famous Harold Shipman case has implications for nurses. The Shipman Inquiry was set up in January 2001 following the conviction of Harold Shipman for the murder of 15 of his patients. Shipman was able to 'divert large quantities of potentially lethal controlled drugs ... without detection' (**www.dh.gov.uk**).

Following the publication of the fourth report of the Shipman Inquiry, published in July 2004, which highlighted these 'serious shortcomings', the UK government is working with professional and regulatory bodies, including the NMC, to develop good practice in relation to the prescribing of controlled drugs and monitoring 'their movement from prescriber to dispenser to patient' (**www.dh.gov.uk**).

The Inquiry found no evidence to impose restrictions on the administration of controlled drugs by nurses (**www.rcn.org**).

The changes to date include:

- computer-generated prescriptions but with handwritten signatures;
- computerised controlled drug registers for drugs listed in Schedules 1 and 2;
- extended list of controlled drugs prescribable by independent (extended formulary) nurse prescribers;
- limiting the prescription period of Schedule 2, 3 and 4 controlled drugs to 28 days;
- collection of controlled drugs in the community; nurses involved in collection will have to provide proof of identity;
- standard operating procedures (relating to stocks of controlled drugs);
- changes to the NHS prescription forms in order to allow all controlled drugs to be allocated to the individual prescriber (and, subject to confidentiality safeguards, to the individual patient) (DH, 2007).

More information, reports and recommendations can be accessed from the DH website (**www.dh.gov.uk**).

Personal and professional development 5.3
Nursing responsibilities

Access your local policy for the administration of medicines and check the requirements for ordering, storing, administering and destruction of controlled drugs.

ORDERING AND STORAGE

Medicines are supplied to patient care environments (whether from NHS or private) from pharmacies. Most clinical areas, wards and departments have a stock supply of the commonly used medicines within that area; this list is determined by the local trust's drugs and therapeutics committee (now often called a medicines management committee). These committees are responsible for all decisions taken in relation to how medicines are used within the trust, thus fulfilling the requirements of the DH (DH, 1988, 2003).

Systems for ordering

Most trusts operate a top-up system that is maintained by a member of the pharmacy department, who makes sure stock is kept within agreed levels.

Specific directions are in place for controlled drugs. For this group of medicines, information regarding the name, form, strength and quantity of medicines must be specific and written in words and numbers.

Storage

Medicines used in patient and clinical areas must be stored in a secure fashion. All medicines have the potential to be harmful and are therefore stored in locked containers, such as cupboards, immobilised trolleys, fridges and, more recently, patients' bedside lockers. There are some exceptions, such as medicines used in emergency situations (see later in this chapter).

The type of locked container used depends upon:

- the purpose of the drug (internal or external use);
- the type of drug (medicines, controlled drugs);
- the formulation and stability (e.g. the need to be stored at a specific temperature) of the medicine.

Personal and professional development 5.4
Safe storage of medicines

We have identified some examples in relation to storage requirements. You might find it useful to locate the following in your workplace:

- medical gases;
- urine-testing reagents;
- intravenous fluids;
- substances used for cleansing purposes.

In order to store medicines safely and appropriately, what information would you expect to find on the label? Answers can be found at the back of the book.

Some tablets are required to be kept in a particular type of container, such as a brown bottle for glyceryl trinitrate because this medicine is unstable in direct light, and ribbed bottles for poisons such as cleansing agents.

Guidance for the design of medicine labels and packages has been updated (Committee on Safety of Medicines, 2001) in order to improve safety. These guidelines include recommendations for layout, text size and colours used (**www.mca.gov.uk**).

Why do we need to consider aspects such as these? Answers can be found at the back of the book.

In an attempt to make the administration of medicines safer and to minimise risks, other systems of administration, ordering and storage have been developed (Greenstein and Gould, 2004), such as the following:

- Dosette boxes (monitored dose systems; compliance/adherence aids) (NMC, 2007; Wiffen *et al.*, 2007)
- Electronic prescribing, which provides immediate and up-to-date information and minimises risks involved with inaccurate or illegible handwritten prescriptions; a doctor's signature is still required (Audit Commission, 2001)
- Self-administration (see page 132)
- Original pack dispensing, to comply with new European directives; there has been an increase in dispensing oral medications in individualised packs
- Using the patient's own medicines (one-stop dispensing) in hospital (previously these would have been destroyed); this provides an opportunity for assessment and review of treatment; it also cuts costs
- Barcoding to allow scanning of patients' identification bands and prescription sheets (Eisenhauer *et al.*, 2007).

One-stop dispensing

One-stop dispensing is recommended by the Audit Commission (2001). It involves using the patient's own prescribed medicines while in hospital. The NMC (2007) recommends that this practice can be used providing the medicines 'contain a patient information leaflet and are labelled with full instructions for use'. The NMC also urges that on discharge, the patient's discharge prescription is checked carefully, as these new prescription medicines may be different from those that the patient was taking on admission.

ADMINISTRATION OF MEDICINES

Most of the legislation related to drugs is quite old. It is important, therefore, that you are familiar with advice related to how to interpret this legislation in contemporary care settings, local policies and professional guidance.

The NMC (2007) has produced *Standards for Medicines Management*, that replaces its previous *Guidelines for the Administration of Medicines*. The purpose of the NMC is to protect the public by producing professional standards and by offering advice and guidance to qualified nurses. The NMC standards provide advice concerning safe practice in relation to legislation and to clarify issues arising from practice. The NMC states that the standards are 'broad principles for practice and registrants will need to apply the principles to their own area of practice'. Although they are produced for registrants (qualified nurses), the advice is also useful for unqualified nurses to reflect upon.

Dimond (2005) states: 'The nurse is personally accountable for [his or] her actions in administering any drug'. There are several sources of advice and information available for nurses so that both they and the patients in their care may feel confident. There are also some more informal guidelines that appear in much of the literature relating to the nurse's role in medicine administration. For example, there are said to be five 'rights' related to medicine administration, which nurses often use as a checklist:

- Right patient
- Right medicine
- Right dose
- Right time
- Right route
  (NMC, 2007; Preston, 2004).

Dimond (2005) also identifies the need for correct procedure and record-keeping.

One of the problems in using a checklist such as this is that medicine administration may become a task, often done against the clock in a busy patient care environment, with the nurse relying on the checklist rather than giving adequate consideration to all aspects involved (Chapelhow *et al.*, 2005). The NMC (2007) makes it quite clear that medicine administration is 'not just a mechanistic task ... it requires thought and professional judgment'. The NMC (2007) identifies the breadth of knowledge required as 'the therapeutic uses of the medicine to be administered, its normal dosage, side effects, precautions and contra-indications'. However, nurses as employees and as part of a professional group also need other types of information, such as the legislation relating to, for example, ordering, storing and recording of medicines. We can therefore see how complex medicine administration can be: nurses thus need a breadth of knowledge and skills in order not only to administer medicines safely but also to promote positive outcomes for the patient. From the discussion so far, we can identify that the key aspects of the nurse's role in relation to administration are (Eisenhauer *et al.*, 2007):

- interpretation of the prescription;
- recording;
- observing the patient's response.

The nurse therefore needs to understand the reason for the prescription and the action and usual dose of the medicine. When administering medicines, the nurse needs to be able to apply their knowledge of the medicine in order to judge whether the prescription is correct. Dimond (2005) states: 'where the nurse is not satisfied with some aspect of the drug [he or] she is instructed to administer, [he or] she must ensure the prescription is checked'.

> ## Personal and professional development 5.5
> ### Recognising a correct prescription
>
> In order to administer medicines safely, you need to be able to interpret the written prescription. What information should be provided?
> Answers can be found at the back of the book.

Nurses in hospitals have no authority to administer medicines unless under the direction of a medical practitioner or independent/supplementary prescriber (Greenstein and Gould, 2004; NMC, 2007), and therefore a prescription sheet is essential. These prescription sheets, now also referred to as 'patient-specific directions' (PSDs) (NMC, 2007) in patient areas, usually consist of a variety of medicine charts that have been developed by the trust to meet its own needs in relation to a clinical specialty. This increases the opportunity for error during administration, when a number of charts and sections of charts have to be checked, such as regular prescription, reducing medicine dose, once-only and as-required charts (Figure 5.1). Staff moving between trusts also have to familiarise themselves with a new set of charts and adapt their working practices (Healthcare Commission, 2007).

Since the introduction of independent nurse prescribing in 2002, there are situations in which some nurses can prescribe, but within most hospital areas the prescriber is usually a doctor. Nevertheless, there are some situations where nurses can administer medicines to 'groups of patients who may not be individually identified before presenting for treatment' (NMC, 2007). This refers to patient group directions (PGDs), locally agreed written instructions signed by a doctor (or dentist) and a pharmacist and approved by the healthcare body (NMC, 2007). This is not a form of prescribing but allows some qualified nurses to administer named medicines to specific groups of patients with particular clinical conditions (Healthcare Commission, 2007). Consider the nurse specialist carrying out an assessment on a newly admitted patient who has some obvious difficulty in breathing: if a PGD is in place, the nurse specialist could administer a named medicine in order to relieve the patient's distress without having to wait for the doctor; this has clear benefits for the patient.

---------------------------------- Hospital   Chart No. ---------------------- of ----------------------

CODES FOR NON-ADMINISTRATION OF PRESCRIBED MEDICINE	Name of Patient

CODES FOR NON-ADMINISTRATION OF PRESCRIBED MEDICINE

In situations where a dose of a medicine is not administered and the matter cannot be resolved immediately the nurse must:-
a) Record on the medicine chart the appropriate code number for the reason why the dose was not administered and initial this code.
b) TAKE APPROPRIATE ACTION to resolve the matter PROMPTLY so that patient treatment is not compromised. For further details refer to the 'Purple Booklet'

Patient refuses	1	Unable to swallow	8	
Patient not present on ward	2	Vomiting/nausea	9	
Medicine not available (obtain as soon as possible)	3	Time varied on Dr's instructions	10	
Instructions not clear or legal	4	Once only/PRN medication given	11	
Patient self-administered medicine	5	**To be specified in the Administration Care Plan**		
Nil by mouth	6	Possible drug reaction/ side effects	12	
Asleep/drowsy	7	Other reasons	13	

Name of Patient	
Patient Number	
Ward	
DOB	
Date of Admission	
Consultant	
Weight	Surface Area

Pharmacy Use only		
	By	Date
Drug History Taken		
Drug Chart Written		
Discharge Prescription Written		

DRUG and OTHER SENSITIVITIES*	Completed by signature
	Name

* If there are no known allergies, write 'None known' in box

ONCE ONLY

Date	Time	Pharmacy	Drug (Approved Name)	Dose	Route	Prescriber's Signature NAME	Time Given	Given by	Checked by

OTHER CHARTS IN USE

Date	Type of chart	Details	Signature NAME

Figure 5.1 Examples of medicine administration charts used routinely in patient care areas. (nuth.nhs.uk)

Name ....   Number ....   **REGULAR THERAPY**

Please state DURATION OF THERAPY for short course treatment e.g. antibiotics				Date												Date	Administration Comments	Initials
DRUG (Approved Name)																			
Dose	Route	Start date	Duration of therapy	0800															
				1200															
Prescriber's Signature		Notes		1800															
Name				2200															
Date Stopped	Initials		Pharmacy use																

DRUG (Approved Name)																			
Dose	Route	Start date	Duration of therapy	0800															
				1200															
Prescriber's Signature		Notes		1800															
Name				2200															
Date Stopped	Initials		Pharmacy use																

DRUG (Approved Name)																			
Dose	Route	Start date	Duration of therapy	0800															
				1200															
Prescriber's Signature		Notes		1800															
Name				2200															
Date Stopped	Initials		Pharmacy use																

DRUG (Approved Name)																			
Dose	Route	Start date	Duration of therapy	0800															
				1200															
Prescriber's Signature		Notes		1800															
Name				2200															
Date Stopped	Initials		Pharmacy use																

DRUG (Approved Name)																			
Dose	Route	Start date	Duration of therapy	0800															
				1200															
Prescriber's Signature		Notes		1800															
Name	'			2200															
Date Stopped	Initials		Pharmacy use																

Figure 5.1 Continued

VARIABLE DOSE MEDICATION

DRUG (Approved Name)	Route	Target INR	Indication/instructions	Start date	Signature	Name	Pharmacy
Date							
Time							
Dose							
IBR*							
Prescribed by (initials)							
Given by							

DRUG (Approved Name)	Route	Target INR	Indication/instructions	Start date	Signature	Name	Pharmacy
Date							
Time							
Dose							
IBR*							
Prescribed by (initials)							
Given by							

DRUG (Approved Name)	Route	Target INR	Indication/instructions	Start date	Signature	Name	Pharmacy
Date							
Time							
Dose							
IBR*							
Prescribed by (initials)							
Given by							

* Only to be used when required for recording INR in patients taking oral anticoagulants

AS REQUIRED THERAPY

DRUG (Approved Name)			Date	
Dose	Route	Start date	Time	
			Dose/route	
			Given by	
Frequency & instructions		Signature	Date	
		Name	Time	
Stop date	Initials	Pharmacy	Dose/route	
			Given by	

DRUG (Approved Name)			Date	
Dose	Route	Start date	Time	
			Dose/route	
			Given by	
Frequency & instructions		Signature	Date	
		Name	Time	
Stop date	Initials	Pharmacy	Dose/route	
			Given by	

Figure 5.1 Continued

Nurse prescribing is discussed in detail in Chapter 17.

In administering medicine to patients, there are some important principles that need to be observed.

Administration sequence

1 *Identify the patient.* This includes checking the patient's name, date of birth and number (patient identity bracelet). *Consent* (based upon education) is usually established.

2 *Check for any drug sensitivity/allergy.* This should be recorded on the prescription sheet.

3 *Check that the prescription is clear and valid.* The prescription should be written clearly, unambiguous and signed.

4 *Check that the dose has not been given already.* This includes regular, as-required and once-only prescription charts.

5 *Select the medicine and dispense into an appropriate measure/cup. Consider the route, dose and form.* Compare the prescription sheet and medicine bottle label. Check the expiry date. Measure or count the correct dose. Avoid contact with the medicine (in order to avoid allergy). This requires a knowledge of the medicine.

6 *Administer the medicine to the patient.* Assess the patient's ability to take the medicine. Check that the medicine has been taken.

7 *Record the administration.* A signature is required. Include non-administration, with the reason, e.g. refused.

8 *Report any adverse reactions/change in appropriateness to prescriber.* Consider the context, e.g. patient's pulse, contraindications.

This sequence is only a guide. A more comprehensive overview is provided in Standard 8 on page 8 of *Standards for Medicines Management* (NMC, 2007).

Administration systems

The traditional method of administering medicines to patients involves the use of a medicines trolley when the nurse undertakes the medicines round. This can be time-consuming given the increasing number and complexity of contemporary medicines. Another problem with this system includes missed doses if a patient is not at their bed (Healthcare Commission, 2007). The Audit Commission (2001) states clearly that this method 'can no longer support safe or efficient medicines administration'.

Bedside lockers are used in some patient areas to enable dispensing for discharge; the use of individual and sufficient patient medicines in labelled packs, to accommodate the use of patients' own medicines and facilitate self-administration (Healthcare Commission, 2007).

Administration of medicines was previously carried out by two nurses, but for some time it has been done by only one nurse. The Duthie Report (1988) suggests that there are some situations where two practitioners should be involved, including controlled drug administration, when administering medicines to children under the age of 12 years and when a calculation is involved, such as for weight-related doses. This information has now been incorporated into many medicine policies within patient areas. The NMC (2007) recommends that the second signatory can be another registered healthcare professional, a student nurse or another person who has been assessed as 'competent'.

As-required medication

An area that needs special consideration is that of as-required or whenever necessary medication (*pro re nata*, which may be identified on medicine charts as PRN - although note that as a general principle, abbreviations should be avoided as they can be misinterpreted). PRN prescriptions enable the nurse to use their discretion as to when to give the medicine, for example in relation to pain relief or night sedation. This means that the medicine can be given when the patient requires it. However, in order for this prescription to be safe and valid, it must contain some specific information, including the dose, the minimum interval between doses and the maximum amount allowed within a 24-hour period. The administration of the medicine should be recorded clearly. This specific advice should be incorporated within medicines policies (Dimond, 2005; NMC, 2007).

SELF-ADMINISTRATION

Self-administration of medicines is the term used when patients in clinical areas administer their own prescribed medicines. This is different from self-medication, which implies that the individual chooses the medication, for example paracetamol for a headache. However, the two terms are often used interchangeably, usually to mean self-administration. Self-administration is viewed as a positive step in enabling patients to manage their medicines. The Audit Commission (2001) states that failure to take medicines as directed is as high as 50% in patients with chronic illness, but self-administration would enable patients to be 'independent' and promotes their involvement in, and management of, their own care. Self-administration and also administration of medicines by carers are 'welcomed and supported' by the NMC (2007).

The NMC emphasises the need for such medicines to be stored safely and access to them limited. The Healthcare Commission (2007) reiterates this, recommending investment in 'suitable storage near to the patient', for example in a bedside locker or portable medicines bag.

It is important that patients self-administering are well informed about their medication. This implies knowledge of both their condition and their medication. The patient must be assessed in relation to their ability to self-administer, for example, a confused patient may not be able to self-administer. Discharge planning is enhanced by self-administration (NMC, 2007) as patients are better informed and problems relating to administration may be identified and dealt with before discharge.

Patients who self-administer often prefer this method, suggesting that it helps to improve their knowledge and therefore confidence about taking medicines (Lowe *et al.*, 1995). Self-administration has other advantages; for example, patients can take pain relief when they need it, it is easier to fulfil directions regarding taking tablets before or after food, and it can result in treatment regimes being simplified (Audit Commission, 2001).

However, some nurses are concerned about their own accountability and responsibility in relation to patient self-administration. The NMC (2007) Standard 9 suggests that registered nurses are still responsible for the ongoing assessment of the patient in order to be able to act upon changes in the patient's condition. Clear policies should be in place so that issues such as safety can be addressed (Dimond, 2005).

PATIENT COMPLIANCE

Understanding and promoting compliance is important for nurses. A fundamental part of the medicines management initiative is concerned with improving patient care by getting the patient more involved in the process and, therefore, treatment decisions.

Richman (2002) suggests that up to 30–60% of patients fail to comply fully with taking medicines, but with some medicines this proportion can be as high as 90%. The reasons for non-compliance can be complex and may be due to the patient simply forgetting to take a dose or consciously deciding not to take a medicine. Other reasons for non-compliance have been identified as complicated treatment regimes, difficulty in coming to terms with a diagnosis, unpleasant side effects, complicated lifestyle, certain health beliefs and manual dexterity (Cheesman, 2006; Wiffen *et al.*, 2007). There are a range of other factors with the potential to influence compliance that need to be considered by the health professional, including:

- the patient's social support networks;
- the cost of medicines;
- breakdown in communication between services, e.g. hospital and home;
- poor knowledge levels (Cheesman, 2006).

The most commonly used definition of compliance is that offered by Haynes *et al.* (1979):

> ... the extent to which a person's behaviour (in terms of taking medications, following diets or executing other lifestyle changes) coincides with medical or health advice.

However, concerns have been expressed by some authors (Wiffen *et al.*, 2007) that this understanding of compliance reflects a paternalistic and authoritarian approach to treatment plans, the implication being that 'doctor knows best' and that the patient's role is passive – that is, the patient does not have a contribution to make.

In order to comply, patients need to both understand and accept the treatment (Greenstein and Gould, 2004). This assumes a more active role for the patient. The term 'adherence' is considered better than 'compliance' (Luker and Wolfson, 1999), because this recognises the patient's role in their medication regime. It also acknowledges that a patient's deviation from treatment should not be regarded as a failure to understand medical advice but may reflect the patient's values and belief systems. Some authors suggest that even the term 'adherence' seems to imply that the patient might be blamed for not taking medications as prescribed and that a better term might be 'concordance'. The Royal Pharmaceutical Society (1997) and the National Prescribing Centre (2007) suggest that the term 'concordance' should replace both 'compliance' and 'adherence', as it encompasses a broader view of patient involvement and negotiation and suggests 'a negotiation between equals'. This acknowledges that patients' beliefs about their medicines are likely to be the most important consideration in whether to take medication, despite best medical evidence about the importance of the treatment. Concordance involves 'respect for the patient's agenda'. If we accept these definitions, we can see that it is possible to have a non-compliant, non-adherent patient, but non-concordance can refer only to the process and not the patient (Weiss and Britten, 2003). In other words, if concordance involves respecting patients' decisions, then the prescriber concurs with what the patient wants, thus eliminating the need for non-adherence.

Reddy (2007) suggests that, despite evidence about the size of the problem, and reasons why it occurs, we have little understanding about how to overcome non-adherence. The current drive for medication review (Healthcare Commission, 2007) is one strategy that could encourage discussions between patients and health professionals and offer patients an opportunity to ask questions.

Medication review is defined as

> ... a structured, critical examination of patients' medicines by a healthcare professional, reaching an agreement with the patient about treatment, optimising the use of medicines, minimizing the number of medication-related problems and avoiding waste.
>
> (Wiffen *et al.*, 2007)

The process involves working with the patient to review all the medicines that the patient is taking, both prescribed and OTC. This enables an investigation of potential and actual interactions, such as adverse reactions that the patient may have experienced. The process should include an assessment of the patient's understanding and ability to take their medicines effectively and a review of the effectiveness of the medication. The outcome should involve the patient being better informed about their medicines and may also include a simplification of the treatment regime and use of compliance aids (Wiffen *et al.*, 2007).

Personal and professional development 5.6
Assessing and managing risk

From the information above, identify the patients most at risk of adverse effects of their medication and therefore those who will benefit the most from a medication review.

Answers can be found at the back of the book.

An essential intervention to be undertaken by healthcare practitioners in order to improve patient adherence is patient education. The nurse has an opportunity during administration of medicines to educate patients (NMC, 2007).

In reality

If we consider the rationale provided for moving from the term 'compliance' to 'adherence', we can see the importance of embracing the concept of adherence, which places such importance on the patient's involvement and the potential for more positive outcomes for the patient. However, the term 'compliance' is still referred to in many key documents, including those of the Audit Commission (2001) and the NMC (2007).

PATIENT EDUCATION

According to the Patients' Charter (DH, 1991), 'every citizen has a right to a clear explanation of any proposed treatment'. Rycroft-Malone (2000) suggests that patient education is gradually assuming more importance in relation to increasing self-care, including enabling patients to manage medicine regimes that can be both continuous and complex. Medicine education is also identified as a key aspect of the nurse's health promotion role in some key government documents (DH, 1992, 1999). This should include education to enable the patient to make an 'informed choice' and to manage their medicines.

The Healthcare Commission (2007) states clearly that patients have a right to:

- time spent explaining medicines from an 'appropriate' professional (this may be a pharmacist);
- an opportunity to raise issues;
- appropriate information to manage their treatment;
- access to their medicines.

Rycroft-Malone (2000) suggests the process of patient education should:

- involve assessment of the patient's beliefs and knowledge;
- be given in stages in relation to the patient's learning needs;
- avoid 'technical jargon';
- allow for clarification;
- have verbal information supported by written information (e.g. patient information leaflets).

Griffith (2006) offers specific details relating to information needs, adverse effects and how to deal with them, evaluation of the effectiveness of treatment, and risks and benefits.

Personal and professional development 5.7
Patient education needs

Identify the information required by patients on discharge in order to manage their medicines. What skills would the nurse need to do this effectively?
Answers can be found at the back of the book.

ISSUES RELATING TO THE ADMINISTRATION OF MEDICINES

Covert prescribing and administration

Dimond (2005) states clearly that 'It is a basic principle of law that the consent of an adult to treatment ... is required'. There are situations in practice where treatments are considered necessary but the patient is unable to give consent, possibly because they are confused or unconscious. Concerns about consent also apply to patients who are judged not to have 'the mental capacity to make his or her decisions' (Dimond, 2005). This does not apply in situations where a patient has the mental capacity but has refused treatment.

The term '**covert administration**' is used to describe the act of disguising medicines in food or drink. This is a very complex issue. It involves the use of deception and therefore should never be used in the care of an adult capable of making decisions about their own treatment. This would contravene the rights of that individual enshrined within the Human Rights Act regarding principles of patient autonomy and consent to treatment. It is therefore 'legally and ethically unacceptable' (Welsh and Deahl, 2002).

The terms 'covert administration', 'surreptitious prescribing' and 'covert prescribing' are used interchangeably within the literature. However, we consider covert administration to be the disguising of medicines as identified above, but covert prescribing as that undertaken knowing that it 'will likely be concealed' (Whitty and Devitt, 2005). Whitty and Devitt (2005) argue that practitioners give medicines in emergency situations and to young children without consent, which is 'accepted practice', whereas Welsh and Deahl (2002) ask why disguising medicines is 'covert' if the patient is unable to give consent.

Perhaps the real concern is not how the medicine is administered but why it is prescribed. An example is the use of tranquillisers in residential settings to 'manage' patients when staffing levels are low. The overriding principle has to be that the medicine is in the best interests of the patient, but we need to reassure ourselves what this means (Dimond, 2005). So, 'if a treatment is right, does it truly matter how it is given?' (Welsh and Deahl, 2002).

If it is felt that the medication is important to the person who cannot consent because of confusion or conscious state, for example, then it would be important to consider several issues before a decision is made, including that:

- the best interests of the patient are the driver: that is, the medication is considered essential;
- the patient lacks the capacity to consent or refuse;
- other methods of administration have been unsuccessful;
- the product licence is considered (see note below).

It is important to recognise that there are situations defined within the Mental Health Act when a patient can be given medication against their wishes, and that non-adherence in certain situations may be considered as a symptom of mental ill-health.

If covert administration is considered, then the following process should be observed:

- It must be based upon an individual assessment of the patient.
- Relatives/carers and appropriate members of the multidisciplinary team must be involved in the decision; it must not be the decision of one person only.
- There should be a local policy in place to support the decision-making process.
- Appropriate documentation should be made of the decision, including details of the staff involved.
- The method of administration should be agreed with the pharmacist.
- Attempts should still be made on an ongoing basis to encourage the patient to take their medication (Dimond, 2005; NMC, 2006, 2007).

Remote prescriptions (directions to administer)

Medicines to be administered to patients should be prescribed in patient areas. This usually involves a medicine administration chart. However, in some circumstances a medicine may be prescribed by fax, text message or email; some literature still refers to this as a 'verbal prescription'.

For example, if a patient unexpectedly and suddenly develops chest pain during the early hours of the morning, and the doctor on call is busy elsewhere, is this a situation where a medicine such as an analgesic could be prescribed by another method? There are situations that the NMC (2007) describes as 'exceptional' in which remote prescribing instructions are acceptable, but only if certain criteria are followed. Trusts usually identify these criteria within protocols and policies, and it is important that employees are familiar with these.

Some general principles underpin these policies:

- Remote prescriptions should not be used for controlled drugs.
- A new prescription must be written by the prescriber within 24 hours.
- Fax or email is the preferred method (NMC, 2007).

Where a medicine has been prescribed previously but a change to the dose is required, the use of fax, text message or email may be used to confirm the change. This must be stapled to the patient's medication administration chart and a new prescription generated within 24 hours (NMC, 2007).

Personal and professional development 5.8
Accessing local policy

Access a copy of your local medicines policy and compare the advice with the recommendations given by the NMC. Note that as an employee, you are required to adhere to the policy documents provided by your employees; the NMC simply provides guidance.

Unlicensed medicines

Medicines should be used in accordance with a product licence or manufacturing authorisation (Medicines Act 1968) that defines the therapeutic purpose of the medicine. The Medicines Act (1968) dictates that only doctors and dentists can authorise the use of unlicensed medicines. Nurses who administer medicines should be aware of the licensed use of the medicine and therefore have enough knowledge to administer it safely. An unlicensed medicine is one that has no product licence; therefore, the risks associated with its use might not have been evaluated. The prescriber, and not the manufacturer, carries the accountability for prescribing the unlicensed medicine if any harm occurs to the patient. In children's nursing, many of the medicines prescribed are not licensed to be given to children. The NMC (2007) guidance in relation to this issue is that the qualified nurse administering the medication should 'be satisfied ... wherever possible, that there is acceptable evidence for the use of that product for the intended indication'. It is strongly recommended that clinical areas have policies relating to the use of unlicensed medicines that state the responsibilities of all involved (Wiffen et al., 2007).

Crushing tablets or opening capsules to put the contents in food may constitute using a medicine outside its licensed use and should always be authorised in writing by the prescriber and a pharmacist's advice sought (Wright, 2002). The NMC (2007) also recommends caution here, as crushing tablets or opening capsules can potentially change the therapeutic properties of the medication, including rendering the medication ineffective. Crushing should occur only in 'the patient's best interest' (NMC, 2007).

Prescribing by nurses

The Medicinal Products: Prescription by Nurses Act (1992) is legislation within the Medicines Act that permitted nurses to prescribe for the first time. This was followed by secondary legislation: Medicinal Prescription by Nurses (1994). This legislation allowed community nurses who had undertaken a recommended programme and recorded this on the NMC register to prescribe from the Nurse Prescribers Formulary. Independent and supplementary nurse prescribers undertake a different programme and have different 'prescribing powers' (see Chapter 17).

Errors

According to the DH (2004), medication errors cost the NHS between £200 million and £400 million per year. A variety of reasons are offered for these errors including prescription errors, increasing workload and poor environment. The Audit Commission (2001) offers the following definition of a medication error:

> ... any preventable event that may cause or lead to inappropriate medication use or patient harm.

Greenstein and Gould (2004) suggest that medication errors can be explained by considering the following factors:

- Patient factors, such as adherence and shorter hospital stays
- Nurse factors, such as not following trust guidelines
- Organisational factors, such as labelling errors, increasing pace of work and staff shortages.

Whatever the reasons for a medication error occurring, it is important that the error is reported to the medical staff managing the patient so that the patient can be assessed and any necessary actions taken in order to avoid or minimise the harmful effects upon the patient (Fegan, 2000). This is supported by the NMC (2007), which stresses the need for an 'open culture ... to encourage the immediate reporting of errors and incidents', moving away from a culture of blame to a culture of learning. These errors and incidents should then be investigated and managed sensitively. One initiative recommended by the Audit Commission (2001) is that we should learn from the practices of other industries and explore near-miss reporting. This topic is discussed further in Chapter 17.

Kapborg (1995) suggests that the administration of medicines makes both the nurse and patient 'very vulnerable' and that it requires mathematical knowledge and skill, as errors can have tragic consequences. Much of the literature relating to medication errors identifies problems in relation to calculation of doses. Medication errors can include miscalculation, overdosing and underdosing (Copping, 2005). This has led to a drive to assess and improve the numeracy skills of staff involved in the administration of medicines. Chapelhow and Crouch (2007) suggest that the numeracy skills used in nursing are 'sophisticated' and that many nurses have concerns about numeracy. Some reasons they offer to explain this are:

● Our perceptions about our ability can impact upon our confidence.
● Number skills are not required in healthcare to the extent that they used to be, due to the emerging technology in clinical areas, which, for example, calculates intravenous fluid rates for us.

Chapelhow and Crouch (2007) suggest that nurses need to consider their numeracy skills in the context of patient care and offer some strategies for developing skills, competence and confidence.

Medicines used in emergency situations

Medicines used within emergency situations such as respiratory and cardiac arrest need to be accessible but also safe. Because of the nature of emergencies, written prescriptions are not used, and so it is important that a careful note is made of the medicine administered, including its dose, route and frequency, so that this can be recorded at the earliest opportunity. This often involves allocating roles within the emergency team, one of which is related to medicines management (Skinner and Vincent, 1993).

Within any patient care environment, it is important to note where emergency medicines are kept. This usually involves a secure (but not locked) pack, so that the medicines can be accessed quickly (e.g. on an emergency/resuscitation trolley). It is important that the pack is designed so that it is easy to identify whether it is intact, because in an emergency situation we need to be confident that the medicines we need are available for use. An emergency medicine pack contains a limited number of medicines, as medicines have only a limited role in resuscitation (Jevon, 2002; Wiffen *et al.*, 2007; **www.resus.org.uk**). A used pack should be replaced as soon as possible, and packs should be checked regularly (usually daily) to make sure they are complete and that the medicines have not expired.

Different routes are used for administration in emergency situations, including intravenous or intraosseous injection and via a tracheal tube. The medicines are usually presented in minijets or prefilled syringes. Minijets require some assembly. The NMC (2007) suggests that if a nurse is required to prepare medicines for injection in an emergency situation for someone else to administer, the person administering the medicine should make the same checks as when administering any other medicine and the nurse preparing the medicine should make sure that these checks have been done. Preparing substances for another professional to administer is usually unacceptable but if required in emergency should be carried out in the presence of the person administering the medicine (NMC, 2007).

Another important responsibility of the nurse is to monitor the effect of the medicines on the patient in the period following the emergency.

Personal and professional development 5.9

You might wish to remind yourself about the various routes used for administering emergency medicines, including intravenous, intraosseous and tracheal.

Answers can be found at the back of the book.

Personal and professional development 5.10
Preparation for placement

According to Wiffen *et al.* (2007), the medicines most commonly found in emergency boxes/packs are:

- Epinephrine (adrenaline)
- Atropine
- Amioderone.

You may also see:

- Lidocaine
- Sodium bicarbonate
- Adenosine
- Magnesium sulphate
- Calcium chloride
- Sodium chloride
- Oxygen.

You may wish to research these medicines in preparation for your clinical placement.

Identify where the emergency medicines are kept, and any specific emergency medicines that differ from those identified above used within your clinical area.

PROFESSIONAL REQUIREMENTS

Clinical governance

All NHS hospital trusts and care homes are required to provide audit trails to confirm that appropriate safety mechanisms are in place in relation to ordering, storage and administration of medicines, in order to avoid abuse (DH, 2007). Clinical governance is a government initiative introduced in 1997 intended to ensure quality in the NHS. It was part of a larger quality agenda intended to balance the quality of care delivery with cost-effectiveness. The DH defines clinical governance as follows:

> Clinical governance is the system through which NHS organisations are accountable for continuously improving the quality of their services and safeguarding high standards of care, by creating an environment in which clinical excellence will flourish.

The purpose of clinical governance is to safeguard the quality of the systems and processes that contribute to the care of patients. Clinical governance should therefore include:

- clinical effectiveness activities, such as auditing;
- clear lines of responsibility and accountability;
- risk management, including patient safety;
- patient involvement.

Clinical governance is therefore an overarching strategy that encompasses initiatives such as:

- NICE, which was set up to provide the NHS with guidance on the clinical management of conditions and on pharmaceuticals, medical devices, diagnostic techniques and procedures;
- the National Patient Safety Agency (NPSA), a 'special health authority that coordinates the efforts of all those involved in healthcare to learn from patient safety incidents occurring in the NHS' (**www.dh.gov**).

Quick reminder

✔ Administration of medicines is a complex activity.

✔ The nurse should be familiar with how the medication works, its actions and side effects, and its usual dose and route.

✔ The nurse should always work within legislation, professional guidance and employer policies.

✔ The nurse should consider safety issues in relation to the prescription, ordering and storage of medicines.

✔ Guidance changes in relation to contemporary issues and knowledge; it is the responsibility of the individual to keep abreast of such changes.

✔ Individual administration using patients' individual prescribed medicines, which are stored in patients' lockers, is now recommended.

✔ Some patient situations are more complex and require extra considerations.

✔ The patient is central to medicines administration and should play an active role in decisions made about their own treatments. The patient should be given an appropriate level of information on which to base their informed consent.

✔ Clinical governance is a governement initiative to ensure safe and effective care.

REFERENCES

Audit Commission (2001) *A Spoonful of Sugar: Medicines Management in NHS Hospitals.* Wetherby: Audit Commission Publications.

Chapelhow C and Crouch S (2007) *Nursing Numeracy: A New Approach.* Cheltenham: Nelson Thornes.

Chapelhow C, Crouch S, Fisher M and Walsh A (2005) *Uncovering Skills for Practice.* Cheltenham: Nelson Thornes.

Cheesman S (2006) Promoting concordance: the implications for prescribers. *Nurse Prescribing* **4**, 205-208.

Committee for the Safety of Medicines (CSM) (2001) *Clearer Labelling of Medicines: Further Action in the Patient Safety Programme.* **www.open.gov.uk/mca**.

Copping C (2005) Preventing and reporting drug administration errors. *Nursing Times* **101**, 32.

Department of Health (DH) (1988) *The Way Forward for Hospital Pharmaceutical Services.* London: The Stationery Office.

Department of Health (DH) (1991) *The Patients' Charter.* London: The Stationery Office.

Department of Health (DH) (1992) *Our Healthier Nation.* London: The Stationery Office.

Department of Health (DH) (1999) *Saving Lives: Our Healthier Nation.* London: The Stationery Office.

Department of Health (DH) (2002) *Advisory Council on the Misuse of Drugs Report: The Classification of Cannabis Under the Misuse of Drugs Act 1971.* London: The Stationery Office.

Department of Health (DH) (2003) *A Vision for Pharmacy in the New NHS.* London: The Stationery Office.

Department of Health (DH) (2004) *Building a Safer NHS for Patients: Improving Medication Safety.* London: The Stationery Office.

Department of Health (DH) (2007) *Safer Management of Controlled Drugs: Early Action.* London: The Stationery Office.

Dimond B (2005) *Legal Aspects of Nursing*, 4th edn. Harlow: Longman.

Duthie R B (1988) *DoH Guidelines for the Safe and Secure Handling of Medicines*. London: The Stationery Office.

Eisenhauer L A, Hurley A C and Dolan N (2007) Nurses' reported thinking during medication administration. *Journal of Nursing Scholarship* **39**, 82-87.

Fegan J (2000) in Prosser S, Worster B, MacGregor J, Dewar K, Runyard P and Fegan J, *Applied Pharmacology: An Introduction to Pathophysiology and Drug Management for Nurses and Healthcare Professionals*. London: Mosby.

Greenstein B and Gould D (2004) *Trounce's Clinical Pharmacology for Nurses*, 17th edn. Edinburgh: Churchill Livingstone.

Griffith R (2006) Adverse drug reactions and non-compliance with prescribed medication. *Nurse Prescribing* **4**, 69-72.

Griffith R, Griffith H and Jordan S (2003) Administration of medicines part 1: the law and nursing. *Nursing Standard* **16**, 47-53.

Haynes R B, Taylor D W and Sackett D L (1979) *Compliance in Health Care*. London: Johns Hopkins Press.

Healthcare Commission (2007) *The Best Medicine: The Management of Medicines in Acute and Specialist Trusts*. London: Commission for Healthcare Audit and Inspection.

Jevon P (2002) Resuscitation in hospital: Resuscitation Council (UK) recommendations. *Nursing Standard* **16**, 41-44.

Kapborg I D (1995) An evaluation of Swedish nurse students' calculation ability in relation to their earlier educational background. *Nurse Education Today* **15**, 69-74.

Lowe C J, Raynor D K, Courtney E A, Purvis J and Teale C (1995) Effects of self-medication programme on knowledge of drugs and compliance with treatment in elderly patients. *British Medical Journal* **310**, 1229-1231.

Luker K and Wolfson D (1999) *Medicines Management for Clinical Nurses*. Oxford: Blackwell Science.

National Prescribing Centre (2007) *A Competency Framework for Shared Decision-Making with Patients: Achieving Concordance for Taking Medicines*. Keele: NPC Plus.

Nursing and Midwifery Council (NMC) (2006) A-Z *Advice Sheet: Covert Administration of Medicines*. **www.nmc-uk.org**.

Nursing and Midwifery Council (NMC) (2007) *Standards for Medicines Management*. London: Nursing and Midwifery Council.

Preston R M (2004) Drug errors and patient safety: the need for a change in practice. *British Journal of Nursing* **13**, 72-78.

Prosser S (2000) in Prosser S, Worster B, MacGregor J, Dewar K, Runyard P and Fegan J *Applied Pharmacology: An Introduction to Pathophysiology and Drug Management for Nurses and Healthcare Professionals*. London: Mosby.

Reddy B (2007) Medication review as a route to optimising treatment. *Nurse Prescriber* **4**, 464-468.

Richman J (2002) Keep taking your medication or you will not get better. Who is the non-compliant patient? In Humphries J L and Green J (eds) *Nurse Prescribing*, 2nd edn. Basingstoke: Palgrave.

Royal Pharmaceutical Society (1997) *From Compliance to Concordance: Achieving Shared Goals in Medicine Taking*. Report of a Working Party. London: Royal Pharmaceutical Society.

Rycroft-Malone J (2000) Nursing and medication education. *Nursing Standard* **14**, 35-39.

Skinner D V and Vincent R (1993) *Cardiopulmonary Resuscitation*. Oxford: Oxford University Press.

The Medicines Act (1968). London: HMSO.

The Misuse of Drugs Act (1971). London: HMSO.

The Misuse of Drugs Regulations (2001). London: HMSO.

Weiss M and Britten N (2003) Concordance: what is concordance? *Pharmaceutical Journal* **271**, 493.

Welsh S and Deahl M (2002) Covert medication: ever ethically justifiable? *Psychiatric Bulletin* **26**, 123-126.

Whitty P and Devitt P (2005) Surreptitious prescribing in psychiatric practice. *Psychiatric Services* **56**, 481-483.

Wiffen P, Mitchell M, Snelling M and Stoner N (2007) *Oxford Handbook of Clinical Pharmacy*. Oxford: Oxford University Press.

Wright D (2002) Swallowing difficulties protocol; medication administration. *Nursing Standard* **17**,

Chapter 6

Complementary medicinal products

The use of complementary and alternative therapies is increasing in the UK and the rest of the world. Murcott (2005) suggests that $US60 billion is spent on alternative medicines each year worldwide. In 2000, it was estimated that six million people in the UK used complementary and alternative therapies (House of Lords Committee on Science and Technology, 2000). Many people turn to complementary and alternative therapies to help them to maintain good health and manage ill-health. However, there are positive and negative aspects of such therapies, and this chapter identifies some of them in relation to the common complementary and alternative therapies that are used in the UK. This chapter also explores the small number of complementary therapies that have been and are being integrated into mainstream NHS care. Such therapies includes homeopathy, herbal medicines, aromatherapy and massage. The concepts of allopathic and non-allopathic medicines are also introduced, and the underpinning principles of each are highlighted. This chapter highlights the recommendations made by the NMC (2006) in relation to what it terms 'complementary medicinal products' and goes on to consider the major issues that this presents for qualified nurses. Three examples of herbal medicines are used: St John's wort, echinacea and garlic. A brief overview of each of these is given, along with the key issues for each that must be considered by nurses.

Learning outcomes

By the end of this chapter you should be able to:

✔ Explain the difference between allopathic (conventional) and non-allopathic (non-conventional) medicines

✔ Clarify the difference between complementary and alternative therapies and complementary medicinal products

✔ List the complementary and alternative therapies identified by the NMC (2006) as complementary medicinal products

✔ Discuss the advantages and disadvantages of complementary medicinal products

✔ Discuss the actions and effects of two commonly used herbal medicines

✔ Identify the nursing knowledge needed relating to the use of complementary medicinal products

✔ Discuss the key dilemmas for nurses raised by the use of complementary medicinal products.

Chapter at a glance

Factors influencing the increasing use of complementary medicinal products
The key debates
Regulating the industry
Belief about complementary medicinal products
Massage and aromatherapy
Herbal medicine: an overview
Homeopathy
Quick reminder
References

Personal and professional development 6.1

Think about your beliefs in relation to complementary and alternative therapies. Write down the first three words that came into your mind when you think about them. Reflect on what this tells you about your values and beliefs. Are you non-judgemental?

FACTORS INFLUENCING THE INCREASING USE OF COMPLEMENTARY MEDICINAL PRODUCTS

In the UK today, as in most of the Western world, healthcare is commonly underpinned by Western medicine with its emphasis on 'scientific' or allopathic medicine. However, more and more people are coming to recognise that the various healthcare professions are a blend of the art of healing (non-allopathic) with the science of medicine (allopathic). The values and beliefs that many other cultures hold about healthcare, particularly in Asia, sometimes appear to be the opposite of those in the West. Asian cultures value more highly the art of healing, the non-allopathic, rather than valuing only the science (allopathic) as people in the West often do. Table 6.1 below lists the major values and beliefs of allopathic and non-allopathic therapies. Over the years, a number of movements have tried to drive a change in the UK's long-held belief in allopathic medicine and the dominance of the medical profession that arose as a result of this belief. Kelleher and colleagues (2006) suggest that there has been a slow realisation that allopathic medicine, despite its promise, does has some major limitations. They claim that this awareness has come about over the past couple of decades and suggest that these limitations are seen particularly in the area of long-term conditions.

At the same time, British society has seen a rise in consumerism and a move towards what Taylor and Field (2007) have called 'individualisation'. Allied with this, during the last 30 years of the twentieth century, many people developed new ideologies, such as hippy, new age and self-help principles. As the twentieth century wore on, these 'alternative' movements became more and more mainstream and began to influence politicians, healthcare professionals and the users of the NHS. As we began to uncover a greater understanding of how the body works, more and more evidence came to light in mainstream science that the allopathic model of medicine, which seemed to be

Table 6.1 Major philosophies of allopathic and non-allopathic therapies (a summary)

Allopathic (conventional)	Non-allopathic (non-conventional)
Illness has a specific cause, such as a diseased organ, a faulty gene or an infection	Illness comes from within, and results from imbalances in thoughts, feelings or lifestyle
Treatment is focused on drugs, surgery or irradiation	A variety of therapies exist, of which only a few rely on drugs in some way
The doctor frequently has a paternalistic attitude towards patients and staff	The practitioner works in a collaborative manner with the patient
The body needs outside help in order to be healed	The body can heal itself given the right conditions
The body is viewed as a machine and the mind is separate from the body	The body is considered as whole

driven by the Cartesian view that the mind functions separately from the body (dualism), was inadequate. Scientists, in the newly formed field of psychoneuroimmunology, are finding more and more evidence that demonstrates a clear link between the mind and the body. This connection seems so evident that it has been called the 'bodymind' (Pert, 1999), a word coined because the author felt that there was no other word that could be used to describe the inseparable relationship between the physiological functioning of our body and our thoughts and feelings. On the other hand, our everyday language suggests that perhaps we have known this all along: think about the terms 'gut instinct' and 'gut reaction'.

THE KEY DEBATES

By the end of the first half of the twentieth century, the discipline of medicine had become a very powerful force in the UK. One of the results of this powerful influence was that the dominant Cartesian view was the belief of many doctors, healthcare professionals and members of the public. From the 1970s onwards, the discipline of medicine was frequently criticised for its reductionist approach (Fitzpatrick, 2000; Illich, 2001; Porter, 2002). One of the key reasons for such criticism today is because the discipline of medicine has been seen to strongly ally itself to the positivist end of the research spectrum, although this has now started to change. Medicine's demand for 'hard' reliable and valid evidence that treatment is effective is often accompanied by many medical doctors dismissing treatments that have been used successfully by many people for many years. This has led to considerable debate, both within and without medicine, about the efficiency and effectiveness of both allopathic and non-allopathic medicines and therapies. Those who support the use of non-allopathic medicines alongside allopathic medicines find it difficult to understand the demands for reliable and valid research evidence (such as from randomised controlled trials) for non-allopathic medicines when even many allopathic medicines used today have little in the way of robust evidence to support their use. For example, digoxin (used to slow and strengthen heart rate) has little evidence from randomised controlled trials to support its use. However, what we do have is years of use, with evidence from the observations of patients and doctors, which in mainstream positivist science would be called 'anecdotal evidence'. Alongside this debate, there has surfaced another, closely linked debate: that related to the increasing power that pharmaceutical companies are thought to hold not only over ill-health but also increasingly over good health (Avorn, 2005; Moynihan and Cassels, 2005). Some authors criticise the large pharmaceutical companies for their development and marketing of 'lifestyle' drugs such as bupropion (to aid smoking cessation) and sildenafil (to aid impotence), and the resulting 'medicalisation' of life (Illich, 2001; Moynihan and Cassels, 2005).

REGULATING THE INDUSTRY

There are a multitude of complementary and alternative therapies available. However, unlike healthcare professionals, the practitioners who offer these therapies have no statutory regulation of their practice, and many of the practitioners offering these services do not have any nationally recognised qualifications. The therapies that do have professional regulation and require qualification in the discipline include homeopathy and medical herbalism (phytomedicine). In order to improve the situation for consumers, the House of Lords Committee on Science and Technology (2000) identified three main categories of therapy and required both the licensing of herbal products and the regulation of practitioners (Table 6.2).

Table 6.2 Varieties of complementary and alternative medicines recognised by the House Lords Science and Technology Committee (2000) report

Professionally organised alternative therapies:
  Acupuncture
  Chiropractic
  Herbal medicine
  Homeopathy
  Osteopathy

Complementary therapies:
  Alexander technique
  Bach and other flower remedies
  Body work therapies, including massage
  Counselling stress therapy
  Hypnotherapy
  Meditation
  Reflexology
  Shiatsu
  Healing
  Maharishi Ayurvedic medicine
  Nutritional medicine
  Yoga

Alternative disciplines:
  Long-established and traditional systems of healthcare:
    Anthroposophical medicine
    Ayurvedic medicine
    Chinese herbal medicine
    Eastern medicine
    Naturopathy
    Traditional Chinese medicine
  Other alternative disciplines
  Crystal therapy
  Dowsing
  Iridology
  Kinesiology
  Radionics

Nursing implications

Rather than trying to explore the rights and wrongs of allopathic or non-allopathic medicine, this chapter presents sufficient information and raises a number of issues so that student nurses can develop their medicine management skills more fully. Whether, as healthcare professionals, we share the values and beliefs of our patients in relation to either allopathic or non-allopathic treatment is irrelevant. Mainstream medicine can often fail to live up to some people's expectations, and consequently those people turn to other types of medicine.

▶

▶ *(continued)*

As a nurse involved in medicines management, it is important to remain non-judgemental and to be armed with the necessary information and communication skills in order to ensure that you fulfil your role as best you can.

Personal and professional development 6.2

List three types of complementary therapy where medicines are one of the key forms of treatment or management. Write a short description of each of these complementary therapies that could form the basis of information that you could give to a patient.

Personal and professional development 6.3

Which profession do you value more: medical herbalists or medical doctors? Which profession seems to be more highly regarded by British society? Would this influence how a patient viewed the information given by each of the practitioners? Write some short notes to support your views.

The House of Lords Committee on Science and Technology (2000) report is useful as it highlights the large range and variety of complementary and alternative therapies that are used in the UK today. However, very few of these therapies are based on the use of medicines. In order to explore the impact of complementary and alternative therapies on medicines management for nurses, we use the groups of therapies identified by the NMC (2006), as these separate therapies that use medicines from those that do not. This chapter considers herbal medicines, homeopathy and essential oils; it uses the collective term 'complementary medicinal products' for these (NMC, 2006). As increasingly more people use complementary medicinal products, it is becoming evident that all healthcare professionals, including nurses, will have to have an appreciation of these products.

BELIEFS ABOUT COMPLEMENTARY MEDICINAL PRODUCTS

Increasing numbers of people are taking one or more complementary medicinal products, frequently in addition to allopathic medicines (Barnes, 2003; Ernst and White, 2000; House of Lords Committee on Science and Technology, 2000; Kemper *et al.,*

2006; Lewith *et al.*, 2001). Complementary medicinal products come in a variety of forms; they may be inhaled, rubbed on the skin or taken orally. Many of these products are derived from natural sources such as flowers and herbs; for this reason, many people, nurses included, view these products as completely safe and refrain from telling their healthcare practitioners that they are using them (Kemper *et al.*, 2006). Cockayne *et al.* (2004) concluded from their observational study that neither doctors nor nurses tend to to ask patients whether they use any complementary medicinal products.

The reasoning behind the belief that these products are 'safe' is somewhat simplistic and assumes that if something is natural, then it will not do harm and indeed may be good for you. Viewed from a modern perspective, it is not easy to see how such beliefs have become established, not only within the general public but also by healthcare professionals. It has been suggested that this is because many of us seem to have lost our closeness with nature. An example to highlight this argument uses one of the oldest known drugs, and which is still very commonly used today: digoxin. Digoxin is derived from digitalis, an extract of the purple foxglove plant. Digitalis has long been renowned for its potential as a herbal remedy that affected the heart's rate and rhythm and helped to drain oedema (fluid in the tissues of the legs and other organs). It was, and still is, used to treat a condition once known as dropsy, a condition that we call heart failure today. Although today digoxin is manufactured synthetically, originally it was derived from the purple foxglove plant, considered a weed by many people in the UK.

Although there are older records of its use, Rang *et al.* (2003) cite Withering, writing in 1775, about using foxglove to control the heart rate. Initially foxglove was used with little or no understanding of how it worked or why some people did not respond to it in the way that was expected. However, we do know from historical writings that people knew that its use could be dangerous in some situations, even though they did not know why. As a result, people consulted with herbalists before taking the medicine. We now know that the therapeutic range of digoxin is very narrow, meaning that there is a fine line between an effective dose and a toxic dose (Rang *et al.*, 2003); this is why much smaller doses are used to treat babies, children and older people.

Using digoxin as an example helps us to appreciate how a herbal medicine can be both useful and dangerous and gives us an opportunity for reflection. Perhaps as a society we have lost our understanding of the benefits and dangers of using many herbs as medicines. However, herbalists do still practise in the UK and in many other Western countries, although they are probably fewer in number these days. Medical herbalists belong to a long-standing profession, and are qualified to first-degree level in the same way that medical doctors are. However, few of these practitioners achieve the level of reward that Western society gives to the majority of medical doctors, such as power, status and financial recompense.

The side effects of digoxin, which result from overstimulating the heart, are extremely common and are serious for many individuals, especially children and frail older people. These side effects have been known about for a long time. In spite of this, many older people are still admitted to hospital as a result of digoxin overdose because of poor prescribing practices (Huang *et al.*, 2002). The unwanted effects of medicines, both allopathic and non-allopathic, can also happen as a result of an interaction between two drugs or between a drug and the chemical constituents of some common foods and drinks. It is important that as nurses we understand these potential effects, whether they involve allopathic medicine or non-allopathic medicines or interactions between chemicals in particular medicines or between the ingredients of a medicine and food/drink.

Having such an understanding is becoming more and more important as healthcare today is generally more successful than it was even just 5 years ago, with the result that many people regularly take two or more prescribed medicines a day. These medicines are most commonly taken for chronic diseases such as diabetes, hypertension and coronary heart disease. The greater the number of medications taken, whether conventional or alternative, the higher the risk that there will be some kind of drug interaction.

Fortunately, the conditions that produce either pharmacodynamic or pharmacokinetic interactions do not happen very often. There are some drugs where major problems can occur because of pharmacokinetic interaction, and Rang *et al.* (2003) cite a variety of commonly used drug groups: the antithrombotics, antidysrhythmics, antiepileptics, some of the antineoplastic and immunosuppressant drugs, and lithium.

An example of a potential interaction

Many foods and drinks interact with conventional and herbal medicines. Although uncommon, some interactions can have potentially disastrous results. For example, the cytochrome P450 system is an enzyme system responsible for the metabolism of many drugs in the liver. An enzyme present in grapefruit and grapefruit juice interferes with the cytochrome P450 system, with the result that drug metabolism is reduced (Rang *et al.*, 2003). A number of studies have highlighted the potential risks of eating grapefruit or drinking grapefruit juice at the same time as taking certain medicines used for the prevention and treatment of cardiovascular disease such as hypertension (high blood pressure) and hypercholesteraemia (high blood levels of cholesterol) (Bailey and Dresser, 2004; Breckenridge, 2000; Miscellaneous, 2005; Rang *et al.*, 2003). In a review of the studies available, Williamson (2003) highlights the potential risk of taking St John's wort alongside many commonly used allopathic medicines, such as digoxin and warfarin.

In the UK, the NMC (2006), mindful of the increasing numbers of people using complementary medicinal products, propose the following:

> Nurses and midwives need to be familiar with a range of complementary medicinal products that their patients may be using, or may wish to be used, in their treatment. These include homeopathic remedies, herbal remedies, aromatherapy oils, flower essences and the broad area of vitamin and mineral supplements.

Nurses should not prescribe any complementary medicinal products unless they have undertaken appropriate recognised training to do so. Where a nurse or midwife considers that complementary medicinal products could be a substitute for, or a complement to, conventional medication then patients or clients should be referred to appropriately qualified practitioners to receive such treatment.

Ernst (1998) and Schmidt and Ernst (2004) highlight that lay books and websites can mislead people about complementary and alternative therapies and sometimes endanger people's health. This can be as a result of the information that these unregulated sources of information either give or do not give. When individuals are seeking help for their symptoms or a cure for their disease, they are potentially very vulnerable and may find sources of information about medicines and therapies that promise too much.

When an individual is ill, it is easy to dampen or ignore normal caution, resulting in impulsive behaviour and preventing further enquiry. It is often easy to see that something seems too good to be true, but patients with life-threatening conditions or severe intractable chronic symptoms such as pain may grasp at straws. In addition, the Internet makes it much easier for people to buy medicines and therapies that until recently they would not have had easy access to.

Nursing implications

Nurses and other healthcare practitioners should be able to minimise the risks to patients of using complementary medicinal products by routinely asking questions about such products when assessing patients. Such data-gathering should be linked to the information that is sought about the patient's use of allopathic medicines. These data should be collected in the same way, so as well as asking patients about their allopathic medicines, routinely ask whether they have taken or are taking any complementary medicinal products and, if so, which ones, why and for how long.

MASSAGE AND AROMATHERAPY

Some complementary and alternative therapies are now being offered by the NHS; aromatherapy massage is highlighted as the therapy most frequently provided (Fellowes *et al.*, 2004). Massage uses the hands to apply pressure and motion to areas of the patient's body to improve their wellbeing. It involves techniques such as rubbing and kneading to stimulate the underlying muscles; this is thought to improve the blood supply to the muscles. A small amount of oil is usually used as a lubricant, reducing friction and making the massage more pleasurable.

Aromatherapy is the use of essential oils, concentrated essences distilled from all flowers, herbs or other plants either for inhalation or as massage oil, Aromatherapy is said to induce relaxation of the body and the mind, stimulate endorphin production and invigorate the immune system (Cassileth, 1998; Froemming, 1998; Goldberg, 1999). Many people believe that aromatherapy allied with massage can be beneficial to all, particularly for people with cancer. Beneficial effects include 'reduced anxiety levels, relief of emotional stress, pain, muscular tension and fatigue' (Fellows *et al.*, 2004).

However, there is little reliable valid research evidence that supports the claims that are made, not only for aromatherapy massage but also for any of the complementary and alternative therapies. Following a systematic review of all of the available studies, Fellowes *et al.* (2004) suggest that although massage seemed to be helpful in the short term for many people in reducing anxiety, there was little evidence that it achieved much else. Even when essential oils were added to the massage – aromatherapy massage – the difference that this made to patient outcomes was barely noticeable. The authors go on to suggest that further studies, especially long-term trials, are needed in order to identify a variety of outcomes for patients, including the benefit of massage, whether adding essential oils makes any difference, how many massages are needed to produce both short-term and long-term effects, which areas of the body should be massaged and, importantly, whether essential oils are safe. Although this systematic review explores studies examining only two types of complementary and alternative therapies in individuals with cancer, the issues it raises highlight some common themes across the literature about complementary and alternative therapies. These themes centre on the effectiveness and safety of complementary and alternative therapies. This is not surprising, given that these are also major concerns for many people taking allopathic medicines. Regardless of the disease or disorder, individuals seeking treatment are hoping to improve their health by using some forms of therapy. So, for nurses supporting patients in their journey through ill-health, there seems to be a key message here: healthcare professionals should ensure that patients have all the necessary information required to use all therapies and medicines safely and effectively, whether those medicines are allopathic or non-allopathic. In other words, nurses must ensure that patients are truly informed consumers of healthcare.

Personal and professional development 6.4

You are Ms Freda Small's primary nurse and it is mid-morning. It is Ms Small's second postoperative day, following a left hip replacement. Ms Small has taken the nifedipine LA (a calcium channel blocker) 60 mg for long-standing primary hypertension that you have administered. Towards the end of the conversation that you initiated with Ms Small about her analgesia (pain control) and postoperative mobility, she tells you that she had some grapefruit juice brought in last evening and had a small glass this morning with her breakfast, as she has heard it's good for reducing blood cholesterol levels.

Later, Ms Small's call bell rings. When you go to answer the call bell, the physiotherapist is there. He tells you that when he helped Ms Small to stand up and walk, she complained of feeling weak, dizzy and nauseated. As a result, the physiotherapist helped Ms Small sit down in the chair and rang the call bell. What has happened to Ms Small? What actions should you take, and why?

Answers can be found at the back of the book.

HERBAL MEDICINE: AN OVERVIEW

Many of the herbs that are used as medicines in the UK today have an age-old anecdotal knowledge base for their use. There are two main reasons why herbal medicines have a very limited research base either for their ingredients or for their pharmacodynamic or pharmacokinetic activity. First, herbs have been used since before written records were kept; Newall *et al.* (1996) suggest that the earliest written descriptions of herbs used as medicines in the Western world were made by the ancient Greeks, and that there is written evidence of herbal medicines being used in China even earlier than this. Much of the early use of herbs as medicines was consequently before we began to demand rigorous scientific investigation of all medicines. Second, most herbal preparations are not patented and therefore are produced by individuals or small companies, as a result, they find it almost impossible to attract funding for research compared with the huge amounts of money that major pharmaceutical companies have at their disposal.

In the UK, interest in herbal medicines has risen dramatically (Murcott, 2005). People use herbal products for a variety of reasons, including the following:

- Many people, particularly those with long-term conditions, find that allopathic medicines are not always successful in managing their symptoms, and so they look for alternatives.
- The consumer does not need to consult a healthcare professional in order to buy herbal products. They can select many products from health food stores, pharmacies, supermarkets and the Internet, both in the UK and when they travel abroad.
- Herbal medicines are perceived by many of the general public to be 'natural' and therefore risk-free.

This final point in this list seems to be a widely held belief among the public (Ang-Lee *et al.*, 2001; Hudson *et al.*, 2001; Murcott, 2005). However, herbal remedies are not always as safe as many people believe. Just as food and drink can interact with conventional medicines, so it can with herbal products. In addition, herbal products can also affect the pharmacokinetics of allopathic medicines. These effects are not always well publicised, however.

Although all prescription medicines supplied by the NHS must by law (Medicines Act 1968) have a product licence, the majority of herbal products sold to the public in the UK are not licensed as medicines. Products licensed as medicines are subject to strict labelling requirements, and manufacturers of licensed medicines are not allowed to make claims about the medicine without both robust evidence and Medical and Healthcare Regulatory Agency approval. As most herbal products are not licensed as medicines, some individuals and companies make what seem to be extremely deceptive claims for their products.

For the nurse, knowing that many people, including some healthcare professionals, choose to use complementary and alternative therapies can raise a number of dilemmas. The field of complementary and alternative therapies is riddled with inconsistencies. These discrepancies arise due to the wide range of terminology used, the large variety of therapies available, the lack of any regulated standards of care, the existence of a variety of practitioners, some with suspect qualifications, and the medical profession's regular dismissal of such therapies as a charade (Ross *et al.*, 2007). This cynicism of many medical staff means that some have judgemental attitudes about patients who use such therapies. For the nurse trying to empower patients and advocate for patients, such an environment can present its own difficulties.

Nursing implications

Many herbal medicines have the potential to interact with many prescribed allopathic medicines, and so it is important that all patients are given specific verbal and written advice about this in a format that they understand and that is readily accessible. As individuals can easily self-select a variety of allopathic and non-allopathic medicines from high-street outlets and over the Internet, patients should be advised to discuss with a healthcare professional any allopathic or non-allopathic medicines that they may think about taking. Nurses need to become proactive during their patient assessments and ask patients whether they are or have been taking any allopathic or non-allopathic medication, documenting this information and acting appropriately.

St John's wort

St John's wort (*Hypericum perforatum*) is a herbal medicine that is being used increasingly (Henderson *et al.*, 2002; Izzo and Ernst, 2001; Tesch, 2002; Zhou *et al.*, 2004). St John's wort is used to alleviate the symptoms of mild to moderate depression. The drug is also not without its problems, however. Among the active constituents identi-fied by Newall and colleagues (1996) in the unprocessed herb are hypericin, flavinoids, phenols, tannins and volatile oils, the latter of which are thought to irritate the skin.

St John's wort is one of the few herbal medicines to have been subjected to many years of robust research studies, and it is well known to increase the availability of a number of neurotransmitters, namely serotonin, norepinephrine (noradrenaline) and dopamine (Linde and Mulrow, 2000). It is thought to work by preventing these neuro-transmitting chemicals from being reabsorbed by the nerve cells once the chemicals have passed on their chemical messages (Di Carlo *et al.*, 2001). As a result, more neuro-transmitting chemicals are available within the nerve cell synapse, and this is thought to reduce the symptoms of anxiety, depression and anorexia.

St John's wort is available in a number of forms depending on the source of the prod-uct. It is available from medical herbalists as a concoction of leaves, which are brewed as a tea to be drunk at specific times of the day, as a liquid extract and as a tincture. It is also available from health food stores and supermarkets in tablet form; the disadvan-tage of this self-selection is that although many medical professionals realise that St John's wort interacts with a number of allopathic medicines, this is not widely known among the general public (Henderson *et al.*, 2002; Izzo and Ernst, 2001; MHRA, 2002). Fugh-Berman and Ernst (2001) identify the interaction between St John's wort and allopathic selective serotonin reuptake inhibitors (SSRIs) that are commonly used to treat mental health disorders; they suggest that this is most likely because of the addi-tive effects of the two drugs, which have similar modes of action. As the popularity of St John's wort increases, its ability to interact with other medicines is becoming clearer. Milton and Abdulla (2007) identified, in a letter to the editor of the *British Journal of Clinical Pharmacology*, an interaction between buproprion and St John's wort that caused an orofacial dystonia (involuntary facial muscle spasms). Although originally manufactured as an antidepressant, buproprion is most commonly pre-scribed to help people stop smoking by reducing the individual's desire to smoke.

Personal and professional development 6.5

During a visit to Mr Jack Robson, a patient discharged from hospital a few days ago, the district nurse notices that he has a box of St John's wort (*Hypericum perforatum*) tablets on the table next to his medicines: digoxin 62.5 μg daily and warfarin 3 mg daily.

What advice should the district nurse give to Mr Robson, and why?

Answers can be found at the back of the book.

Garlic

Garlic contains a number of sulphur compounds, such as allicin, that have been credited with a variety of different pharmacological actions. Newall *et al.*, (1996) suggest that many studies highlight the value of garlic as a herbal medicine in a variety of situations. They describe its properties as 'useful' and list its pharmacological actions:

- *Hypocholesterolaemic*: Garlic reduces serum cholesterol, triglycerides and low-density lipoprotein (LDL) and increases high-density lipoprotein (HDL). Garlic reduces the LDL/HDL ratio.
- *Anti-thrombotic*: Garlic inhibits the sticking together of platelets, which reduces the formation of thrombi (blood clots).
- *Hypotensive*: Garlic may lower blood pressure.
- *Antimicrobial*: Garlic inhibits the growth of a number of bacteria, including *Staphylocococus*, *Escherichia*, *Proteus* and *Salmonella* species.

Kayne (2006) and Newall *et al.* (1996) point out that although numerous studies in both animals and humans demonstrate that garlic has these properties, it has not yet been identified which of the chemicals in garlic, and in what concentrations, are responsible for the effects. They do accept, however, that the evidence suggests that eating a lot of garlic regularly seems to bestow some beneficial health effects on the eater. Another uncertainty that is yet to be answered is whether the therapeutic ingredients in garlic are a component of the chemicals that produce garlic's unique pungent odour; if they are, then this begs the question of whether odourless garlic medicines actually contain any active ingredients. It is difficult to calculate how much fresh garlic someone would have to eat in order to produce a pharmacological effect, given that the compounds are not distributed evenly among different plants.

Echinacea

Another commonly used herbal medicine is echinacea, which is commonly used to boost the immune system. Some people use echinacea to prevent them getting, or to reduce the symptoms of, a cold or other infection.

Echinacea has been long thought to possess a number of useful properties. It is valued as an antiseptic, an antiviral and for its ability to cause peripheral vasodilitation (Newall *et al.*, 1996). Because of these qualities, echinacea has been used as a herbal medicine to treat a variety of infections, from tonsillitis to abscesses (Newall *et al.*, 1996; Shah *et al.*, 2007). A number of animal studies have supported this use of echinacea, but this has not been replicated in the human studies reviewed, possibly because these studies were too small and not scientifically rigorous. In a review of a number of human studies, Shah and colleagues (2007) suggest that echinacea is effective for both the prevention and the treatment of the common cold, however.

The results of these studies have fuelled the belief that echinacea stimulates the immune system. This appears to be the most likely reason that many people with cancer consider taking echinacea, perhaps feeling that echinacea is a 'safer' and more 'natural' way to invigorate their immune system and to treat their disease.

There have been some reports of sensitivity reactions in people taking echinacea (Izzo and Ernst, 2001; Newall *et al.*, 1996; Shah *et al.*, 2007).

> ## Personal and professional development 6.6
>
> As part of your role as an occupational health nurse, you are running annual health reviews. The first client today is Mick, who is 24 years old. He has asthma and is a fitness enthusiast. He swims twice a week and goes to the gym three times a week. He has what he thinks is a fungal infection on his foot. During the consultation, he tells you that he has recently bought some echinacea because he has heard that it is good for treating and preventing infections. What advice would you give him?
>
> Answers can be found at the back of the book.

HOMEOPATHY

Homeopathy is a long-used therapy that does not appear to cause any sensitivity reactions. Homeopathy is a complementary therapy, but many people believe that it is a science in its own right, despite this being hotly disputed by many mainstream scientists and the medical profession.

The word 'homeopathy' means 'similar suffering' and is derived from two Greek words *homeos* (similar) and *pathos* (suffering or tragedy). The origin of homeopathy as a science can also be traced back to the ancient Greeks: it is acknowledged that Hippocrates, the ancient Greek philosopher often considered the 'father of Western medicine', proposed what he called the 'laws of similars'. These ideas were built on by a group of people led by Hahnemann over 200 years ago to become what we know today as homeopathy. Homeopathy has two underpinning principles:

- *Like cures like*: If taken in large doses by a healthy individual, the treatment will produce similar symptoms to that produced by the disease. Kayne (2006) uses the example of the herb arnica. This is thought to have some anticoagulant properties because the drug coumarin (commonly used in traditional medicine as an anticoagulant) is found in its makeup (Newall *et al.*, 1996). This could cause a reduction in platelet aggregation, leading to bruising and bleeding. In homeopathy, arnica is used orally and as a skin cream to prevent bruising and bleeding - that is, an opposite reaction to that expected.

- *Greater dilution equals greater potency*: The more dilute the remedy, the more potent it is. Many healthcare professionals feel uncomfortable with this principle, as it seems to fly in the face of current understanding of allopathic medicines. A major belief underlying conventional medicine is that the greater the concentration of a drug, the greater will be its response. In homeopathy, the remedies are prepared using a process that dilutes the substance repeatedly until it is extremely weak – so much so that many mainstream scientists believe that there is nothing left in the mixture. This is considered dubious science by those with an allopathic philosophy. The consensus among many sceptics is that any effects that are acheived as a result of homeopathy remedies are as result of the placebo effect (**www.badscience.net**; Moerman, 2002). However, homeopaths and their followers argue that such mixtures leave some kind of 'signature', or undetectable trace in the solution, that is recognised by the cells in the body and has very few negative effects when taken internally or applied externally (Barnes, 1998; Kayne, 2006).

Although many homeopathic medicines are made from substances that are plant-based, they are very different from herbal medicines, herbal tinctures, herbal extracts and dried herbs. As in allopathic medicine, some of the substances used to prepare homeopathic medicines have an animal or mineral compound as the source material.

One of the key concerns for people choosing to use homeopathic medicines is that the individuals and companies making homeopathic remedies have little money available for research and development; consequently, few homeopathic products have a product licence.

Unless consumers buy such products from a very reliable source, it is very difficult to be sure that what is in the medicine is what the package states is in the medicine. Most pharmacists advise that because of the very dilute nature of most homeopathic products, they are safe to use in combination with allopathic medicines, with little risk of interactions or adverse effects, providing the medicine is from a reliable source.

It is possible to receive homeopathic treatment on the NHS. Many GPs will refer individuals to homeopaths if requested, and there are five homeopathic NHS hospitals in the UK, although they are often threatened with closure, particularly when NHS budgets come under increasing pressure. Following such a threat in 2007, more than 100 members of Parliament supported an Early Day Motion in the House of Commons, where they:

> ... welcomed the positive contribution made to the health of the nation by the NHS homeopathic hospitals; notes that some six million people use complementary treatments each year; believes that complementary medicine has the potential to offer clinically-effective and cost-effective solutions to common health problems faced by NHS patients, including chronic difficult to treat conditions such as musculoskeletal and other chronic pain, eczema, depression, anxiety and insomnia, allergy, chronic fatigue and irritable bowel syndrome; expresses concern that NHS cuts are threatening the future of these hospitals; and calls on the Government actively to support these valuable national assets.
> (House of Commons, 2007)

This demonstrates the importance of homeopathy to many people in the UK today.

As this chapter has highlighted, homeopathy is only one of a great number of comple-mentary and alternative therapies available to individuals today. With the use of complementary medicinal products predicted to rise even further, and some comple-mentary medicinal products now being provided by the NHS (Fellowes *et al.*, 2004), it is imperative that nurses comprehend the principles underpinning the action of these products and how these products relate to allopathic medicines. Nurses in the NHS have an increasingly important role in medicines management, and a greater understanding of all medicinal products, both allopathic and non-allopathic, can only enhance their effectiveness and increase patient understanding, safety and concordance.

Quick reminder

✔ A large variety of complementary and alternative therapies are available in the UK today, and their use is increasing.

✔ Complementary and alternative therapies are based on a different value system from that of conventional UK medicine.

✔ Few of these therapies use recognised medicines as part of their practice.

✔ The NMC has defined the products used in complementary and alternative therapies as complementary medicinal products. These include herbal medicines, homeopathic medicines, essential oils, flower essences, and vitamin and mineral supplements.

✔ The NMC recommends that nurses should 'be familiar with a range of complementary medicinal products', but it reminds nurses that they should not prescribe any of these medicines unless they have completed 'appropriate and recognised training to do so'.

✔ There are advantages and disadvantages to the use of all medicines, whether allopathic or non-allopathic.

✔ All medicines, other than perhaps homeopathic medicines, may interact with other medicines, foods, vitamin and mineral supplements, and drinks.

✔ All medicines supplied by the NHS are legally required to be licensed, but this does not apply to the majority of non-allopathic medicines. A disadvantage of this for the consumer is that the label on the medicine may give misleading claims.

REFERENCES

Ang-Lee M K, Moss J and Yuan C-S (2001) Herbal medicines and perioperative care. *Journal of the American Medical Association* **286**, 208-216.

Avorn J (2005) *Powerful Medicines: The Benefits, Risks and Cost of Prescription Drugs*. New York: Vintage Books.

Bailey D and Dresser G K (2004) Interactions between grapefruit juice and cardiovascular drugs. *American Journal of Cardiovascular Drugs* **45**, 281-297.

Barnes J (1998) Homeopathy. *Pharmaceutical Journal* **260**, 493.

Barnes J (2003) Quality, efficacy and safety of complementary medicines: fashions, facts and the future. Part 1: regulations and quality. *British Journal of Clinical Pharmacology* **55**, 226-233.

Breckenridge A (2000) *Important Interactions between St John's Wort (Hypericum perforatum) Preparations and Prescribed Medicines*. London: Medicines Control Agency.

Cassileth B R (1998) *The Alternative Medicine Handbook: The Complete Reference Guide to Alternative and Complementary Therapies*. New York: W W Norton.

Cockayne N L, Duguid M and Shenfiels G M (2004) Health professionals rarely record history of complementary and alternative medicines. *British Journal of Clinical Pharmacology* **59**, 254-258.

Committee on Safety of Medicines (2004) Statins and cytochrome P450 interactions. *Current Problems in Pharmacovigilance* **30**, 1-2.

Di Carlo G, Borello F, Ernst E and Izzo A A (2001) St John's wort: Prozac from the plant kingdom. *Trends in Pharmaceutical Sciences* **22**, 292-297.

Ernst E (1998) Lay books on complementary/alternative medicine: a risk factor for good health? *International Journal of Risk and Safety* **11**, 209-215.

Ernst E and White A (2000) The BBC survey of complementary medicines in the UK. *Complementary Therapies in Medicine* **8**, 32-38.

Fellowes D, Barnes K and Wilkinson S (2004) Aromatherapy and massage for symptom relief in patients with cancer (review). *Cochrane Database of Systematic Review* **3**, CD002287.

Fitzpatrick M (2000) *The Tyranny of Health: Doctors and the Regulation of Lifestyle*. London: Routledge.

Froemming P (1998) *The Best Guide to Alternative Medicine*. Los Angeles CA: Renaissance Books.

Fugh-Berman A and Ernst E (2001) Herb-drug interactions: review and assessment of report reliability. *British Journal of Pharmacology* **52**, 587-595.

Goldberg B (1999) *Alternative Medicine: The Definitive Guide*. Tiburon, CA: Future Medicine Publishing.

Henderson Q Y, Yue C, Bergquist B, Gerden P and Arlett P (2002) St John's wort (*Hypericum perforatum*): drug interactions and clinical outcomes. *British Journal of Clinical Pharmacology* **54**, 349-356.

House of Commons (2007) *Complementary Therapies*. Early Day Motion, 28 March 2007. **www.publications.parliament.uk/ cgi-bin/newhtml_hl?DB=semukparl&STEMMER= en&WORDS=complementari%20therapi&ALL= &ANY=&PHRASE=&CATEGORIES=&SIMPLE= complementary%20therapies&SPEAKER=&COLOUR =red&STYLE=s&ANCHOR=muscat_highlighter_ first_match&URL=/pa/cm/cmedm/70620e01.htm# muscat_highlighter_first_match**.

House of Lords Committee on Science and Technology (2000) *Complementary and Alternative Medicines*. Session 1999-2000. Sixth report.

Huang B, Bachmann K A, He X, Chen R, McAllister J S and Wang T (2002) Inappropriate prescriptions for the aging population of the United States. *Pharmacoepidemiology and Drug Safety* **11**, 127-134.

Hudson K, Brady E and Rapp D (2001) What you and your patients should know about herbal medicines. *Journal of the American Academy of Physician Assistants* **14**, 27-33.

Illich I (2001) *Limits to Medicine: Medical Nemesis - The Expropriation of Health*. London: Marion Boyars Publishers.

Izzo A A and Ernst E (2001) Interactions between herbal medicines and prescribed drugs: a systemic review. *Drugs* **61**, 2163-2175.

Kayne S (2006) *Homeopathic Pharmacy: Theory and Practice*, 2nd edn. London: Elsevier Churchill Livingstone.

Kelleher D, Gabe J and Williams G (2006) *Challenging Medicine*, 2nd edn. London: Routledge.

Kemper K J, Gardiner P, Gobble J and Woods C (2006) Expertise about herbs and dietary supplements among diverse health professionals. *BMC Complementary and Alternative Medicine* **6**, 15.

Lewith G T, Hyland M and Gray S F (2001) Attitudes to and use of complementary medicine among physicians in the United Kingdom. *Journal of Alternative and Complementary Medicine* **9**, 167-172.

Linde K and Mulrow C D (2000) St John's wort for depression. *Cochrane Database of Systematic Reviews* (2), 448.

Medicines Control Agency (2002) Safety of herbal medicinal products. **http://www.mhra.gov.uk/home/idcplg?IdcService=SS_GET_PAGE&nodeId=96**.

Medicines and Healthcare Products Regulatory Agency (MHRA) (2002) *Report on the Safety of Herbal Medicinal Products*. London: Medicines and Healthcare Products Regulatory Agency.

Milton J C and Abdulla A (2007) Prolonged oro-facial dystonia in a 58 year old female following therapy with buproprion and St John's wort (letter to the editor). *British Journal of Clinical Pharmacology* **64**, 717-718.

Miscelleneous (2005) Avoid even normal consumption of grapefruit juice if potential interaction with oral cardiovascular drugs. *Drugs and Therapy Perspectives* **21**, 9, 21-24.

Moerman D E (2002) *Meaning, Medicine and the Placebo Effect*. Cambridge: Cambridge University Press.

Moynihan R and Cassels A (2005) *Selling Sickness: How Drug Companies are Turning Us into Patients*. London: Allen & Unwin.

Murcott T (2005) *The Whole Story: Alternative Medicine on Trial?* Basingstoke: Macmillan.

Newall C, Anderson L A and Phillipson J D (1996) *Herbal Medicines: A Guide to Health Care Professionals*. London: Pharmaceutical Press.

Nursing and Midwifery Council (NMC) (2006) *Standards of Proficiency for Nurse and Midwife Prescribers*. London: Nursing and Midwifery Council.

Pert C (1999) *The Molecules of Emotion*. London: Pocket Books.

Porter R (2002) *Blood and Guts: A Short History of Medicine*. London: Allen Lane.

Rang H P, Dale M M, Ritter J M and Moore PK (2003) *Pharmacology*, 5th edn. Edinburgh: Churchill Livingstone.

Ross S, Simpson C and McLay J (2007) Author's response: homeopathy is safe and does not lack positive evidence in clinical trials/Scottish GP's use of homeopathy (letter to the editor). *British Journal of Clinical Pharmacology* **64**, 398-399.

Schmidt K and Ernst E (2004) Assessing web-sites on complementary and alternative medicine for cancer. *Annals of Oncology* **15**, 733-742.

Shah S A, Sander S, White C M, Rinaldi M and Coleman C I (2007) Evaluation of echinacea for the prevention and treatment of the common cold: an analysis. *Lancet Infectious Diseases* **7**, 473-480.

Taylor S and Field D (2007) *Sociology of Health and Health Care*, 4th edn. Oxford: Blackwell Publishing.

Tesch B J (2002) Herbs commonly used by women: an evidence-based review. *American Journal of Obstetrics and Gynaecology* **188**, S44-S55.

Williamson E M (2003) Drug interactions between herbal and prescription medicines. *Drug Safety* **26**, 1075-1092.

Zhou S, Chan E, Pan S-Q, Huang M and Lee E J D (2004) Pharmacokinetic interactions of drugs with St John's wort. *Journal of Psychopharmacology* **18**, 262-276.

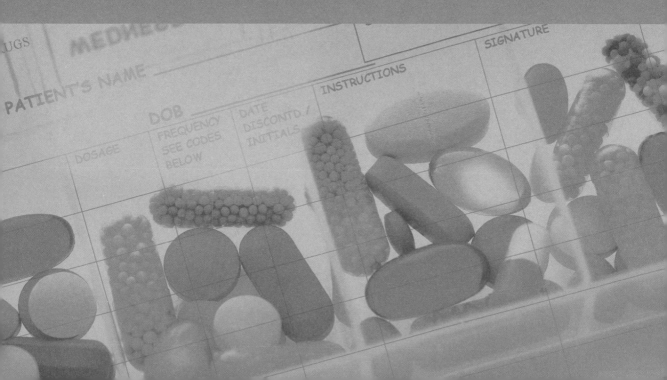

Part 3

Starting to apply the information

Chapter 7

Cancer care

According to the Department of Health (2004), more than one in three people develops **cancer** at some time in their life, and one in four people dies from cancer. We can access a range of sources to help us understand cancer. A dictionary may tell us that cancer is 'any malignant tumour' (Martin, 2004), while a nursing textbook may offer a similar definition but develop this further, to explain signs, types and treatments. Patients may describe cancer quite differently (websites such as **www.cancerhelp.org.uk** carry patients' stories); they often describe 'cancer' as an emotive word and the process of coping with the diagnosis and treatments as a 'journey', which some people cope with better than others.

This chapter provides an overview of cancer and introduces the range of treatment options available to patients with cancer. Understanding the causes of cancer, and its development, can help nurses understand the many approaches to treatment. This chapter considers current approaches to treatments, including specific treatments for specific cancers. We have included radiotherapy within this group of treatments; although not a medicine, radiotherapy is a commonly used treatment, either alone or in conjunction with other treatment. The chapter also considers the medicines prescribed in relation to the effects of the cancer, such as pain, and medicines prescribed to alleviate problems associated with cancer therapies, such as nausea.

Learning outcomes

At the end of this chapter you should be able to:

✔ Provide an overview of cancer, including types, spread and associated problems

✔ Suggest a range of treatments available for use for patients with cancer

✔ Describe the adverse effects of cancer treatments on patients

✔ Recognise the range of medications used to manage problems related to cancer and its treatments

✔ Identify the government initiatives that have influenced cancer care

✔ Demonstrate an awareness of future strategies for treating cancer.

Chapter at a glance

The nature of cancer
The cell
The development of cancer
Approaches to treatment
Specific therapies for cancer
Medicines used to treat problems associated with cancer
Professional guidance and issues
The future?
Quick reminder
References

THE NATURE OF CANCER

Essential terminology

The word 'cancer' comes from the Latin for crab. Crabs are said to behave unpredictably, and this can describe cancerous tumours, which are irregular and uncontained, behaving much differently from the normal body tissue in which they develop.

Morgan (2001) states that 'cancer is a universal disease', meaning that it can occur in any body tissue. The World Health Organization (WHO, 2006) suggests that 'cancer' is a term used to describe more than 100 diseases. Cancer may also be referred to as a 'carcinoma', 'malignant tumour' or 'neoplasm'.

Cancer cells, although originally normal cells, change and become uncontrollable. They behave differently from the original cell and destroy tissue, resulting in some loss of function of the original tissue.

THE CELL

The human body is made up of eukaryotic cells, which are responsible for different functions within the body. These cells are organised and interact. Cells that perform the same function are grouped into tissues, which are then grouped together to form organs such as the heart and the lungs. Each organ consists of different types of tissue such as nervous tissue, and muscle tissue (James *et al*., 2002).

All cells have the same basic structure. Each cell has an outer membrane that encloses protoplasm, a jelly-like substance that is made up of approximately 70% water, enzymes (manufactured by the cell), amino acids, minerals such as potassium, glucose molecules and adenosine triphosphate (ATP; a substance that the cell uses to provide energy) (Wickens, 2005).

The cell contains a nucleus, which contains genetic material, and organelles (mini-organs) such as mitochondria (the site of energy production within the cell) and ribosomes (involved in protein synthesis). Organelles have specific functions and perform the metabolic processes of the cell (Figure 7.1). Organelles have membranes that keep them separate from each other, thus assisting them to function differently. However, they are able to communicate with each other via pores in the membranes (James *et al*., 2002).

Eukaryotic cells contain genetic material, deoxyribonucleic acid (DNA), which is packaged into chromosomes that carry our genetic blueprint within the nucleus. The nucleus also contains ribonucleic acid (RNA), which transmits genetic instructions from the nucleus to the cytoplasm (Downie *et al*., 2003).

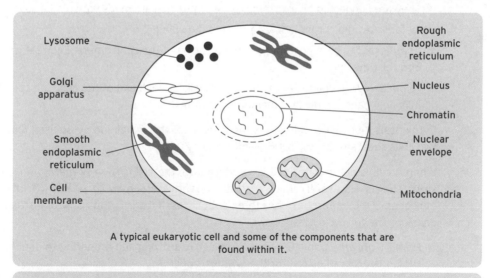

A typical eukaryotic cell and some of the components that are found within it.

Figure 7.1 **Organelles found in a typical eukaryotic cell** (after Gabriel, 2004 © John Wiley & Sons Limited. Reproduced with permission)

Related knowledge Pathophysiology

Any cell has the potential to undergo malignant changes. The transformation of a normal body cell into a cancer cell is a multistage process (WHO, 2006). The function and division of normal body cells are controlled by genes. Cancerous cells divide by the same process as normal cells, but unlike normal cells their division is uncontrolled and their numbers increase. Cancer arises from the build-up of several genetic mutations, which disrupt normal cell development and growth (Brice and Sanderson, 2006).

The cell cycle is an ordered set of events culminating in cell growth and division into two daughter cells (Marieb, 2000).

The cell cycle

The number of cells in the body is regulated by cell division and cell death. The cell renewal cycle is regulated carefully; this is a sequence of activities resulting in the formation of two daughter cells, with each new cell receiving an identical full set of chromosomes and DNA as the original cell. The new cells are exact replicas, structurally and functionally; this process is known as **differentiation**. The cell cycle begins and ends with **mitosis**, a period of cell division to replace old, dead cells.

Mitosis (nuclear cell division) has four phases (Figure 7.2):

1 *Prophase*: The chromosomes become shorter and thicker to become chromatoids. They are connected by centromeres. Microtubules are made for spindle assembly.

2 *Metaphase*: The chromosomes attach to the spindle.

3 *Anaphase*: The chromosomes are pulled apart at the centromere. Each set moves into the new cell.

4 *Telophase*: A complete set of chromosones is at each end of the cell. The spindle falls apart and the nuclear membrane reforms.

Cytokinesis, not part of mitosis, is the division of the remaining cytoplasm. Finally, the two cells separate (Blows, 2005; James *et al.*, 2002).

When a cell is not in mitosis, it is in interphase; the cell is then preparing for cell division. This is also referred to as the 'metabolic' or 'growth phase' (Gribbon and Loescher, 2000). Interphase has three subphases; mitosis is thus only one stage of cell division. The full cycle is as follows:

● *Primary growth - gap 1 (G1) phase*: The cell is growing and preparing to double its DNA. RNA is synthesised for the synthesis of DNA.

● *Synthesis (S1) phase*: The amount of DNA is doubled in order to supply the two new cells.

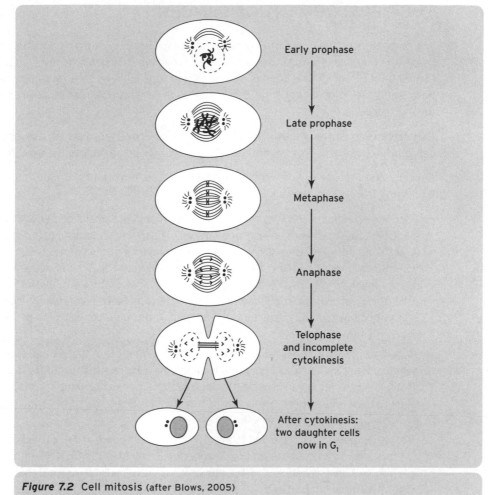

Figure 7.2 Cell mitosis (after Blows, 2005)

- *Gap 2 (G2) phase*: The cell prepares for mitosis. G2 is a short phase in which the proteins required for mitosis are synthesised.

- *Mitosis (M) phase*: The two new cells are produced.

- *Gap 0 (G0) phase*: Resting phase for stem cells.

Of the two identical daughter cells that are the result of mitosis, one cell will take on the function of the tissue from which it is developed; the other cell remains as a **stem cell**, awaiting a stimulus to reproduce and take the place of the other.

THE DEVELOPMENT OF CANCER

The genome (the basic set of chromosomes that contain genes) of all living cells is made up of double-stranded DNA. DNA is the molecule that contains the genetic code. If the genetic code of any gene is altered in any way, such as by a mutation, this can have significant consequences for gene expression, for example leading to the development of cancers.

Cancer-causing mutations usually affect genes that are responsible for cell growth or cell death (apoptosis). This provides an opportunity for uncontrolled cell growth.

Cancer genes can be divided into three main groups: oncogenes, tumour suppressor genes and DNA repair genes:

- *Oncogenes (activate cellular proliferation)*: The first cancer-causing genes to be identified, these activate cellular proliferation, which leads to unregulated cell growth and differentiation (Ponder, 2001). The majority of oncogenes result from a non-mutant version of the gene known as a proto-oncogene. Proto-oncogenes are usually involved in normal cell growth; they act as accelerators of growth by promoting cell division, regulated by appropriate signals from outside the body so that only damaged and dead cells are replaced. Proto-oncogenes become oncogenes when a mutation occurs within them.

- *Tumour suppressor genes (anti-oncogenes)*: It is thought that these gatekeeper genes prevent uncontrolled growth and cancer development: They act as the cell's *brakes* by preventing cell division. Damage to these genes opens up the potential for cancers to develop. These genes are frequently inactivated by loss-of-function mutations in cancer development.

- *DNA repair genes*: Also referred to as mismatch repair genes (MMR), these repair any mistakes that occur during DNA replication. Defects in the DNA repair mechanisms lead to genomic instability, which in turn leads to chromosomal abnormalities and mutations.

A way of understanding this is to consider the words used to describe the effects of these genes – 'accelerate' and 'brake' – and to think about these in relation to a car. If the accelerator (proto-oncogene) becomes jammed, the car will move very fast and become out of control. If the brakes (tumour suppressor genes) fail, the car may move forward and it may be impossible to stop it. We can liken DNA repair genes to the service engineer in the garage, responsible for maintaining the accelerator and brake (Prior, 2007).

'Cancer is not one disease, nor is the course of the illness the same for all patients' (DH, 2004). Some cancers are curable, but for other people the cancer is incurable even from diagnosis.

The main groups of cancer are:

- lung cancer (responsible for 1.3 million deaths per year);
- stomach cancer (responsible for about one million deaths per year);

- liver cancer (responsible for 662 000 deaths per year);

- bowel cancer (responsible for 655 000 deaths per year);

- breast cancer (responsible for 502 000 deaths per year);

- prostate cancer (responsible for 9000 deaths per year) (DH, 2004; WHO, 2006).

Cancer is believed to be caused by a number of substances (**carcinogens**), such as physical carcinogens (e.g. ultraviolet and ionising radiation), chemical carcinogens (e.g. asbestos and tobacco smoke) and biological carcinogens (e.g. viral infections) (WHO, 2006). Additional risk factors include excessive alcohol use, poor diet and family history.

Cancers can be classified as solid tumours, such as those that occur in lungs, and liquid, such as blood and lymph cancers. They can also be classified according to the tissue of origin, such as breast or lung (Downie *et al.*, 2003).

In order to decide on the most appropriate treatment, we need to know the extent of the cancer. Cancer develops in phases, depending upon the tissues affected, moving from dysplasia (abnormal development of tissue), to cancer in situ, localised invasive cancer, regional node involvement and distant **metastases** (the spread of cancer cells from the primary site to other parts of the body) (**www.who.int/entity/cancer/media**).

Most solid-tumour cancers are staged using a classification system. The TNM (tumour, node, metastases) classification system identifies the tumour size, lymph node involvement and presence of metastases (secondary growth of the cancer) (International Union Against Cancer, UICC, 1997). Using this classification system provides an indication of the prognosis for the patient (Gabriel, 2004). There are also other classification systems that can be used to classify cancers that occur within blood/lymph and bone marrow, such as the Rai classification for chronic lymphocytic leukaemia.

Nursing implications Teaching patients

Patients may have to undergo several diagnostic tests in order to confirm a diagnosis of cancer and to determine the spread of the cancer. These tests may involve:

- history-taking;

- radiology: X-rays, computed tomography (CT), magnetic resonance imaging (MRI), ultrasound, mammography;

- pathology: blood tests, monoclonal antibodies, tumour markers, biopsy, cytology;

- endoscopy.

You might wish to find out more about these tests in order to provide useful explanations to patients.

APPROACHES TO TREATMENT

The fact that 'cancer is a diverse group of assorted disorders' (Meisheid, 2005) means that there are also a diverse range of treatment approaches for cancers. Three of these approaches have been available for some time: surgery, radiotherapy and chemotherapy. These treatments can be directed against the tumour itself or used to target metastases.

> ## Personal and professional development 7.1
> ### Teaching colleagues
>
> Consider whether you could explain to a new colleague what the terms 'radiotherapy' and 'chemotherapy' mean.

Metastases are the result of the spread of the primary (original) cancer. The fact that cancerous cells spread so easily to other parts of the body means that it is difficult to assess the extent of the cancer. Where diagnosis is difficult or complicated, inevitably treatment is also difficult or complicated (Whittaker, 2004)

Essential terminology

Palliative

Palliative is derived from the Latin for 'cloak'. Palliative refers to care that is aimed at promoting comfort – that is, it 'cloaks' symptoms such as pain.

The aims of treatment are to:

- achieve a cure;
- palliate – that is, reduce the impact of the associated problems and improve quality of life;
- prolong life by increasing the likelihood of a cure or prolonging remission (Prosser *et al.*, 2000; WHO, 2006).

Surgery is the only treatment that physically removes the tumour. This is a useful approach if the cancer is localised and easy to access. Surgical removal of the tumour is often accompanied by chemotherapy and/or radiation, the goal being to eradicate any cancerous cells that might have been left behind or to target areas to which the cancer may have spread. Newer techniques allow the use of minimally invasive surgery.

Unfortunately, there is potential for the surgery to be responsible for the spreading of cancerous cells. The surgical instruments or the surgeon's hands can inadvertently transfer cancerous cells from one area of the body to another. Cancerous cells survive being detached from each other and therefore can be transferred to other sites. When a normal body cell is detached, on the other hand, the cell usually stops growing (Whittaker, 2004).

Both chemotherapy and radiotherapy may be used to shrink tumours before surgery.

Radiotherapy involves the use of radiation (high-energy rays) – X-rays or gamma rays – directed at the tumour to damage the cells' ability to reproduce. Unfortunately, radiotherapy is not selective, and so it damages both the healthy and the cancerous cells (Morgan, 2003).

Chemotherapy involves the administration of chemical agents (cytotoxic therapy) to prevent or treat disease. More recently, the term has become associated mainly with the eradication of or limiting the growth of cancers (Morgan, 2003).

Cancerous tumours are often classified according to the type of tissue in which they develop. This can be established by sending a sample of the tumour (biopsy) for laboratory analysis. Identifying the tissue of origin is important; it helps us target therapies, because different tissues respond differently to different treatments (Whittaker, 2004). The stage and grade of tumour are also taken into consideration when deciding treatment options. Treatments for cancer are often combinations of several therapies.

Radiotherapy

Radiotherapy involves the use of ionising radiation to destroy cancer cells. Radiotherapy can also be used palliatively to relieve symptoms such as pain by reducing the size of the tumour.

Radiotherapy is given in a variety of ways related to the size and stage of the cancer and the patient's condition. Radiotherapy is given by placing a radioactive material internally, close to the tumour, or by placing the material outside the body (Macmillan Cancer Support, 2004).

Factors taken into account when considering radiotherapy include:

- the type, location and stage of the cancer;
- how far the radiation needs to infiltrate;
- the known effectiveness of radiation in relation to the type of cancer;
- the patient's state of health and medical history;
- the availability and suitability of other cancer treatments.

External radiotherapy uses high-energy X-ray beams, cobalt irradiation, or particle beams such as protons and ions. External radiotherapy also damages healthy cells. Conformal radiotherapy (3DCRT) involves the use of metal blocks in the path of the radiation beam to change the shape of the beam so that it conforms closely to the shape of the tumour and therefore there is less risk of damaging healthy cells. This is useful for tumours that are close to important organs and other body structures. A course of conformal radiotherapy can last for up to 8 weeks, usually administered on week days in order to allow the weekend for recovery. The dose of radiation is given in fractions (small doses) to reduce adverse effects (Macmillan Cancer Support, 2004).

Internal radiation involves the placing of radioactive material in, or close to, the tumour, using implants, liquids, tubes, wires or seeds. Some forms, such as gold seeds, are permanent; others, such as wires, are always removed. Liquids can be delivered via a drink or injection; examples include phosphorus for blood disorders, strontium for secondary bone cancers and iodine for benign thyroid conditions and cancer.

Adverse effects of radiotherapy are related to the location and amount of tissue being eradicated, the dose of radiation and the patient's physical condition. Adverse effects include fatigue, skin reactions, alopecia, damage to the mouth, loss of voice, cough, nausea, vomiting, diarrhoea, cystitis and altered sexual function.

Chemotherapy

Cancer cells have particular characteristics. Cancer cell reproduction is not governed by the control mechanisms that influence normal cells. Growth of cancer cells varies depending upon the type of cancer; some types of lung cancer, for example, are described as 'aggressive' because of their fast development. The replicating cancer cells, unlike normal cells, do not become exact replicas and do not have a clear purpose and so this can result in some loss of function; this is referred to as 'differentiation'. As a rule, poorly differentiated cancers grow quite fast and therefore carry a poor prognosis.

Normal body cells 'respect' each other; in other words, they co-exist. Cancer cells on the other hand invade neighbouring tissues and have the capacity to develop second-ary tumours (metastases); they are spread by being carried in blood or lymph and being deposited in body cavities.

Chemotherapy is directed at controlling this abnormal cell growth to reduce the number of actively dividing cells. Most current chemotherapy targets the replication of the cancer cell; chemotherapy drugs have an antiproliferative action (Rang et al., 2003). The term 'cytotoxic' is used to describe this antiproliferative action. All cells (both normal and cancer cells) are in different stages of the cell cycle. Chemotherapy can be phase-specific (more effective during a specific phase of the cell cycle), or cycle-specific (equally effective at any stage of the cell cycle). Combinations of chemotherapy agents are often used, so that all cancer cells, even though they may be at different stages of cell division, are targeted. Chemotherapy does not destroy cells in the G0 phase (resting stem cells). Chemotherapy is also more effective when the number of cancer cells is small; this is the rationale for combining chemotherapy with other therapies, such as surgery and radiotherapy.

Chemotherapy agents are administered systemically; that is, they can target cancer cells in any part of the body, the tumour and the metastases (Morgan, 2003). However, one of the problems associated with this is that the drugs target healthy as well as cancerous cells; the result for the patient is the experience of side effects. Much cur-rent research and development in cancer treatments is therefore invested in making existing treatments targetable, so that they target cancer cells but not healthy cells.

Cytotoxic therapies (those that target cell division) can be divided into the following categories: alkylating agents, antimetabolites, cytotoxic antibiotics and vinca alkaloids (Figure 7.3).

Each type of cytoxic drug affects a separate stage of the cancer cell's development, and each type of drug kills the cell by a different mechanism of action. The action of some of the principal classes of cytoxic drugs is described below.

Alkylating agents and cytoxic antibiotics
These act within the cell's nucleus to damage the cell's genetic material, DNA. This prevents the cell from growing and dividing.

Antimetabolites
These drugs prevent the cell from metabolising (processing) nutrients and other substances that are necessary for normal activity in the cell.

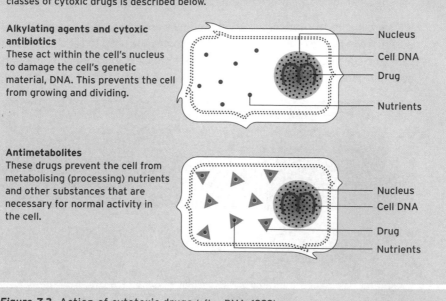

Figure 7.3 Action of cytotoxic drugs (after BMA, 1992)

Cell-cycle specific chemotherapy

Antimetabolites resemble molecules that the cell needs to complete cell division. They substitute or compete with intracellular metabolites. They are incorporated into new nuclear material (www.bnf.org) and act by preventing the cell from metabolising the nutrients essential for normal cell activity, ultimately interfering with DNA synthesis so that the cell dies. Examples include fluorouracil, methotrexate and mercaptopurine.

Phase-specific chemotherapy

Vinca alkaloids and related compounds (M phase)

These agents inhibit cell mitosis by interfering with a protein involved in nuclear spindle activity. They bind to the microtubular proteins required for formation of the spindle. Examples would include vincristine, vindesine and vinorelbine. They are used to treat leukaemias, lymphomas, breast cancer and lung cancer (Gabriel, 2004).

Alkylating agents (M phase)

This is the most widely used group. They were the first non-hormonal drugs used to treat cancer effectively (Gabriel, 2004). They act by damaging the DNA, thus interfering with cell replication. They work within the cell nucleus to damage the cell's genetic material, causing breaks in the strands of DNA; cell division is therefore faulty or prevented, resulting in cell death. This destroys both dividing and resting cells. Examples of this group are cyclophosphamide, chlorambucil and chlormethine (mustine) (Gabriel, 2004; **www.bnf.org**).

Cytotoxic antibiotics (S phase)

This group of drugs produce their effects mainly by direct action on the DNA. They act by binding to the DNA, which prevents its synthesis and reproduction. Examples include aclarubicin, doxorubicin and bleomycin (Downie *et al.*, 2003; Rang *et al.*, 2003).

We have identified that combination therapies are often used to treat cancer (Morgan, 2003). Initial letters of the drug names are commonly used to represent combinations of cytotoxic agents used in these situations, for example, CVP represents the combination of cyclophosphamide, vincristine and prednisolone in the treatment of breast cancer.

Personal and professional development 7.2
Patient education

What would you need to explain to the patient about to have their first cycle of chemotherapy?

Nursing implications

In order to protect healthcare professionals and patients when handling cytotoxic agents, NHS trusts have developed guidelines that cover

- extravasation;
- staff protection;
- handling of body fluids.

Access your local policy and make brief notes relating to these issues.

SPECIFIC THERAPIES FOR CANCER

Hormone therapy

A number of hormones, such as progestogens, oestrogens and androgens, are used in the treatment of cancers that develop in hormone-sensitive tissues and are therefore described as 'hormone-dependent'. The cancer tumour can be treated by hormones or hormone analogues that have an inhibitory effect upon the tissue in which the tumour has grown. Oestrogens such as fosfestrol can be used to block the effect of androgens in prostrate cancers, which are androgen-dependent, or used to recruit resting breast cancer cells, which are then more susceptible to other anticancer drugs (Rang *et al.*, 2003).

Another approach is the use of a hormone antagonist, such as tamoxifen. Tamoxifen is an oestrogen antagonist used in breast cancer when the tumour is oestrogen-positive. The majority of breast cancers retain oestrogen receptors, which means their growth is stimulated by the presence of oestrogen (Chapman and Goodman, 2000). Tamoxifen competes with oestrogen to bind to the oestrogen receptors in breast cancer cells. It is used in both pre- and postmenopausal women.

Hormone therapy can also be used in prostate cancer. Anti-androgens such as flutamide act by blocking androgen receptors on cells in the target tissues.

Immunotherapy

Also called biological therapy, immunotherapies exert their effects by stimulating the immune response within the patient. Modjtahedi and Clarke (2004) suggest that a fully functioning immune system can prevent the incidence of cancer. However, as cancer cells are similar to other healthy body cells, the immune system is less able to deal with tumours than with infective agents. It is suggested that tumour cells escape immune recognition and destruction. As a consequence, strategies have been developed to enhance the immune response or reduce the tumour tolerance to the immune response.

The two main immunotherapeutic strategies are monoclonal antibody based therapies and cancer vaccines.

Monoclonal antibody therapy

Monoclonal antibodies (MoAbs) are usually produced in response to antigenic (capable of stimulating antibodies) stimuli. Monoclonal antibodies are immunoglobins that have the ability to bind to tumour antigens with high specificity and selectivity. Our increasing understanding of tumour biology and the anti-tumour properties of antibodies, which inhibit growth by binding to growth factors essential for tumour development, has enabled the development of monoclonal antibodies such as trastuzamab (Herceptin®) for use in breast cancer. It is thought that monoclonal antibodies block the binding of ligands (specific signalling chemicals such as hormones, or in this case drugs that bind to cell receptors to influence cell function) to growth factors (Rang *et al.*, 2003).

Vaccines

Vaccines are used to provide antibodies to stimulate the immune system. The underlying principle is that introducing a quantity of an antigen (any substance, usually a protein, capable of producing an immune response) into the body can stimulate the immune system without causing disease.

In 2007 the UK government announced a campaign to vaccinate girls aged 12–13 years against the human papilloma virus (HPV), which is sexually transmitted and is thought to cause cervical cancer. Vaccination is due to commence in 2008 (**www.dh.gov.uk**).

Cytokine-based therapies

Cytokines are small protein hormones that stimulate or inhibit many cell functions. They include interferons and interleukins (Gabriel, 2004).

Interferon

Interferon has two key actions when used to treat malignancy:

- Interferon has an antiproliferative effect on the normal and malignant cells. The decrease in cell growth rate may be great enough to result in a cytotoxic effect.
- Interferon modulates the activity of the immune system, enhancing the host's response and thus increasing the response of the immune system.

There are three types of interferon; alfa, beta and gamma. They are complex molecules with slightly different structures, but they have very similar actions. Interferon alfa is used in anti-tumour regimes, particularly in some lymphomas and solid tumours (Downie *et al.*, 2003).

Interleukins

Interleukins enhance the immune response. The body produces many interleukins, which have different functions. Interleukin 2 (aldesleukin) is produced by genetic engineering and used in the management of metastatic renal cell carcinoma (Galbraith *et al.*, 2007). It stimulates the immune system to fight cancer by inducing cell-mediated immunity and the secretion of cytokines.

Cell-based approaches

This approach involves making the cancer cells more immunogenic such that the cells become capable of stimulating a greater immune response. There are two approaches: inserting genes into tumour cells that increase T-cell activation, and by using vaccines.

Bone marrow transplants

Chemotherapy can cause myelosuppression, a reduction in blood cell production. One therapy used to overcome this problem involves removing some bone marrow from the patient before starting chemotherapy. The bone marrow is then replaced after the treatment.

Essential terminology

Myelosuppression

Severe bone marrow suppression. Cytotoxic therapy can result in a reduction of blood cell production by the bone marrow. Erythrocytes (red blood cells), leucocytes (white blood cells) and platelets may be affected. A reduction in leucocytes can lead to infection. White blood cells, because of their rapid rate of turnover, are damaged most readily. Because of their role in response to infection, the patient is then at risk of developing infections. Anaemia can occur due to a lack of erythrocytes. Spontaneous bleeding can occur due to a deficiency of platelets (Gabriel, 2004; Prosser *et al.*, 2000).

MEDICINES USED TO TREAT PROBLEMS ASSOCIATED WITH CANCER

It is important when caring for a patient with cancer that the whole patient experience is considered. It is often certain features associated with the cancer that cause the most distress, such as the destruction of normal tissues; for example,

- obstruction; oesophageal cancer can cause difficulty in swallowing;
- pressure; a rectal tumour can put pressure on and damage a kidney.

The adverse effects of cancer treatment often cause much distress to the patient. Some body cells, such as those lining the gastrointestinal tract and hair follicles, are rapidly dividing cells and so are constantly in the process of division; therefore, they are particularly vulnerable to chemotherapy agents. Adverse effects can impact significantly on the patient's quality of life and worsen the patient's existing problems, such as pain. There are a great number of adverse effects associated with cancer and its treatment; they include the following:

- Pain
- Psychological problems, e.g. anxiety, depression and insomnia
- Bone marrow suppression, which increases the risk of infection and bleeding
- Anaemia as a consequence of the tumour invading nearby blood vessels, causing chronic blood loss
- Cough due to tumour mass, lung metastases or pleural effusion (excessive fluid between the pleura, the membranes that line the chest wall and cover the lungs)
- Mouth problems
- Damage to the gastrointestinal tract, resulting in anorexia, nausea, vomiting, constipation and diarrhoea
- Extravasation (damage to the surrounding tissues following leakage of the cytotoxic therapy from a vein)
- Hair loss
- Cachexia (chronic state of malnutrition and debility, associated with weight loss and weakness) (Downie *et al.*, 2003; Kaye, 1994).

For some of these problems, no medications are available.

**Personal and professional development 7.3
Nursing interventions**

For each of the problems identified above, can you identify some strategies to improve the situation for the patient?

Pain

Pain is an 'unpleasant subjective sensation' (Polomano *et al.*, 2008). According to Hovi and Lauri (1999), pain associated with cancer is the 'most dominant cause of suffering'. Pain has three main components: sensory, emotional and intensity (MacLellan, 2006). We use lots of terminology to describe and explain pain:

- *Categories*: Acute (sudden and short duration), chronic (lasting for more than 3 months), intractable (chronic pain without any associated disease process, and therefore difficult to treat).
- *Severity*: Mild, moderate, severe.
- *Quality*: Sharp, burning, dull.
- *Length*: Short-lasting, ongoing, intermittent.

Pain may also be superficial or deep, localised or diffuse. Several types of pain exist:

- *Nociceptive*: Transient pain that occurs in response to a harmful stimulus.
- *Somatic*: Occurs in deep structures such as the joints. May be dull and intense.
- *Visceral*: From the body organs and internal cavities. Poorly localised and often radiates to other sites.
- *Neuropathic*: Spontaneous pain in response to damage to the nervous system.

Localised pain is usually due to inflammation caused by irritation or trauma to tissue, such as tumour formation (Blows, 2005).

There are also other types of pain that are not easy to explain, such as phantom limb pain, a sensation of pain from an absent limb.

> **Essential terminology**
>
> **Referred pain**
> Pain felt in an unexpected part of the body. This occurs when sensory nerves from different parts of the body share common pathways in the spinal cord (Martin, 2004).

The processing of pain, although intricate, follows the same process as other sensory information: incoming stimuli are changed into nerve impulses and relayed along nerve fibres to the spinal cord and ultimately brain centres (Godfrey, 2005). The sensory experience of acute pain is mediated by a specialised sensory system called the nociceptive system. This system extends from the periphery through the spinal cord, brain stem and thalamus to the cerebral cortex, where the sensation is perceived. Two types of nerve transmit pain signals to the brain: A-delta fibres enable rapid transmission of pain, which is experienced as a sharp sensation (these are found within the skin and mucous membranes, the moist membranes lining some structures and cavities); C fibres transmit slow pain (these fibres are found in the skin and most other body tissues), which may be difficult to locate, for example headache. Nociception is often used as another word for pain.

The pathway for pain transmission from the periphery to the brain is a three-neuronal system (Blows, 2005):

1 The pain impulse passes from the nociceptor into the posterior part of the spinal cord via a specialised neuron, the posterior root ganglion.

2 The pain impulse is transmitted from the spinal cord to the thalamus in the brain.

3 The pain impulse is relayed to the cerebral cortex of the brain.

Dickman (2007a) describes the pain associated with cancer as 'a complex chronic pain often with multiple causes' and associated with depression, insomnia and anxiety. Addington-Hall and McCarthy (1995) take this further, suggesting that pain is the 'most common and feared' symptom of cancer. Cancer pain is an individual experience and is difficult to treat, requiring multiple approaches, such as medicines and social, spiritual and emotional support. Dickman (2007a) states that cancer pain increases in intensity with progression of the cancer.

Pain related to cancer can occur because of direct invasion of the nerves by a tumour or because of compression of neighbouring tissue by the tumour, which stimulates sensory nerves.

Pain theories are discussed in Chapter 11.

WHO analgesic ladder

The WHO (1986) have produced an 'analgesic ladder' (Figure 7.4) that identifies a three-step approach to treating mild, moderate and severe pain. The ladder recommends a 'hierarchy' of medicines to be used. This analgesic ladder can be applied to all chronic pain, but it is important to remember that the ladder provides guidelines rather than a rigid set of rules for practitioners.

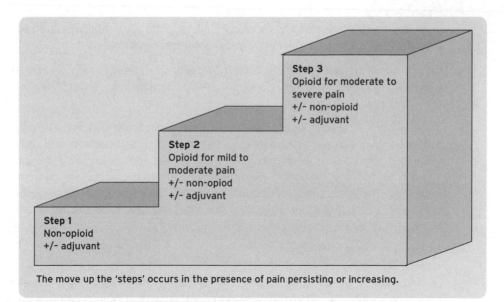

Step 3
Opioid for moderate to severe pain
+/- non-opioid
+/- adjuvant

Step 2
Opioid for mild to moderate pain
+/- non-opiod
+/- adjuvant

Step 1
Non-opioid
+/- adjuvant

The move up the 'steps' occurs in the presence of pain persisting or increasing.

Figure 7.4 The WHO analgesic ladder (WHO, 1986)

Analgesia

Analgesics are more effective in preventing than treating pain and should be given both frequently and regularly (**www.bnf.org**). Figure 7.5 explains the actions of analgesics.

Opioids

Since the development of the WHO analgesic ladder, opioids have been the most commonly used medicines for pain management (Wiffen *et al.*, 2007). Opioids feature in steps 2 and 3 of the analgesic ladder and are particularly indicated for **visceral** pain. The principal medicines in this group are morphine, diamorphine, codeine and fentanyl.

Most opioid medicines exert their effects by interacting with opioid receptors throughout the CNS. They act in a similar way to endogenous opioids (naturally occurring endorphins; a combination of the words 'endogenous' and 'morphine') at one or more of the endogenous opioid receptors that inhibit ascending pain impulses. McCaffrey and Beebe (1997) suggest that endorphins 'lock into' the narcotic receptors at nerve endings in the brain and spinal cord to block the transmission of the pain signal. When opioids bind to these receptors, morphine-like effects are produced: they reduce the excitability of nociceptors, inhibiting nociceptive transmission.

Different opioid analgesics have different effects on different types of receptors, and this helps to explain their range of actions including analgesia, sedation and bradycardia (Rang *et al.*, 2003).

There are three types of opioid receptor: mu (μ), delta (σ) and kappa (κ). The μ receptors are thought to be responsible for most of the analgesic effects and some of the unwanted effects, such as respiratory depression, euphoria, sedation and dependence. The σ receptors are thought to be more important in the periphery, contributing to analgesia. The κ receptors are thought to contribute to analgesia at the spinal level; they have relatively few side effects but may cause sedation and dysphoria (alterations in mood such as anxiety and hallucinations) (Rang *et al.*, 2003).

Morphine

Morphine remains the opioid of choice for moderate to severe pain. It is the standard to which other opioids are compared. It is usually given orally, via a suspension or tablet, to enable the patient to remain in control of their pain relief. However, if the patient is nauseated or drowsy or their condition is deteriorating, it may be necessary to choose another route, such as subcutaneous; in this case, diamorphine (heroin) is

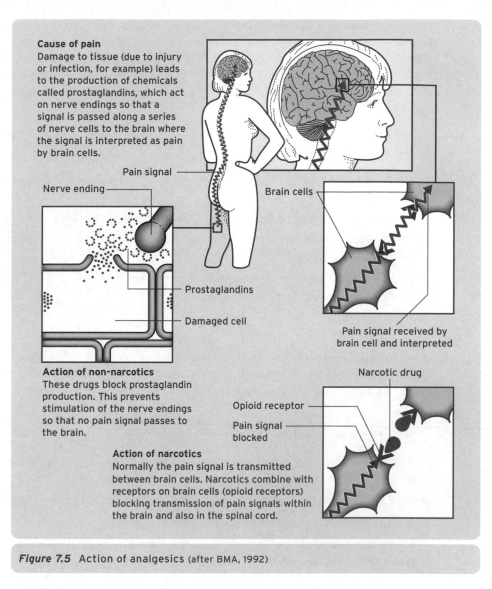

Cause of pain
Damage to tissue (due to injury or infection, for example) leads to the production of chemicals called prostaglandins, which act on nerve endings so that a signal is passed along a series of nerve cells to the brain where the signal is interpreted as pain by brain cells.

Pain signal

Nerve ending

Brain cells

Prostaglandins

Damaged cell

Pain signal received by brain cell and interpreted

Action of non-narcotics
These drugs block prostaglandin production. This prevents stimulation of the nerve endings so that no pain signal passes to the brain.

Narcotic drug

Opioid receptor

Pain signal blocked

Action of narcotics
Normally the pain signal is transmitted between brain cells. Narcotics combine with receptors on brain cells (opioid receptors) blocking transmission of pain signals within the brain and also in the spinal cord.

Figure 7.5 Action of analgesics (after BMA, 1992)

usually given instead, as an effective dose can be given in smaller volumes, which might be important if the patient is emaciated (**www.bnf.org**). Once the patient's pain is controlled and their total 24-hour dose has been established, they can be given the morphine in a modified-release preparation. If not tolerated orally, morphine can be given as a suppository.

The aim is to keep the patient pain-free and alert. Healthcare professionals are often cautious about the use of morphine, expressing concern about the patient becoming dependent (addicted) or suffering respiratory depression. In reality, there is a very small risk (less than 1%) of dependence; however, the patient receiving opioids for pain relief may develop a tolerance (require a larger dose to maintain the same effect). Downie *et al.*, (2003) suggest that 'there is no general limit' to the dose given unless there is a risk of renal impairment. A typical dose is 5–10 mg intravenously, which would provide pain relief for 3–5 hours. Morphine has the advantage of inducing a feeling of euphoria and mental detachment (**www.bnf.org**). It also causes a dry mouth, constipation, sedation and vomiting.

Pharmacokinetics Morphine

Absorption: Absorbed rapidly and completely after oral administration or by injection.

Distribution: Rapidly crosses the blood–brain barrier (see Chapter 4).

Metabolism: Metabolised in the liver to active metabolites. Half-life of active metabolites is 2–3 hours.

Elimination: Through the kidneys (80% within 24 hours)
(**www.bnf.org; www.emc.medicines.org.uk**).

Diamorphine

Diamorphine is a powerful analgesic. It is converted to morphine in the body. It crosses the blood–brain barrier more effectively than morphine, hence its popularity with drug users. It is more soluble than morphine and so can be given in smaller volumes.

Pharmacokinetics Diamorphine

Absorption: Absorbed rapidly and completely, even when taken orally, although absorption from the gastrointestinal tract may be erratic.

Distribution: Diamorphine metabolites rapidly cross the blood–brain barrier.

Metabolism: Rapidly hydrolysed (see Chapter 4).

Elimination: Up to 80% of the dose is excreted in the urine within 24 hours
(**www.emc.medicines.org.uk**).

Codeine

Codeine is a step 2 analgesic, used for mild to moderate pain. It is metabolised to morphine by the enzyme cytochrome, which results in an analgesic effect. Some medicines, such as haloperidol, an antipsychotic, interfere with the action of codeine by inhibiting the action of this enzyme. Also, some patients may lack the active enzyme, and so codeine may have limited benefit (Dickman, 2007b). Codeine is said to exert one-tenth the effect of morphine, and so it needs to be administered in doses larger than 30 mg in this context. However, despite being a weak opioid, codeine still produces some adverse effects associated with the stronger opioids, such as nausea, vomiting, sedation and constipation (Dickman, 2007b). A dose of 240 mg over 24 hours achieves the maximum benefit of codeine; higher doses will result in more adverse effects than benefits, and so another analgesic from step 3 on the ladder should be used if additional pain relief is required (Dickman, 2007b). The BNF (**www.bnf.org**) suggests that codeine should not be used for long-term use because of its potential to cause constipation.

Pharmacokinetics Codeine

Absorption: Well absorbed orally.

Distribution: Distributed widely throughout body tissues.

Metabolism: By the liver.

Elimination: Mainly by the kidneys (60–90%)
(**www.bnf.org**; **www.emc.medicines.org.uk**; Chowdhury, 2006).

Fentanyl

Transdermal fentanyl is an alternative for patients who have difficulty swallowing. It is a strong opioid delivered by patch applied every 72 hours to achieve stable plasma concentrations. The dose can vary between 25–100 micrograms per hour, increasing if the dose does not provide pain relief for 72 hours. Fentanyl has similar adverse effects to morphine, but with less constipation and drowsiness.

Pharmacokinetics Fentanyl

Absorption: After application of the first patch, there is a gradual increase in concentration, levelling after 12–24 hours and then remaining constant for 72 hours. Absorption may vary between sites of patch application.

Distribution: Plasma protein binding approximately 84%.

Metabolism: In the liver; the major metabolite is inactive.

Elimination: Concentrations decline gradually; 78% is excreted in urine, 9% in faeces as metabolites
(**www.bnf.org**; **www.emc.medicines.org.uk**).

Tramadol

Although tramadol is a step 2 analgesic, it exerts its effect in a different way from traditional opioids. It has an opioid effect and enhances serotonergic and adrenergic pathways. It has a weak opioid action, having the same analgesic qualities as codeine but with slower effect. Tramadol may be effective for pain that is usually unresponsive to opioids, such as neuropathic pain. It has adverse effects of nausea, vomiting and dizziness. It is available in a slow-release form for long-term treatment.

> ## Pharmacokinetics Tramadol
>
> *Absorption:* Absorbed rapidly and almost completely after oral administration.
>
> *Distribution:* Plasma protein binding of about 20%.
>
> *Metabolism:* Metabolised extensively after oral administration.
>
> *Elimination:* About 30% of the dose is excreted in urine as the unchanged drug; 60% is excreted as metabolites
> (www.bnf.org; www.emc.medicines.org.uk).

Other treatment options

Methadone, a synthetic opioid, may be used in palliative care, but the response to this drug can be unpredictable. Methadone is less sedating than morphine. It is well absorbed by the oral and rectal routes, but it can cause local irritation when given subcutaneously.

> ## Pharmacokinetics Methadone
>
> *Absorption:* May be dependent upon the site of intramuscular injection.
>
> *Distribution:* 60–90% bound to plasma, and tissue proteins. The distribution in the blood and brain is lower than in the kidney, lung and spleen. The drug diffuses across the placenta, can be found in saliva and sweat, and can be detected in breast milk.
>
> *Metabolism:* Metabolised extensively in the liver.
>
> *Elimination:* Excreted in the urine and bile
> (www.bnf.org; www.emc.medicines.org.uk).

Non-opioids

According to the BNF (www.bnf.org), the use of non-opioids can make the use of opioids avoidable. Examples of non-opioid medicines include paracetamol, aspirin and non-steroidal anti-inflammatory drugs (NSAIDs).

Paracetamol

Paracetamol has analgesic and antipyretic actions. It is useful for mild to moderate pain and has the advantage of being widely available. Its mode of action is not fully understood (Chowdhury, 2006), but it is thought that it inhibits prostaglandin synthesis in the central nervous system, with little effect on peripheral prostaglandin formation; as a consequence, it has a limited anti-inflammatory action. Paracetomol is also thought to act upon peripheral pain chemoreceptors (Chowdhury, 2006).

Paracetamol is relatively free of adverse effects, but when given in overdose it causes hepatitis and liver necrosis. General adverse effects include rashes and blood disorders. Paracetamol is often considered safer, particularly for older adults, than aspirin as it does not cause gastric irritation. Paracetamol can be given in divided doses up to a maximum of 4 g in 24 hours.

Pharmacokinetics Paracetamol

Absorption: Readily absorbed; reaches peak plasma concentrations within 30–60 minutes.

Distribution: Distributed rapidly.

Metabolism: Almost completely metabolised in the liver.

Elimination: Via the kidneys
(www.bnf.org; www.emc.medicines.org.uk).

Aspirin

Aspirin (acetylsalicylic acid) is indicated for mild to moderate pain. It has analgesic properties and is classified as an NSAID, but it is also an antipyretic and decreases platelet aggregation, so reducing clot formation. Aspirin interrupts the synthesis of prostaglandins from arachidonic acid by inhibiting the enzyme cyclo-oxygenase (COX). COX-1 is an isoenzyme of COX found in tissues and responsible for tissue homeostasis. COX-1 regulates platelet aggregation and exerts a protective effect on the lining of the stomach. COX-2 is another isoenzyme; its action results in the production of prostaglandins that mediate inflammation. Tissue trauma that leads to inflammation results in the release of arachidonic acid from cell membranes. Aspirin and NSAIDs such as ibuprofen are believed to reduce inflammation by inhibiting one or both of the COX enzymes (Dickman, 2007a). The gastrointestinal effects of asprin are thought to be as a consequence of inhibiting COX-1 synthesis.

Pharmacokinetics Aspirin

Absorption: Well absorbed orally, primarily in the small intestine. Food in the stomach slows absorption.

Distribution: Distributed widely throughout body tissue; highly protein-bound.

Metabolism: Converted in the liver to water-soluble conjugates.

Elimination: Via the kidneys
(www.bnf.org; www.emc.medicines.org.uk).

Non-steroidal anti-inflammatory drugs (NSAIDs)

NSAIDs do not cause dependence, depress respiration or lead to constipation and so they can be a useful alternative or adjuvant to opioids (Wiffen *et al.*, 2007). They are the most common group of prescribed analgesics (Dickman, 2007a). They act by decreasing prostaglandin production by inhibiting the production of the enzyme cyclo-oxygenase (see above). NSAIDs are considered a useful choice for pain associated with inflammation, such as arthritis and dysmenorrhoea (see also Chapter 9). NSAIDs are particularly useful for bone pain, but they may exacerbate fluid retention. The pharmacokinetics of NSAIDs are very similar to those of aspirin.

Pharmacokinetics NSAIDs

Absorption: Rapid following oral dosing.

Distribution: Distributed widely throughout body tissue; NSAIDs are weak acids that are highly protein-bound.

Metabolism: Metabolised in the liver.

Elimination: Excreted unchanged in the urine
(www.bnf.org; www.emc.medicines.org.uk).

Adjuvants

These are defined by Dickman (2007a) as medicines that 'have analgesic properties but have a primary indication other than alleviating pain'. Examples of medicines in this class include the following:

- *Amitriptyline*: A tricyclic antidepressant used in neuropathic pain.
- *Carbemazepine*: An anticonvulsant also used in neuropathic pain; interferes with neuronal activity (see Chapter 12 for more information on anticonvulsants).
- *Diazepam*: A benzodiazepine used in musculoskeletal pain.
- *Dexamethasone*: A corticosteroid useful for relieving pain by reducing inflammation.

As well as relieving pain in conjunction with analgesics, adjuvants may also encourage relaxation and induce a sense of wellbeing (Downie *et al.*, 2003).

Problems associated with treatments

The medicines used to treat cancer can cause many unwanted adverse effects for the patient. Because of the importance of the treatment, stopping the treatment to eliminate these unwanted effects is not an option. In this case, we can 'cover' the medicines used as treatments with medicines that relieve the unwanted effects; there are many examples of this in patient care. For example, morphine can cause nausea and vomiting, and so we routinely administer it with an anti-emetic (a medicine that prevents vomiting).

Nausea and vomiting

Causes of nausea and vomiting in patients with cancer fall into two main categories: related to the cancer and its effects such as anxiety, and related to the cancer treatments (adverse effects). It is important that the cause is established by careful nursing and clinical assessment so that appropriate nursing interventions can be identified. It may be possible to eliminate the cause of nausea and vomiting. If not, then a review of the patient's current medication should be undertaken, with consideration of the route of administration, in case the medication can be given in a way that is better tolerated.

Wiffen *et al.* (2007) claim that nausea and vomiting are two of 'the most feared adverse effects of chemotherapy'. They suggest that anti-emetics should be given on a regular basis to prevent the patient experiencing nausea and vomiting.

Anti-emetic therapy

A principle underpinning prescribing is to try to identify the cause in order to determine the most appropriate anti-emetic. In many situations, it is not possible to identify the cause of the nausea and vomiting, which makes the 'choice of an appropriate anti-emetic ... almost haphazard' (Thompson, 2004). With a patient experiencing nausea and vomiting, we also need to consider carefully the most appropriate route of administration.

There are several groups of anti-emetics, including the following:

- *Phenothiazines*: These are dopamine antagonists. They act centrally by blocking the chemoreceptor trigger zone thought to be involved in cancer and sickness associated with radiotherapy, chemotherapy and opioids (**www.bnf.org**).
- *Metoclopramide*: This effective anti-emetic closely resembles the phenothiazines. It aso acts directly on the gastrointestinal tract.
- *Domperidone*: This acts at the chemoreceptor trigger site. It is used to relieve the nausea and vomiting associated with cytotoxic therapy. It is less likely to cause sedation and dystonia (muscle dysfunction, e.g. spasms, contraction) than metoclopramide or the phenothiazines.
- *Dexamethasone*: This has anti-emetic effects and is used when vomiting is associated with chemotherapy.

A combination of anti-emetics is often more effective than anti-emetic monotherapy (Wiffen *et al.*, 2007). Figure 7.6 shows the actions of anti-emetics.

Personal and professional development 7.5
Nursing interventions

Although this book is primarily about pharmacological knowledge, patient problems such as nausea and vomiting can be helped by nursing as well as pharmacological interventions.

Identify some non-pharmacological strategies that you might employ to help the patient with nausea and vomiting.

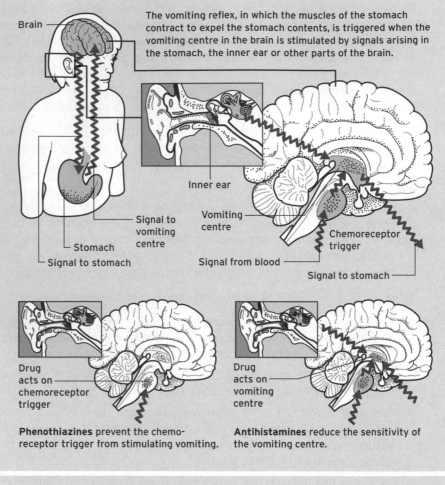

The vomiting reflex, in which the muscles of the stomach contract to expel the stomach contents, is triggered when the vomiting centre in the brain is stimulated by signals arising in the stomach, the inner ear or other parts of the brain.

Brain

Inner ear

Vomiting centre

Signal to vomiting centre

Stomach

Signal to stomach

Signal from blood

Chemoreceptor trigger

Signal to stomach

Drug acts on chemoreceptor trigger

Phenothiazines prevent the chemo-receptor trigger from stimulating vomiting.

Drug acts on vomiting centre

Antihistamines reduce the sensitivity of the vomiting centre.

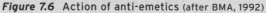

Figure 7.6 Action of anti-emetics (after BMA, 1992)

If nausea and vomiting do not respond to anti-emetics 48 hours after commencing treatment, or if vomiting persists for more than 24 hours, Coakley and Skinner (2003) suggest that anti-emetics should be given via the subcutaneous route.

Constipation

Constipation can be both 'common and debilitating' in patients with cancer, but this is often overlooked (Perdue, 2005). The most common cause of constipation in the patient with cancer is the treatment that the patient is receiving, but constipation can also occur as a result of reduced fluid intake and tiredness. Opioids delay transit through the large intestine by increasing smooth muscle tone, suppressing forward peristalsis, increasing anal sphincter tone and reducing sensitivity to rectal distension (Perdue, 2005); ultimately, the stool becomes drier and harder. Constipation may cause other problems, such as abdominal pain, anorexia, bowel obstruction, overflow diar-rhoea and urinary retention. When a medicine associated with constipation, such as morphine, is commenced, it is important that the patient is also prescribed a **laxative**. General advice for the patient should include eating more foods rich in fibre and ensur-ing an adequate intake of fluid. Most constipated patients benefit from a stool softener; alternatives include giving a bulking agent (with fluids) to stimulate peristalsis or an osmotic laxative such as lactulose.

Stool softeners

Stool (feacal) softeners such as docusate sodium allow water to penetrate faeces that have become dry and hard. They also have some stimulant activity. Co-danthrusate is a combination of docusate sodium and dantron (a stimulant laxative that directly stimu-lates colonic nerves) and is indicated for constipation linked to the use of opioids in palliative care.

Bulking agents (bulk-forming laxatives)

These add mass to faeces to stimulate peristalsis and are useful for patients who have small, hard stools. Examples include methylcellulose (available as a tablet; this is also a stool softener) and sterculia (available as granules to mix with water). This group of medicines are relatively slow-acting.

Osmotic laxatives

This group work within the colon to attract and retain fluid into the intestine by osmo-sis. Osmotic laxatives either draw fluid from the body into the bowel or retain the fluid they were administered with. Lactulose is an example of an osmotic laxative (Allen, 2007; **www.bnf.org**).

Bowel obstruction

Sometimes it is difficult to differentiate between constipation and bowel obstruction. Bowel obstruction can be a consequence of primary or metastatic bowel cancer or pelvic disease. The patient has a gradual history of worsening constipation, colic, loss of appetite, nausea, fatigue and vomiting (Rawlinson, 2001). Treatment aims are to relieve the pain, nausea and constipation. Traditionally, treatment involved insertion of a nasogastric (NG) tube and administration of intravenous fluids. However, as bowel obstruction is usually associated with advanced cancers, more recently care has become more supportive and based upon the patient's wishes, rather than the auto-matic use of the 'aggressive' NG tube and fluids (Yarbro et al., 2000). Pharmacological interventions include dexamethasone (a corticosteroid) to relieve inflammation around the tumour, diamorphine (an opioid) and hyoscine butylbromide (an antimuscarinic, which acts by reducing intestinal motility and so relieving muscle spasm) to relieve the pain, and an anti-emetic such as cyclizine (an antihistamine anti-emetic) or haloperidol (an antipsychotic medicine that also has a powerful action against nausea and vomit-ing) (Thompson, 2004).

The patient may also receive octreotide (see below) to reduce gastric secretions, but this is incompatible with diamorphine.

Diarrhoea

Chemotherapy can be destructive to the gastrointestinal mucosa, resulting in the production of intestinal secretions and vomiting. As a consequence, the patient may develop severe secretory diarrhoea (**www.bnf.org**). The treatment for this is a medicine such as octreotide. This drug inhibits growth hormone and other hormones in the gastrointestinal tract. It stimulates water and electrolyte absorption and inhibits secretion of water in the small bowel. It also has some value in reducing vomiting.

Anaemia and fatigue

According to Foubert (2006), anaemia and fatigue, although occurring frequently in patients with cancer, are not always recognised and therefore are not treated effectively, despite their potential to affect the patient's quality of life. Foubert suggests that **anaemia** and fatigue are some of the most important issues for patients, but this does not always coincide with the perception of healthcare professionals.

> **Essential terminology**
>
> **Anaemia**
> A reduction in the quantity of the oxygen-carrying pigment haemoglobin in the blood.

In common with other problems in patients with cancer, effective assessment of anaemia and fatigue is the key. The degree of anaemia can be related to the type of tumour, the stage of the cancer, the age of the patient and the type of treatment. Unfortunately, the subtle symptoms of anaemia are easily missed. Treatments for cancer can depress the bone marrow, affecting the development of red blood cells, compromising the kidneys' ability to produce erythropoietin, or damage the stem cell pool (Mughal, 2001) resulting in nutritional deficiencies. The consequence for the patient is fatigue, which can interfere with their ability to perform tasks and interact with others and cause them to focus on negative aspects of their condition, due to the overwhelming tiredness.

Treatments include transfusions of red cells (the effects of which can be temporary) and the use of medicines that copy the body's naturally occurring erythropoietin (erythropoietic protein therapy), thus improving haemoglobin levels. Patients with haemoglobin levels of 8 g/dl (normal ranges of haemoglobin are 11.5–16 g/dl for women and 13.5–18 g/dl for men) are usually transfused.

> **Nursing implications** Management of problems
>
> There are a range of other problems that patients receiving chemotherapy might experience but that are managed by nursing strategies rather than pharmacological interventions.
>
> Can you identify some supportive nursing strategies for patients with mouth problems?
>
> Answers can be found at the back of the book.

Targeted therapies

As identified earlier, the traditional chemotherapy agents used in the treatment of cancer are toxic to healthy cells as well as cancer cells, and so much research is being carried out to produce targeted therapies that target only cancer cells. These therapies work by attacking specific cell molecules or pathways, inside and outside the cancer cell. Monoclonal antibodies and cancer vaccines are examples.

Prodrugs

Prodrugs are used to target potentially toxic medication at specific body sites. Prodrugs are 'inactive precursors that metabolise to active metabolites' (Rang *et al.*, 2003). Some medicines, such as cyclophosphamide, have been identified as prodrugs only with hindsight. It is hoped that prodrugs could eliminate some of the problems with current approaches to medication by making cancer treatments more specific.

Essential terminology

Toxic
Having a poisonous effect

Concerns have been expressed about prodrug use related to the individual patient response. There may be a variation in the way that the body metabolises prodrugs and therefore increased potential for toxicity in some people.

A new cytotoxic therapy is being developed that is claimed to overcome tumour resistance and drug toxicity (Bryan, 2005). This is described as a 'hypoxic cell-activated anti-tumour therapy' that is activated within the low-oxygen conditions of cancer cells. If cancer cells are able to survive low-oxygen conditions, then they can become resistant to cytotoxic therapies and radiotherapy (Bryan, 2005).

Other therapies

Corticosteroids

Corticosteroids are a complex group of naturally occurring hormones (and therefore may be used as hormone therapy). Their key use in therapeutics is in response to inflammation and/or allergy. Corticosteroids produce a range of different effects in different tissues, for example glucocorticoids are used in conditions characterised by allergy, inflammation or are autoimmune. The other group of corticosteroids used therapeutically are mineralo-corticoids (Simonsen *et al.*, 2006).

For example, **asthma** is a condition where **bronchospasm** (narrowing of the bronchi) occurs in response to an allergen. The response to this allergen is inflammation, which narrows the airways further, and so corticosteroid medicines are a useful approach to treatment. However, in cancer, corticosteroids are often administered for other reasons. The anti-inflammatory effects of corticosteroids are complex. They are thought to be a consequence of increasing lipocortin, a substance that results in reduced production of leukotrienes (a group of regulatory lipids that mediate the immune response) and prostaglandins. Increasing the production of lipocortin results in reduced vasodilation and reduced oedema in the inflamed area (Simonsen *et al.*, 2006).

There is a suggestion that the anti-inflammatory effect of corticosteroids can help shrink a tumour by reducing any accompanying inflammation. One of the effects of treatment by corticosteroids is euphoria, enhancing the sense of wellbeing of the patient, which can also result in an increase in appetite (Whittaker, 2004).

Nursing implications Pain management

Cancer pain is described as 'a complex chronic pain with multiple causes' (Dickman, 2007a). It is likely to be accompanied by depression and anxiety. For these reasons, approaches to pain relief should involve providing information and reassurance as well as analgesia. Using a combination of analgesics and non-pharmacological approaches is thought to be the most effective approach.

Nursing knowledge Approaches to pain relief

WHO (1986) recommends that pain relief should be given 'by the clock'; in other words, pain relief should be managed by administering pain relief at regular intervals to prevent the need for the patient to experience pain.

Breakthrough pain

Cancer pain often presents as continuous pain with incidents of more serious pain. This breakthrough pain is 'an exacerbation of pain that occurs despite relatively stable and adequately controlled background pain' (Dickman, 2007a). Breakthrough pain can occur as a consequence of an action, such as coughing or having a wound dressed, or it may have no apparent cause. The rescue treatment for this type of pain should be based upon the characteristics of the pain, the existing treatment and the patient.

Personal and professional development 7.6 Nursing interventions

There are a range of approaches to pain management in cancer care. Try to identify some non-pharmacological approaches that may be used concurrently to relieve pain.

Answers can be found at the back of the book.

Routes of administration

- *Oral*: Oral medication is usually acceptable, but the route may be difficult to use as the patient's condition worsens. Other routes of administration should then be considered.
- *Transdermal*: An example is fentanyl skin patches.

- *Injection*: Pain relief can be administered by intravenous, intramuscular or subcutaneous injection, but in palliative care it is usually delivered by continuous administration using syringe drivers.

- *Subcutaneous administration*: Advantages of the subcutaneous route versus other routes are that the medicines can be administered continuously, it is less painful than other injections, it is easier to manage from the patient's perspective, and it is less intrusive than other routes of infusion. The medication is usually delivered by a syringe driver either at an hourly or daily rate. Medications given in this way are maintained at constant levels within the plasma (MacLellan, 2006). Combinations can be delivered by this method, although it is recommended that no more than three or four medicines are given together.

  Only a few cytotoxic drugs can be given in this way because of the potential damage to the tissues. It is advised that the smallest-calibre needle is used. The compatibility of medications when mixed can also be a problem, such as acidic and alkaline medications.

- *Spinal analgesia*: Intermittent or continuous local neural blockade such as local anaesthetics may be used (MacLellan, 2006).

> **Personal and professional development 7.7**
> **Nursing implications**
>
> Identify the potential problems that may occur as a consequence of subcutaneous administration.
> Answers can be found at the back of the book.

Patient-controlled analgesia

Patient-controlled analgesia (PCA) enables the patient to be actively involved in the management of their own pain. The patient receives a basal or background level of analgesia via intravenous infusion, but this can be topped up by the patient pressing a button, which delivers a preset dose of the medicine. Most systems contain a timing (lock-out) device, which controls the number of top-up doses within a period and the intervals between doses so that overdose does not occur. Medicines used via this route include morphine and fentanyl (MacLellan, 2006).

Potential gene therapies

Newer gene therapies are currently being developed to treat cancer, including the following:

- Replacement of missing or altered genes that may lead to cancer: substituting these genes could prevent cancer from developing
- Stimulating the patient's immune response
- Using 'suicide genes' to destroy the cancer.

More information about these strategies can be found at **www.cancer.gov**.

PROFESSIONAL GUIDANCE AND ISSUES

A Policy Framework for Commissioning Cancer Services (DH, 1995) (The Calman-Hine Report)

This document recommended the establishment of specialist cancer networks in England and Wales to coordinate care and the use of primary, secondary and tertiary services in order to ensure high standards and equity of care. However, because there was no additional funding to support the project's implementation, there were variations in provision – the 'postcode lottery of care'. Despite its shortcomings, the report did bring cancer to 'the forefront of the health agenda' (Bungay, 2005).

NHS Cancer Plan (DH, 2000)

The NHS Cancer Plan (DH, 2000) identified the need for 'fast, convenient, high quality care with patients at the centre' (Bosanquet and Sikora, 2003), and involving the 'best treatments' available. The DH (2004) suggests that the rationale for the NHS Cancer Plan was that many patients with cancer were not receiving appropriate treatment. Its aims were to:

- save lives through prevention, early detection and improved treatment;
- improve patients' experience of care;
- reduce inequalities;
- improve outcomes in the future.

The DH (2003) notes that one of the most important developments has been the development of specialist multidisciplinary cancer teams. Also cancer networks that coordinate care between primary, secondary and tertiary services have introduced better ways of working, including the use of new treatments. The DH (2003) notes, however, that waiting times for radiotherapy are still too long and that the 'postcode lottery' still exists.

Postcode prescribing

There is much media attention about 'postcode prescribing' – that is, the difference in prescribing patterns in different GP practices, related to the cost of the medicine. There is a suggestion that senior health ministers in Scotland are trying to introduce a national system to enable patients to have the same level of access to medicines, regardless of where they live. However, the DH (2003) notes that NICE guidelines in relation to treatments are still not being implemented fully and that there is still a 'postcode lottery of care'.

THE FUTURE?

- Innovative strategies: patient-controlled transdermal analgesia (MacLellan, 2006)
- Highly specific and individualised medicines as a consequence of gene therapy (Dickman, 2007a)
- Electronic prescribing (DH, 2004) from 2006 to identify and address underprescribing
- Case management roles for nurses (DH, 2004).

Quick reminder

✔ Cancer is a complex disease that can occur in any body tissue.

✔ The three mainstays of therapy are surgery, radiotherapy and chemotherapy.

✔ These therapies are toxic to healthy and cancer cells, and therefore they may cause associated problems, which may themselves require medication.

✔ Special precautions need to be taken when administering chemotherapy.

✔ In most situations, a variety of therapies is used.

✔ There are a number of distressing problems that occur as a consequence of cancer, e.g. pain, constipation, vomiting.

✔ WHO has produced an analgesic ladder to guide decisions regarding pain relief.

REFERENCES

Addington-Hall J and McCarthy M (1995) Dying from cancer: results of a national population-based investigation. *Palliative Medicine* **9**, 295-305.

Allen S (2007) How to deal with constipation. *Pharmaceutical Journal* **279**, 23-26.

Blows W T (2005) *The Biological Basis of Nursing: Cancer*. London: Routledge.

Bosanquet N and Sikora K (2003) Cancer care in the United Kingdom: new solutions are needed. *British Medical Journal* **327**, 1044-1046.

Brice P and Sanderson S (2006) Genetics, health and medicine. *Pharmaceutical Journal* **277**, 53-56.

British Medical Association (BMA) (1992) *British Medical Association Guide to Drugs and Medicines*. London: Dorling Kindersley.

Bryan J (2005) How new drug technologies might overcome toxicity from chemotherapy. *Pharmaceutical Journal* **274**, 397.

Bungay H (2005) Cancer and Health Policy: The Postcode Lottery of Care. *Social Policy and Administration* **39**, 1, 35-48.

Chapman D and Goodman M (2000) Breast cancer. In Yarbro C. *Cancer Nursing: Principles and Practice*. Sudbury, MA: Jones and Bartlett.

Chowdhury S (2006) An exploration into the pharmacology of analgesics. *Nurse Prescribing* **4**, 32-37.

Coakley A and Skinner J (2003) *Guidelines for the Management of Nausea and Vomiting in Palliative Care: The Liverpool and Cheshire Palliative Network Audit Group – Standards and Guidelines*, 2nd edn. Liverpool: Marie Curie Centre.

Department of Health (DH) (1995) *A Policy Framework for Commissioning Cancer Services: The Calman–Hine Report*. London: The Stationery Office.

Department of Health (DH) (2000) *NHS Cancer Plan: A Plan for Investment and Reform*. London: The Stationery Office.

Department of Health (DH) (2003) *NHS Cancer Plan: A Progress Report*. London. The Stationery Office.

Department of Health (DH) (2004) *NHS Cancer Plan and the New NHS: Providing a Patient-Centred Service*. London: The Stationery Office.

Dickman A (2007a) Pain in palliative care: a review. *Pharmaceutical Journal* **278**, 679–682.

Dickman A (2007b) Opioid analgesics in palliative care. *Pharmaceutical Journal* **278**, 745–748.

Downie G, Mackenzie J and Williams A (2003) *Pharmacology and Medicines Management for Nurses*, 3rd edn. Edinburgh: Churchill Livingstone.

Foubert J (2006) Cancer-related anaemia and fatigue: assessment and treatment. *Nursing Standard* **20**, 50–57.

Gabriel J (2004) *The Biology of Cancer*. London: Whurr Publishing.

Galbraith A, Bullock S, Manias E, Hunt B and Richards A (2007) *Fundamentals of Pharmacology: An Applied Approach for Nursing and Health Care*, 2nd edn. Harlow: Pearson Education.

Godfrey H (2005) Understanding pain. Part 1: physiology of pain. *British Journal of Nursing* **14**, 846–852.

Gribbon J and Loescher L J (2000) Biology of cancer. In Yarbo C H, Frogge M H and Goodman M (eds) *Cancer Nursing: Principles and Practice*, 5th edn. Sudbury, MA: Jones and Bartlett.

Hovi S L and Lauri S (1999) Patients' and nurses' assessments of cancer pain. *European Journal of Cancer Care* **8**, 213–219.

International Union Against Cancer (UICC) (1997) *TNM Classification of Malignant Tumours*, 5th edn. New York: John Wiley & Sons.

James J, Baker C and Swain H L (2002) *Principles of Science for Nurses*. Oxford: Blackwell Science.

Kaye P (1994) *A–Z Pocketbook of Symptom Control*. Northampton: EPL Publications.

MacLellan K (2006) *Management of Pain*. Cheltenham: Nelson Thornes.

Macmillan Cancer Support (2004) *Radiotherapy*. **www.macmillan.org.uk**.

Marieb E (2000) *Human Anatomy and Physiology*, 5th edn. Menlow Park, CA: Benjamin Cummings.

Martin E A (2004) *Oxford University of Nursing*, 5th edn. Oxford: Oxford University Press.

McCaffrey M and Beebe A (1997) *Pain: Clinical Manual for Nursing Practice*. London: Mosby.

Meisheid A M (2005) Targeted therapies in the treatment of cancer. *Journal of Continuing Education in Nursing* **36**, 193–194.

Modjtahedi H and Clarke A (2004) The immune system. In Gabriel J (ed.) *The Biology of Cancer*. London: Whurr Publishing.

Morgan (2001) Making sense of cancer. *Nursing Standard* **115**, 49–53.

Morgan G (2003) Chemotherapy and the cell cycle. *Cancer Nursing Practice* **2**, 27–30.

Mughal T (2001) Anaemia in patients with cancer: an overview. In Bokemeyer C and Ludwig H (eds) *European School of Oncology Scientific Updates*, Vol. 6. Anaemia in cancer. Amsterdam: Elsevier Science.

Perdue C (2005) Managing constipation in advanced cancer care. *Nursing Times* **101**, 36–41.

Polomano R C, Dunwoody C J, Krenzischek D A and Rathmell J P (2008) Perspective on pain management in the 21st century. *Journal of Perianaesthesia Nursing* **23** (suppl. 1), S4–S14.

Ponder B A (2001) Cancer genetics. *Nature* **411**, 336–341.

Prior D (2007) Conservation with Sandra Crouch, 25 October 2007.

Prosser S, Worster B, MacGregor J, Dewar K, Runyard P and Fegan J (2000) *Applied Pharmacology: An Introduction to Pathophysiology and Drug Management for Nurses and Healthcare Professionals*. Edinburgh: Mosby.

Rang H P, Dale, M M, Ritter J M and Moore P K (2003) *Pharmacology*, 5th edn. Edinburgh: Churchill Livingstone.

Rawlinson F (2001) Malignant bowel obstruction. *European Journal of Palliative Care* **8**, 137–140.

Simonsen, T, Aarbakke I K, Collman I and Sinnott R L (2006) *Illustrated Pharmacology for Nurses*. London: Hodder Arnold.

Thompson I (2004) The management of nausea and vomiting in palliative care. *Nursing Standard* **19**, 46–53.

Whittaker N (2004) *Disorders and Interventions*. Basingstoke: Palgrave.

Wickens A (2005) *Foundations of Biopsychology*, 2nd edn. Harlow: Pearson Education.

Wiffen P, Mitchell M, Snelling M and Stoner N (2007) *Oxford Handbook of Clinical Pharmacy*. Oxford: Oxford University Press.

World Health Organization (WHO) (1986) *Cancer Pain Relief*. Geneva: World Health Organization.

World Health Organization (WHO) (2006) *Cancer*. Fact sheet no. 297. Geneva: World Health Organization.

Yarbro C H, Frogge M H, Goodman M and Groenwald S L (2000) *Cancer Nursing: Principles and Practice*. Sudbury, MA: Jones and Bartlett Publishers.

Chapter 8

Older adults and medication

This chapter explores how the process of ageing affects the body and considers how the effects of ageing influence how medicines work. From a nursing perspective, the chapter highlights medicines management issues that arise from ageing, such as recognising and managing dysphagia (difficulty in swallowing). It also considers the concepts of polypharmacy (taking four or more medicines), self-administration of medicines, self-medication and concordance/adherence. The concept of concordance is discussed specifically in this chapter, but it is important to note that the principles apply to all age groups; we have chosen to examine the concept here as older people in general take more medication than any other group in the population.

Learning outcomes

By the end of this chapter you should be able to:

✔ Give an overview of how the ageing process can affect the actions of drugs
✔ Discuss the ways in which ageing can have an effect on the body's ability to absorb, distribute, metabolise and excrete drugs
✔ Identify the nursing implications that arise related to the prescription and administration of medicines for older people
✔ Defend the claim that empowering patients improves concordance/adherence
✔ Differentiate between self-medication and self-administration
✔ Discuss the safeguards that should be in place so that inpatients may self-administer medicines while in hospital
✔ Discuss the advantages and disadvantages of multiple prescriptions
✔ Explain how adverse drug interactions/reactions can be avoided.

Chapter at a glance

RATIONALE FOR UNDERSTANDING THE AGEING PROCESS

The ageing process has to be well understood by nurses as more and more of the patients that use health services are older people (DH, 2001b). Nursing older people is not only skilful but also frequently complex. Knowledge of the process of ageing and the consequent implications that this has when caring for an older person will influence the way in which a nurse practices: The nurse will have to consider carefully whether the ageing process is responsible for aspects of the data collected during the patient assessment and will have to analyse whether any of the proposed nursing interventions will need to be modified in recognition of the ageing process.

THE NATURE OF OLD AGE

For many people, their view regarding when old age begins alters as they age. Many people can recall that as teenagers they thought that being 25 was old. On the other hand, many people in their seventies and eighties may never refer to themselves as old but describe similarly aged members of their family and friends as old. Our perceptions of old age and ageing seem to change as we age, but those perceptions are influenced by how physically fit a person appears to be and their attitudes and outlook on life. Individuals age at different rates, and so using someone's chronological age or appearance may not be a true reflection of the age of their internal organs and cells. Nevertheless, this changing physiological process in older people (biological ageing) means that their organs and cells tend to work less efficiently than those of young people. The implication of this in relation to medicines management is that the effects of medications in older people are sometimes very different from those that one expects to see in younger people.

▲ **Personal and professional development 8.1**

Take a few moments to explore your attitudes to age and ageing. How do the feelings you identified make you feel towards both older people as a group and older people as patients? Perhaps this might be an area that you would like to explore further using your professional portfolio.

How ageing affects the body

Ageing affects the body by bringing about changes in both the body's composition and the way in which its organs work. These changes may affect how older people respond to their medication. Understanding these bodily changes and how they affect the way in which medicines work is becoming increasingly important for nurses in the developed world. More people in the developed world are living longer, and often with chronic diseases (DH, 2001b). Consequently, the majority of the people using health services in the UK are older people (DH, 2001b). It must be borne in mind that although this chapter considers the effects of medication on older people, the term 'older people' is very much one created by society, and it implies some kind of generality. Indeed, the term suggests some kind of sameness among the people to which it refers, but sameness is far from the reality. Just as teenagers are not a homogeneous group, so 'older people' comprise a group in which individuals range in age from 50 years to over 100 years: a span of at least 45 years. No other group of people includes such a wide time span.

Such a grouping can be useful, but it has its disadvantages too. From the perspective of medicines management, these disadvantages centre on the fact that the concern is not chronological age but rather the effects of the ageing process at the cellular level. It must also be remembered that, as in any age group, there is a considerable difference in individuals: some people age 'better' than others – some individuals are athletes well into their nineties while others are infirm in their sixties. In relation to medicines management, the importance is placed not on the person's appearance but on how their cells and organs change with age and the impact these changes may have on the medications that they take. Unfortunately, as people get older, any deterioration in the way that their organs function physiologically may not be immediately obvious. Alongside this is the increasing prevalence of chronic diseases in the older age group (DH, 2001b); the older the individual, the more likely they are to have ill-health or disability. This means that older people may well have tissues and organs that are not only affected by the ageing process but also are affected by disease; as a result, their organs may function inadequately, and therefore they are more likely to also have had organs or parts of organs surgically removed.

These issues are clearly recognised by the National Service Framework for Older People (DH, 2001b). In order to highlight the group of people who have the most morbidity and mortality, this report classifies older people into three main groups:

- Entering old age – these are the people who have finished paid employment and/ or bringing up children and are active and independent frequently into late old age.

- Transitional phase – this phase recognises that this group of people is in the process of moving from being active and independent to having health problems and the frailty that this can bring. This frequently seems to happen in the person's seventies or eighties but can happen earlier or later than this.

- Frail older people – these are older people who have developed problems with their health. They have increasing poor health as they go into late old age (DH, 2001b).

Although the latter group, frail older people, comprises the minority of older people, these are the majority users of the NHS. Every time a frail older person has an episode of ill-health, they become less able to recover fully from the strain that the illness places on the body. Frequently, situations that in a young person might be considered minor insults to the body, such as a fall, set off a train of events in the frail older person. This chain reaction results in a slow, steady decline, with the person becoming more and more disabled before dying from the complications of old age. There are a number of studies and a white paper (DH, 2005; Ershler, 2007; Hart *et al.*, 2002; Xue *et al.*, 2008) that demonstrate a clear link between frailty and the risk of falling, disability, iatrogenic disease and being admitted to hospital.

Despite the media's obsession with the drive to remain eternally young, none of us can escape the fact that ageing is an inevitable result of living. The process of ageing affects all body cells but, although they all degenerate, not all cells age in the same way or at the same time. Indeed, cells seem to age in very different ways (Kirkwood, 1999). Walsh (1997) states that the criteria of ageing are:

- Universal, in that it occurs in all members of the population (unlike disease).

- Progressive, it is therefore a continuous process.

- Intrinsic to the organism.

- Degenerative (as opposed to developmental or 'maturational' changes).

Aspects of physiological ageing relevant to medicines management

As we age, our physiological processes begin to wane, with the result that the body finds it increasingly difficult to maintain homeostasis. One of the consequences of this is a need for greater care when prescribing and administering medicines, because the gap between the wanted and unwanted effects of medication becomes smaller and smaller (Greenstein and Gould, 2004; McGavock 2005; Simonsen *et al.*, 2006).

The effects of ageing bring about a number of physiological changes. Some of these differences affect the body's composition; with age, there is less lean body mass (muscle), less total body water (reduces from 60% of total body weight in a young adult to 40% in an older adult), and an increase in the total fat content of the body.

There are also accompanying changes in the way that organs work, such as reduced glomerular filtration in the kidneys, less efficient liver metabolism and less efficient cardiac output.

The effects on the musculoskeletal system include the loss of calcium from bones, which can lead to osteoporosis and kyphosis (curvature of the upper spine). These latter effects are more common in women than in men and are thought to be linked to the loss of oestrogen that women experience as they age (Mera, 1997). Collagen loss means that the joints, ligaments and tendons become stiffer and less flexible. The erosion of cartilage in the joints results in joint flexion becoming painful.

Changes in the integumentary system (skin, nails and hair) affect the epidermal cells. These are replaced less frequently: approximately every 30 days in an older adult compared with every 20 days in a young adult. There is also a loss of subcutaneous fat.

Any or all of these changes can influence how an older person responds to their medicines. Older people tend to respond differently to most medications compared with younger people (McGavock, 2005; Rang *et al.*, 2003) as the process of ageing may affect the way in which drugs act. This is a result of changes in the body's physiology that affect the way the body takes up drugs and the way that drugs are removed from the body.

HOW THE AGEING PROCESS CAN INFLUENCE PHARMACOKINETICS

Absorption

- Dysphagia (difficulty in swallowing): Deterioration in the ability of the salivary glands to produce saliva, along with changes in the effectiveness of the oesophageal sphincters, makes swallowing more difficult for many people in late old age.

Personal and professional development 8.2

List three forms of medication that could be considered for a patient who is unable to swallow tablets or capsules.

Related knowledge Nursing interventions

Ensuring that the patient's mouth is moist before tablets or capsules are put into the mouth will help the swallowing process. If the individual is able to take fluids, the nurse should encourage them to have a drink or take a few sips of fluid

▷

▶ *(continued)*

before taking their medication. This moistens the upper gastrointestinal tract in preparation for swallowing the tablets or capsules. Other helpful actions that should be considered, particularly if the patient has xerostomia (dry mouth) as a side effect of a medicine (e.g. trycyclic antidepressants), are taking regular sips of cool fluid and/or mouthwashes and sucking on ice chips; if needed, an artificial saliva spray can be prescribed. If these are not successful, then consideration should be given to changing the prescription to another form of medication. Many medications are in liquid form, but gels, patches and inhalers can also be considered.

● The loss of lean body mass (muscle) and reduced blood flow to the muscles may mean that medicines given by the **intramuscular (IM)** route are absorbed unevenly.

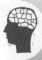

Related knowledge Nursing interventions

When administering medication to an older person by the intramuscular route, close observation of the patient's response to the medicine is needed in order to know whether there is sufficient absorption.

● Consideration should be used when prescribing and administering topically applied medicines, as the changes that occur to the integumentary system (skin, nails, hair) may reduce absorption. The invisible changes that the internal body cells undergo are not obvious to the naked eye. However, the changes in the integumentary system are frequently visible, both to the patient and to others. Although the decreased thickness of the **dermis** that results from the ageing process may enhance absorption, the skin is less well hydrated and so absorption may be reduced.

Essential terminology

Intramuscular
Into the muscle; usually refers to an injection given by this route.

Dermis
The layer of skin that lies underneath the epidermis. The blood and lymph vessels along with sweat glands and nerve endings are all contained within this layer.

Topical
Describes medicines that are applied to the skin or mucous membranes.

Related knowledge Nursing interventions

Topical medicines are used mostly for local conditions. When they are used for their systemic effects, the patient's response to topically applied medicines and transdermal medicines should be observed closely, as the response may be unpredictable.

- The cells that secrete hydrochloric acid in the stomach reduce in number, and therefore the amount of hydrochloric acid produced by the stomach is reduced. The pH of the gastric juice rises, resulting in a less acid environment. The drugs that need an acid environment to be absorbed successfully (e.g. aspirin) are thus not absorbed as effectively.

- The stomach takes longer to empty and so oral medication stays in the stomach for longer. As a result, it takes longer for medication to reach the small intestine, where most absorption takes place.

- Reduced peristalsis in the small intestine means that the contents move along the gut more slowly. This slower transit time increases the time that the drug is in the gut.

- There is reduced surface area in the small intestine; therefore, there are fewer blood vessels available to allow passive diffusion of drugs from the gut into the bloodstream, and so there is less absorption (Swonger and Burbank, 1995).

In reality

The factors described above in themselves may not be problematic, and therefore on their own probably do not interfere with the efficacy of the medication. However, if the older person also has diarrhoea or malabsorption, doses of any prescribed medication may need to be increased (Greenstein and Gould, 2004; Rang *et al.*, 2003).

Distribution

- The production of plasma proteins declines with age. As a result, if the patient is taking a drug that would normally bind with a plasma protein, then more of the drug will be available for use by the body. (Only the drug dissolved in the plasma - unbound portion of a drug - is available for use.) If there are fewer plasma proteins in the serum, lesser amounts of drug will bind, leaving a greater concentration of free drug in the plasma. As a result, the binding of the drug to the plasma proteins can decrease by as much as 15-25%. This means that there could be increased levels of medication in the bloodstream, for example diazepam (an anxiolytic) or warfarin, leading to toxicity (Greenstein and Gould, 2004; Rang *et al.*, 2003; Simonsen *et al.*, 2006).

In reality

The reduction in plasma proteins is only likely to be a problem with drugs that are 90% protein-bound, such as warfarin (a commonly prescribed anticoagulant that prevents blood clotting easily) (Rang *et al.*, 2003).

- Total body fat increases: As the muscle fibres reduce in number, they are replaced by fat; even in thin older people, the proportion of fat to muscle increases (Mera, 1997; Tortora and Derrickson 2006). For fat-soluble drugs, there are then a larger number of fat cells where the drug can be stored, and so a greater amount of the drug is stored in the body. This leads to an increased duration of action and an increased half-life of the drug. Commonly prescribed fat-soluble drugs include benzodiazepines such as flurazepam and temazepam, barbiturates, thiazides, phenytoin and the fat-soluble hypnotics (Greenstein and Gould, 2004; Rang *et al.*, 2003).

- There is also a potential for adverse effects to occur. Many people present with vague symptoms that are frequently disregarded, by both patients and healthcare professionals, such as shakiness, unsteadiness, falling, constipation and confusion.

- The reduction in total body water seen in older people means that there is reduced circulating fluid, and so any medication is in a higher concentration in the bloodstream. As a result, the effects of the drug are potentially more toxic.

Personal and professional development 8.3

Consider what happens when you add one spoonful of sugar to a mug of coffee compared with adding the same amount of sugar to an espresso coffee. Write short notes that you could use to explain to a patient why there will be a higher concentration of drug in the bloodstream of an older adult compared with a younger adult.

Metabolism

The size of the liver decreases with age, although the rate at which this happens varies both within the same individual and between individuals. From the medicines management perspective, the results of this are two-fold. Not only will the liver have less blood circulating through it but it will also have fewer cells to produce the enzymes needed for metabolism and excretion. This affects both the liver's ability and the speed at which it can metabolise (break down) drugs. This means that detoxification of drugs happens more slowly in older people. The result of this is that there is more drug available in the circulation and more opportunity for the drug to be stored in the fat, as happens with tricyclic antidepressants and warfarin. A consequence of this is an increase in the risk of toxicity.

Excretion

As the body ages, the glomerular filtration rate decreases and kidney function becomes less efficient (Mera, 1997). McGavock (2005) explains that this is a result of the nephron numbers falling by 6% a year. Most drugs are eliminated from the body by the kidneys (Greenstein and Gould, 2004; Rang *et al.*, 2003; Simonsen *et al.*, 2006); if less of the drug is excreted via the kidneys, then there is a potential for drugs that are normally excreted in this way to build up in the circulation. This may mean that blood levels rise quickly to be toxic. A glomerular filtration rate of only 60-70% of normal causes accumulation of drugs and their toxic metabolites. Some common examples of drugs to consider in this situation are digoxin, atenolol and cimetidine; these all have a narrow **therapeutic range** and therefore a high toxic potential.

Nursing implications

It is important to ensure that older people have adequate renal function. Fluid balance monitoring may be required. It is also important that nurses make close observation of patients, looking for early signs of toxicity; a routine example of this is the monitoring and recording of a patient's pulse before administering digoxin. Earlier signs and symptoms in older people include anorexia, nausea, vomiting, diarrhoea, abdominal pain, visual disturbances, headache, fatigue, drowsiness, confusion, hallucinations, arrhythmias and heart block.

Drug receptor sensitivity

It is thought that both the number and the efficiency of cell receptors decrease as the body ages. The consequence of this is that some older people become either more sensitive or less sensitive to some drugs (McGavock 2005; Rang *et al.*, 2003). This increase or decrease in responsiveness to some drugs is especially important in the central nervous system, and so prescribers need to bear this in mind before prescribing medicines that act on the brain to older people (Cowan *et al.*, 2002; Livingston, 2003). A number of drug groups show a markedly increased effect on the brain when given to older people; this effect is seen most commonly with opioid analgesics, benzodiazepines, antipsychotics and antiparkinsonian drugs (Livingston, 2003).

Nursing implications

When administering opioid analgesics, benzodiazepines, antipsychotics and antiparkinsonian drugs to the older person, careful observation should be made for any evidence of increased or decreased response to the medicines. For example, increased drowsiness, disorientation or confusion may be seen the following morning after administering benzodiazepines and hypnotics.

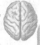

Pharmacological knowledge

A number of studies (Beers, 1997; Fick *et al.*, 2003; Gallagher *et al.*, 2007) have identified a range of medicines that are prescribed commonly for older adults. Given our understanding of how the ageing process affects the body's physiology, and the impact that this can have on pharmacokinetics, it is also possible to identify a range of medicines that should be prescribed only with caution and after careful thought for the older person (**www.bnf.org.uk**; Beers, 1997; Fick *et al.*, 2003; Gallagher *et al.*, 2007). These include diuretics, hypnotics and NSAIDs (non-steroidal anti-inflammatory drugs). Using the example of diuretics, it is possible to highlight the adverse reactions that can ensue.

A patient taking diuretics may lose too much sodium in the urine, leading to hyponatraemia (low blood sodium levels). This can lead to postural hypotension (low blood pressure on standing), which can cause the person to faint when they stand up. The resulting falls may lead to bony fractures in older people, especially older women. Loop diuretics such as furosemide are described in the BNF as 'powerful' and can cause hypokalaemia (low blood potassium). Hypokalaemia can cause cardiac arrhythmias, and so supplements of potassium may be given with furosemide. In men, hypokalaemia may cause urinary retention if the prostate gland is enlarged. The BNF suggests that this can be prevented by using small doses and beginning treatment with less potent diuretics.

POLYPHARMACY

It is well recognised (Audit Commission, 2001; DH, 2001b) that although chronic illness occurs across all age groups, it is much commoner in old age. Because more people are living into old age than ever before, and many chronic diseases such as cancer can be a consequence of ageing, many older people live with some form of chronic disease. In order to manage chronic disease, many people take more than one medication.

Williams' (2002) review of the studies undertaken suggests that of all the Americans prescribed medication, most take an average of three to five different medicines. Although this review highlights what is thought to occur in the USA, and supports the DH's (2001b) assertion about the number of prescribed medicines it is thought that people take in the UK, there is little robust evidence to say how many prescribed medicines people actually take.

Consider a patient with coronary heart disease. If the patient is treated according to the NSF Coronary Heart Disease (DH, 2000) guidelines it is likely that they will be prescribed at least the following medicines:

- Aspirin
- Beta-blocker
- ACE inhibitor
- Statin.

Many older people also have more than one chronic disease, and so the likelihood that they take more than one prescription medication is even higher. Take the fairly common example of a patient with type 2 diabetes mellitus who also has primary hypertension and coronary heart disease. Along with the medicines identified in the list above, this patient may also take lisinopril for hypertension and rosiglitazone to manage the diabetes.

It is easy to see why people with long-term conditions may be prescribed large numbers of medicines. Taking more than one medicine is known as polypharmacy. Until recently, there was little consensus about how many medicines a person had to take concomitantly in order for their regime to be described as polypharmacy. Polypharmacy was simply described as the use of several prescribed medicines by an individual (Larsen and Martin, 1999; LeSage, 1991; Shepherd, 1998). Although there is no widely accepted definition, in the UK the DH (2001a) states that when four or more medicines are prescribed for an individual, then this is to be considered as polypharmacy. It is also evident from the literature that when the term 'polypharmacy' is used, the medicines under consideration are only those that are prescribed, and little consideration is given to either OTCs or herbal medicines that the patient may also be taking.

Taking four or more prescribed medicines at the same time is common among older people. The DH (2001a) acknowledges:

> As people get older, their use of medicines tends to increase. Four in five people over 75 take at least one prescribed medicine, with 36% taking four or more medicines. Alongside this come increasing challenges to ensure that medicines are prescribed and used effectively, taking into consideration how the ageing process affects the body's capacity to handle medicines. Multiple diseases and complicated medication regimes may affect patients' capacity and ability to manage their own medication regime.

Stewart and Hale (1992) referred to polypharmacy as 'an uncontrolled experiment'. They explained that a scientist in a laboratory would never combine eight to ten chemicals in a test tube without preparing for the consequences. Therefore, it would be reasonable to suspect that in the situation where an older person is taking eight to ten medicines concurrently, then the result would be impossible to predict. This is partly because the use of multiple medications predisposes the patient to adverse drug reactions. For example, one medicine can affect the absorption of another, such as iron supplements.

In reality

Often, all that is required is to 'stagger' the timings of the doses, for example by leaving 2–4 hours between the medicines (Livingston, 2003).

Although the risks increase as a patient takes more medicines, polypharmacy in itself is not necessarily a bad thing. Many people have two or more long-term conditions and therefore need to take one or more medications to deal with each of their conditions. What is to be criticised is inappropriate prescribing, but why this happens is often difficult to pinpoint and, like many aspects of healthcare, it is complex and multifactorial. Reasons for polypharmacy include the following:

- *Multiple pathology*: 50% of individuals over age 65 years have more than one chronic condition; 85% have one chronic condition (Swonger and Burbank 1995).
- *Multiple prescribers*: When the patient has more than one long-term condition, they may see several doctors or specialist nurses, each of whom may prescribe medication. Because of the nature of medical specialisms, the patient is rarely seen by a team of healthcare professionals who considers the patient as a whole. For example, an individual with concurrent long-term conditions may be prescribed medicines by a cardiologist, a renal physician, an endocrinologist and a vascular surgeon. Now that polypharmacy has become recognised, perhaps this will change in the future.
- *Self-medication*: Many patients take OTC, herbal and homeopathic medicines in addition to their prescribed medicines.
- *Misuse*: After discharge from hospital, patients may continue taking their previous regime as well as the new regime that they have been prescribed. Some people share medicines with others.
- *Expectations*: Many people expect to leave a consultation with their GP with a prescription. At least 75% of all patient–GP encounters result in the patient receiving a prescription (Britten, 1994; Cutts and Tett, 2005; LeSage, 1991; MacFarlane *et al.*, 1997).

Personal and professional development 8.4

In order to demonstrate how common self-medication actually is, try using the questionnaire below with members of your family, friends and colleagues. First ask yourself the following questions, and then ask members of your family, friends and work colleagues the same questions. It is important to:

- take note of the numbers of people who self-medicate and of those who do not;
- note the types of medicines that people take most commonly.

Remember: you must explain carefully to people the purpose of this exercise and must gain their consent to gather the information. DO NOT keep any information about people without their consent. Any details that you do collect must be temporary and anonymised.

1. Do you take drugs/tablets/medicines prescribed by a doctor?
2. Do you take drugs/tablets/medicines recommended by friends?
3. Do you take drugs/tablets/medicines bought at a chemist?
4. Do you take drugs/tablets/medicines bought at a supermarket?
5. Do you take drugs/tablets/medicines bought at a health food shop?
6. If you answered yes to any of the above questions, name the drugs/tablets/medicines that you take:

7. Do you take the drugs/tablets/medicines for:
   - Constipation
   - Headache
   - Pain
   - Other (please note what for)
8. How frequently do you take these drugs/tablets/medicines?
9. Do you take any herbal or alternative/complementary medicines?
10. If you answered yes to the previous question, please identify what you take and why.

11. Do you know whether these drugs/tablets/medicines have any unwanted effects?
12. If yes, give a brief explanation.

13. Do you take caffeine/alcohol/nicotine regularly?
14. Do you consider caffeine, alcohol or nicotine to be drugs?

If you have used the self-medication questionnaire, is there any indication that people considered caffeine, alcohol or nicotine to be drugs?

If you have used the self-medication questionnaire on a number of people, you may have been able to identify how common self-medication seems to be. Many people take conventional OTC medicines, and doctors and nurses frequently enquire about the use of such medicines. There are no reliable figures that identify how many people take herbal medicines, but a number of studies suggest that in the UK between 12% and 44% of people report taking herbal medicines (Constable *et al.*, 2006; Harrison *et al.*, 2004; Holden *et al.*, 2005). However, few doctors and nurses routinely ask patients about their habits in relation to herbal and complementary self-medication (Cockayne *et al.*, 2004; Constable *et al.*, 2006; Harrison *et al.*, 2004; Holden *et al.*, 2005). Constable *et al.* (2006) find this disturbing and suggest that gathering such information is becoming more and more important, given both the rise in the popularity of herbal medicines and the growing evidence that these preparations can have harmful effects in the same way that prescription medicines can.

Many people do not think of caffeine, alcohol or nicotine as drugs, as they are often seen as socially acceptable. However, these *are* powerful drugs and alcohol is exceptionally toxic to the liver. It is important that nurses bear this in mind when exploring patients' medication (Cockayne *et al.*, 2004; Harrison *et al.*, 2004; Holden *et al.*, 2005). It also seems that many healthcare professionals fail to recognise that many older people have problems with alcohol or other social drugs.

In order to establish how common polypharmacy is, patients over 60 years of age who were taking five medicines or more were invited to take part in a study. As a result of the methods used in the study, it became known as a 'Brown Bag Review' (Nathan *et al.*, 1999). (The term 'Brown Bag Review' describes one of the methods used by pharmacists to collect information from patients about their current medication. The review is carried out in order to improve concordance and reduce adverse drug effects. The methodology originated in the USA: patients were given brown paper bags, and asked to put all their medicines into these bags and bring their filled bags to the pharmacy. A pharmacist would then carry out a medication review with the patient.) Some of the surprising results are presented here:

- From one patient they collected medicines worth £1000.
- Over half of the patients had outdated medicines or medicines that were in excess of their needs.
- When tidying up, one patient emptied the tablets from one medicine bottle into another so the contents of the two medicine bottles were mixed together. This meant that he was taking antihypertensive medicine three times daily instead of once daily.
- One patient was muddling up diuretic tablets with tablets that had been prescribed for dizziness (DOH, 2001a; Yang *et al.*, 2001).

In order to prevent problems like these arising in the future, Denneboom *et al.* (2006) recommend that a medication review should be carried out with the patient both regularly and routinely. This is now also considered to be good practice, as it is one of the quality standards looked for in the Quality Outcomes Framework assessment, which, since 2004, measures and rewards general practitioners in the UK (NHS Information Centre, 2007). However, whether the patient is also self-medicating with OTC, herbal or homeopathic medicines is still frequently not considered in such reviews.

The use of over-the-counter medicines to treat unrecognised side effects of prescription medicines

As we discussed earlier in this chapter, age-related changes in the body's physiology affect the pharmacokinetic process and consequently lead to altered pharmacodynamics in the older person. Because older people respond differently from younger people to many medications, many older people have side effects as a result of their prescribed medications. Unfortunately, many people do not appreciate that these side effects are due to their prescribed medications and try to compensate for the side effects by taking OTC medications. Poole *et al.* (1999) say that, according to the evidence in their study, many older people who are taking antidepressants also take OTC laxatives, probably because constipation is a common side effect of antidepressants, while those taking corticosteroids often also take OTC antacids, probably because dyspepsia is a frequent side effect of corticosteroids.

> ### Essential terminology
>
> **Dyspepsia**
> Sometimes known as heartburn or acid reflux, this is a burning, boring discomfort in the upper abdomen as a result of irritation of the oesophagus. Also known as gastro-oesophageal reflux disease (GORD).

The use of multiple medications predisposes to adverse drug reactions. Swonger and Burbank (1995) estimated that the potential for an adverse drug reaction is:

- 6% when taking two different drugs;
- 50% when taking five different drugs;
- 100% when taking eight or more different drugs.

Drug–drug interactions

Drug-drug interactions are thought to be common; however, many are considered harmless, and the few that are harmful affect only a minority of people (McGavock, 2005). McGavock (2005) suggests that '12% of all acute hospital admissions of elderly patients and 18% of elderly deaths are the direct result of prescribed medicines'. He cites drug-drug interactions as 'one of the commonest causes of these admissions' and suggests that these interactions are frequently not reported when they occur. Interactions can occur between medicines and between medicines and food or drink. Many of these interactions in elderly people can be explained by the effects of the ageing process on the pharmacokinetics of the drug and the resulting altered pharmacodynamics. The effects of drug-drug interactions can be exacerbated by malnutrition and the effects of nicotine and alcohol (Greenstein and Gould, 2004; McGavock, 2005; Simonsen *et al.*, 2006).

It is thought that the risk of having a drug-drug interaction increases exponentially the more drugs the patient takes. For example, with two drugs, there are only two possible interactions; with five drugs, there are 20 possible interactions; and with 10 drugs there are 90 possible interactions (Astrand *et al.*, 2007; Johnell and Klarin, 2007; Kohler *et al.*, 2000; Swonger and Burbank, 1995).

Pharmacological knowledge Drug–drug interactions

One of the most commonly prescribed medications for older patients is digoxin. Adverse reactions between digoxin and other medicines occur fairly frequently. Some of the medicines that are known to cause adverse reactions when taken together with digoxin are:

- *Amiodarone*: This is an anti-arrhythmic (stabilises the heart's rhythm). It increases the plasma concentration of digoxin, so slowing down the heart rate too much. The digoxin dose must be reduced in order to compensate.

- *Antacids*: These are given for dyspepsia. They are thought to reduce the absorption of digoxin, so making it less ineffective.

- *Kaolin*: This is used to treat diarrhoea. It probably reduces the absorption of digoxin.

- *Spironolactone*: This is a potassium-sparing diuretic. It enhances the effect of digoxin.

CONCORDANCE

The words 'concordance', 'adherence' and 'compliance' are used by healthcare profession-als to describe whether patients follow the recommendations that are made to them by healthcare professionals about their care and treatment. The term 'concordance' will be used throughout this book. Another term is beginning to creep into healthcare literature in relation to concordance – therapeutic alliance'; this describes the process that should be engaged in to ensure concordance. These terms are used in relation to taking medicine but also in relation to other treatment, therapies and health promotion generally. Here, we discuss concordance in relation to the nurse's role in medicines management.

Haynes *et al.* (1979) describe compliance as 'the extent to which a person's conduct, in terms of keeping appointments, taking medications and carrying out lifestyle ges, matches with the advice given by healthcare professionals'. This definition s to be well accepted and, although it previously defined compliance, it now to be used to define concordance and adherence. It would seem from the liter- that although it is recommended that the terms 'concordance' or 'adherence', e 'compliance' the words are frequently used to express the same concept: e professional knows what is best for the patient, despite knowing very little

STARTING TO APPLY THE INFORMATION

about the person or their life and lifestyle (Badger and Nolan, 2006; Conrad, 1985; Dickinson *et al.*, 1999; Donovan and Blake, 1992, Stevenson and Scambler, 2005; Vermeire *et al.*, 2001).

However, the term 'compliance' has connotations of professional power, and so in an attempt to give back some autonomy to the patient the Royal Pharmaceutical Society published a report in 1997 that recommended that the term 'concordance' be used when referring to the concept of compliance. This happened in part because society was changing rapidly but healthcare was responding less rapidly (Illich, 2001). Allied to this, there had been considerable debate and discussion in the medical and nursing literature over a number of years attempting to explore why some patients do not follow the treatment prescribed for them (Aronson, 2007; Badger and Nolan, 2006; Dickinson *et al.*, 1999; Donovan and Blake, 1992; Stevenson and Scambler, 2005; Vermeire *et al.*, 2001; Wainwright and Gould, 1997). Much of this literature implies that there are three main issues at stake: terminology, the values and beliefs of the user, and the unequal relationship between patient and healthcare professional, especially between patient and doctor. Many of these papers suggest that many healthcare professionals have strong beliefs in both the efficacy of conventional medicine and the roles and responsibilities of each person in maintaining health and in the healthcare professional–patient relationship. Inherent in this is the idea that the healthcare professionals are the experts, and that the healthcare professional, as an expert, will follow rational and scientific thought while the patient, a non-expert, will be illogical and irrational. As a result, the patient should passively follow the guidance and prescription of the healthcare professional in order to get well.

This role that people were expected to adopt when accessing healthcare was first highlighted in Parsons' seminal work of 1951. Parsons used the term 'sick role'. Although society and healthcare have changed markedly since then, many of these attitudes still exist, both in patients and in healthcare professionals. The healthcare professional may think of themselves as dominant, while the patient is passive; one person gives the orders and the other receives and acts on them. Playle and Keeley (1998) capture this well by arguing that healthcare professionals can support concordance by operating under the umbrella of the ethical principle of beneficence along with their duty of care, so that they can then present a rationale of 'in the best interest of the patient' or 'for the patient's good'. They suggest that when a patient is concordant, this demonstrates to the healthcare professional that the patient understands and has insight into their illness and what can make them well. The patient is then seen to be in a collaborative and trusting relationship; such people are frequently viewed by healthcare professionals as 'popular' or 'good' patients (Stockwell, 1984). Conversely, patients who are non-concordant can be seen to be deviant, wrong or blameworthy.

The rhetoric of much UK government policy (e.g. Audit Commission, 2001; DH, 2001a) goes some way in reinforcing this message. It encourages healthcare professionals to use approaches that will empower patients to make what the state deems to be the 'right' choices. Such tactics include patient education and more sophisticated communication strategies such as establishing therapeutic alliances to encourage patient empowerment.

Conversely, this could be seen to be somewhat underhand. This type of behaviour can be interpreted as using benevolent influencing skills that, far from giving patients choice, are manipulating patients' behaviour, resulting in the patient conforming both to the expectations of healthcare professionals and to the government's agenda.

Personal and professional development 8.5

Consider your attitudes to patients who may be non-adherent. Take five minutes to ponder whether healthcare professionals should judge patients who are non-adherent. Are there more appropriate thoughts and actions, rather than judging patients as 'good' or 'bad', that a nurse could take? If so, what are they? Perhaps you might like to use your professional portfolio to record your ideas.

One advantage of this debate has been to generate a better understanding of why some patients may not follow treatment regimes. It has also highlighted how common non-concordance can be. Some research studies (Britten, 1994; Donovan and Blake 1992; Gamble *et al.*, 2007; Hugtenburg *et al.*, 2006; Vermeire *et al.*, 2001; Wainwright and Gould, 1997) have helped to illuminate the debate from the patient's perspective.

For example, diuretics are frequently prescribed, but patients often stop taking them. This is usually because diuretics often result in an immediate and urgent need to micturate large volumes of urine on more than one occasion. Consequently, the patient needs to be close to toilet facilities and able to access them fairly quickly. Diuretics can thus have a major impact on the patient's lifestyle (Ulfvarson *et al.*, 2007). Allied with this, many patients are given little information about the effects of diuretics and how best to manage them. Healthcare professionals should explore with the patient when they can take their diuretics to fit in with their lifestyle; for example, if they work in the mornings but are at home in the afternoons, then the best time to take their medication may be early afternoon when they first return home.

What all these studies have identified is that the factors that influence concordance are, like the patients themselves, frequently complex and also unique (Table 8.1).

Other factors that may influence concordance include the following:

- Simple forgetfulness is common. If this is a problem, compliance aids can be considered.
- People can view medicines either positively or negatively. If a patient views medicines negatively, it could be because medicines are seen to be unnatural or addictive and therefore perceived as harmful.
- Positive beliefs about medicines can self-motivate people to take them as prescribed, whereas people who hold negative beliefs may alter the dosage or stop taking them.

Table 8.1 Factors that seem to influence concordance

Increasing concordance	Decreasing concordance
Believing that your condition is serious	Having a chronic disease
Accepting that the treatment will be successful	Long and/or complicated treatment
	Treatment that is unpleasant or embarrassing
	Treatment that has a significant effect on everyday life

Source: Britten, 1994; Donovan *et al.*, 1989; Gamble *et al.*, 2007; Hugtenburg *et al.*, 2006; Vermeire *et al.*, 2001; Wainwright and Gould, 1997).

- If the side effects are felt to be worse than the disease, the patient may stop taking the medicine.
- If the routine of taking the medicines does not fit with the patient's lifestyle, they may stop taking the medicine.
- The taste or texture of the medicine may reduce the patient's concordance.
- Inability to swallow tablets will reduce patient concordance.
- The way in which medicines are manufactured may be in opposition to the patient's values and beliefs, for example if the drugs have been tested on animals before they are used by humans or if the medicines contain animal ingredients such as gelatine.
- Many people find the use of more than one name for a particular medicine confusing, for example furosemide and Lasix™.

The many factors involved in patient concordance/adherence are summarised in Figure 8.1.

Assessing whether the patient is concordant

Without testing the patient's blood for the serum levels of a particular drug, it is difficult to assess whether they are taking their medicines as prescribed. Goldberg *et al.* (1998), in their seminal study of physicians, suggested that doctors found it difficult to recognise non-concordance. They accepted that patients were considered concordant if the doctors could 'communicate well with patients and patients appear to be knowledgeable about the medical problem'.

The attitudes reflected by the physicians in Goldberg *et al.* (1998) study suggest that those people who are articulate, good conversationalists, socially adept and well informed are seen to be concordant. These attributes are the very ones that Stockwell (1984) identifies as those of 'the popular patient'. Perhaps the very attributes that are thought to suggest patient concordance are the same as those that influence whether a healthcare professional views a patient as popular or unpopular.

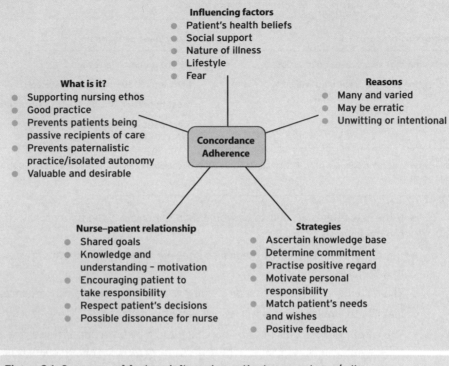

Influencing factors
- Patient's health beliefs
- Social support
- Nature of illness
- Lifestyle
- Fear

What is it?
- Supporting nursing ethos
- Good practice
- Prevents patients being passive recipients of care
- Prevents paternalistic practice/isolated autonomy
- Valuable and desirable

Concordance Adherence

Reasons
- Many and varied
- May be erratic
- Unwitting or intentional

Nurse–patient relationship
- Shared goals
- Knowledge and understanding – motivation
- Encouraging patient to take responsibility
- Respect patient's decisions
- Possible dissonance for nurse

Strategies
- Ascertain knowledge base
- Determine commitment
- Practise positive regard
- Motivate personal responsibility
- Match patient's needs and wishes
- Positive feedback

Figure 8.1 Summary of factors influencing patient concordance/adherence

One of the reasons that concordance is being debated in the public arena is economics (Audit Commission, 2001). The cost of medicines today takes up a third of NHS resources. These costs are likely to soar, given that increasingly expensive drugs are coming on to the market. Alongside this are rising public expectations: many people now expect to have drugs when they need them, regardless of the cost or even how robust the evidence is that they are effective treatment. One method that has been suggested to guarantee cost-effectiveness in relation to medicines is to ensure that older people are able to manage their medicines when they are discharged from hospital by self-administration.

Self-administration

We use the term 'self-administration' to describe the situation in which the patient in hospital is able to administer to themselves their prescribed medication. Note that this is different from self-medication, which we use to refer to a situation where the individual chooses a medication, the dosage of the medication and the form of the medication in order to treat, for example, a headache. Confusingly, some textbooks use the two terms interchangeably.

The principle of self-administration has patient autonomy at its roots. Once the patient is well enough, and deemed to be competent, the responsibility for taking their own prescribed medicines is handed back to them. This means that the patient understands how and when to take the medicines. One advantage of this is it this frees up the nurse to spend more time educating patients about their prescribed medicines. The NMC (2007), in its *Standards for Medicines Management*, supports the principle of self-administration by patients as this enables them to be active partners in their own care. The Audit Commission (2001), however, expresses the need for caution until appropriate procedures and policies are agreed by the NHS trust to protect the healthcare professionals involved. Of particular importance are the action plans that NHS trusts need to have in place in order to ensure safety, security and storage to comply with legislation such as the Medicines Act (1968).

An important factor in relation to self-administration is the need to ensure that the patient is able to carry out the administration appropriately; therefore, assessment is essential. A number of healthcare professionals are involved in the patient assessment, including the pharmacist, doctor, nursing staff and, where appropriate, professionals from other services. They ensure that the patient has the understanding and skill necessary to administer their own prescribed medicines safely and accurately. Evidence suggests that patients who self-administer are more knowledgeable about their illness and their medication; concordance/adherence is improved, as is patient autonomy, because the patient feels more in control and more confident (Lowe *et al.*, 1995).

Related knowledge The role of the nurse in self-administration

- Participate in multidisciplinary team (MDT) assessment of patient
- Enable patient to make informed choice
- Educate patient about their medication
- Supervise and support patient during the implementation of self-administration
- Keep accurate and up-to-date records
- Monitor the process of self-administration
- Evaluate the success and the safety of the process from both the patient's and the nurse's perspective.

Personal and professional development 8.6

Consider whether you assume that people who communicate well are concordant. If you do, which groups of people are you in danger of assuming are not concordant? List two strategies that may help you identify whether a patient is concordant.

Quick reminder

✔ Ageing affects the composition of the body and organ functioning.

✔ Chronological age does not necessarily reflect the person's biological age.

✔ Pharmacodynamics and pharmacokinetics can be affected by the ageing process.

✔ Many more people in the UK live to reach old age than ever before, and large numbers of older people live with one or more chronic diseases.

✔ Many older people with long-term conditions are commonly taking four or five prescribed medicines a day – polypharmacy.

✔ Polypharmacy is not necessarily a bad thing, but it can be the result of inappropriate prescribing. There are multiple reasons for this, including a patient having multiple prescribers and self-medication.

✔ Taking more than one medicine may result in a drug-drug interaction.

✔ Many acute medical admissions of older people are as a result of drug-drug interactions.

✔ Many adults self-medicate with over-the-counter drugs and herbal medicines.

✔ Many healthcare professionals rarely ask about self-medication with herbal medicines.

✔ In order to ensure more effective use of medicines, healthcare professionals should encourage patient concordance and adherence with their prescribed medication.

✔ One way of ensuring concordance is to assist older people to self-administer medicines while in hospital.

✔ Self-administration alters the nurse's role in medicine administration.

REFERENCES

Aronson J K (2007) Compliance, concordance, adherence. *British Journal of Clinical Pharmacology* **63**, 383-384.

Astrand E, Astrand B, Antonov K and Petersson G (2007) Potential drug interactions during a three-decade period: a cross-sectional study of a prescription register. *European Journal of Clinical Pharmacology* **63**, 851-859.

Audit Commission (2001) *A Spoonful of Sugar: Medicines Management in NHS Hospitals.* Wetherby: Audit Commission Publications.

Badger F and Nolan P (2006) Concordance with antidepressant medication in primary care. *Nursing Standard* **20**, 35-40.

Beers M H (1997) Explicit criteria for determining potentially inappropriate medication use by the elderly. *Archives of Internal Medicine* **157**, 1531-1536.

Britten N (1994) Patient's ideas about medicines: a qualitative study in a general practice population. *British Journal of General Practice* **44**, 465-468.

Cockayne N L, Duguid M and Shenfiels G M (2004) Health professionals rarely record history of complementary and alternative medicines. *British Journal of Clinical Pharmacology* **59**, 254-258.

Conrad P (1985) The meaning of medications: another look at compliance. *Social Science and Medicine* **20**, 29-37.

Constable S, Ham A and Pirmohamed M (2006) Herbal medicines and acute medical emergency admissions to hospital. *British Journal of Clinical Pharmacology* **63**, 247-248.

Cowan D, While A, Roberts J and Fitzpatrick J (2002) Medicines management in care homes for older people: the nurse's role. *British Journal of Community Nursing* **7**, 634-638.

Cutts C and Tett S E (2005) Do rural consumers expect a prescription from their GP visit? Investigation of patients' expectations for a prescription and doctors' prescribing decisions in rural Australia. *Australian Journal of Rural Health* **13**, 43-50.

Denneboom W, Dautzenburg M G, Grol R and De Smet P A (2006) Analysis of polypharmacy in older patients in primary care using a multidisciplinary expert panel. *British Journal of General Practitioners* **56**, 504-510.

Department of Health (2000) *Coronary Heart Disease: National Service Framework for Coronary Heart Disease – Modern Standards and Service Models.* London: The Stationery Office.

Department of Health (2001a) *Medicines and Older People: Implementing Medicines-Related Aspects of the National Service Framework for Older People.* London: The Stationery Office.

Department of Health (DH) (2001b) *National Service Framework for Older People.* London: The Stationery Office.

Department of Health (DH) (2005) *Supporting People with Long Term Conditions.* London: The Stationery Office.

Dickinson D, Wilkie P and Harris M (1999) Taking medicines: concordance is not compliance. *British Medical Journal* **319**, 787.

Donovan J L and Blake D R (1992) Patient non-compliance: deviance or reasoned decision making? *Social Science and Medicine* **34**, 507-513.

Donovan J L, Blake D R and Fleming W G (1989) The patient is not a blank sheet: lay beliefs and their relevance to patient education. *British Journal of Rheumatism* **28**, 58-61.

Ershler W B (2007) A gripping reality: oxidative stress, inflammation and the pathway to frailty. *Journal of Applied Physiology,* **103**, 1, 3-5.

Fick D M, Cooper J W, Wade W E, Waller J L, Maclean R and Beers M H (2003) Updating the Beers criteria for potentially inappropriate medication use in older adults: results of a U.S. consensus panel of experts. *Archives of Internal Medicine* **163**, 2716-2724.

Gallagher P, Barry P and Mahoney D (2007) Inappropriate prescribing in the elderly. *Journal of Clinical Pharmacy and Therapeutics* **32**, 113-121.

Gamble J, Fitzsimmons D, Lynes D and Heaney L (2007) Difficult asthma: people's perspectives on taking corticosteriod therapy. *Journal of Advanced Nursing* **16**, 59-67.

Goldberg A I, Cohen G and Rubin A-H E (1998) Physician assessment of patient compliance with medical treatment. *Social Science and Medicine* **47**, 1873-1876.

Greenstein B and Gould D (2004) *Trounce's Clinical Pharmacology for Nurses.* Edinburgh: Churchill Livingstone.

Harrison R, Holt D, Pattison D J and Elton P J (2004) Who and how many people are taking herbal supplements? A survey of 21 923 adults. *International Journal of Vitamin and Nutritional Research* **74**, 83-86.

Hart B, Birkas J, Lachmann M and Saunders L (2002) Promoting positive outcomes for elderly persons in the hospital: prevention and risk factor modification. *Advanced Practice in Acute Critical Care* **13**, 22-33.

Haynes, R B, Taylor D W and Sackett D L (1979) *Compliance in Health Care*. Baltimore, MD: Johns Hopkins University Press.

Holden W, Joseph J and Williamson L (2005) Use of herbal remedies and potential drug interactions in rheumatology outpatients. *Annals of the Rheumatic Diseases* **64**, 790.

Hugtenburg J G, Blom A T and Kisoensingh S U (2006) Initial phase of chronic medication use: patients' reasons for discontinuation. *British Journal of Clinical Pharmacology* **61**, 352-354.

Illich I (2001) *Limits to Medicine: Medical Nemesis - The Expropriation of Health*. London: Marion Boyars Publishers.

Johnell K and Klarin I (2007) The relationship between number and potential drug-drug interactions in the elderly: a study of over 600 000 elderly patients from the Swedish Prescribed Drug Register. *Drug Safety* **30**, 911-918.

Kirkwood T B L (1999) *Time of Our Lives: The Science of Human Ageing*. London: Weidenfeld & Nicolson.

Kohler G I, Bode-Boger S M, Busse R, Hoopemann M, Welte T and Roger R M (2000) Drug-drug interactions in medical patients: effects of in-hospital treatment and relation to multiple drug use. *International Journal of Clinical Pharmacology and Therapeutics* **38**, 504-513.

Larsen P D and Martin J L (1999) Polypharmacy and elderly patients. *American Operating Room Nursing Journal* **69**, 619-628.

LeSage J (1991) Polypharmacy in geriatric patients. *Nursing Clinics of North America* **26**, 273-289.

Livingston S (2003) NSF for older people. 2: the older patient. *Pharmaceutical Journal* **270**, 862-863.

Lowe C J, Raynor D K, Courtney E A, Purvis J and Teale C (1995) Effects of self medication programme on knowledge of drugs and compliance with treatment in elderly patients. *British Medical Journal* **310**, 1229-1233.

MacFarlane J, Holmes W, MacFarlane R, and Britten N (1997) Influence of patients' expectations on antibiotic management of acute lower respiratory tract illness in general practice: questionnaire study. *British Medical Journal* **315**, 1211-1214.

McGavock H (2005) *How Drugs Work: Basic Pharmacology for Healthcare Professionals*. Abingdon: Radcliffe Publishing.

Mera S (1997) *Understanding Disease: Pathology and Prevention*. Cheltenham: Stanley Thornes.

Nathan A, Goodyer L, Lovejoy A and Rashid A (1999) 'Brown bag' medication reviews as a means of optimising patients' use of medication and identifying potential clinical problems. *Family Practice* **16**, 278-282.

NHS Information Centre (2007) *Quality Outcomes Framework*. www.ic.nhs.uk/services/qof.

Nursing and Midwifery Council (NMC) (2007) *Standards for Medicines Management*. London: Nursing and Midwifery Council.

Parsons T (1951) *The Social System*. Glencoe: Free Press.

Playle J F and Keeley P (1998) Non-compliance and professional power. *Journal of Advanced Nursing* **27**, 304-311.

Poole C, Jones D and Veitch B (1999) Relationships between prescription and non-prescription drugs in an elderly population. *Archives of Gerontology and Geriatrics* **28**, 259-271.

Rang H P, Dale, M M, Ritter J M and Moore P K (2003) *Pharmacology*, 5th edn. Edinburgh: Churchill Livingstone.

Shepherd M (1998) The risks of polypharmacy. *Nursing Times* **94**, 60-62.

Simonsen T, Aarbakke J, Kay I, Coleman I, Sinnott P and Lysaa R (2006) *Illustrated Pharmacology for Nurses*. London: Hodder Arnold.

Stevenson S and Scambler G (2005) The relationship between medicine and the public: the challenge of concordance. *Health* **9**, 5-21.

Stewart R B and Hale W E (1992) Acute confusional states in older adults and the role of polypharmacy. *Annual Review of Public Health* **13**, 415-430.

Stockwell F (1984) *The Unpopular Patient*. London: Royal College of Nursing.

Swonger A K and Burbank P M (1995) *Drug Therapy and the Elderly*. London: Jones & Bartlett Publishers.

Tortora G J and Derrickson B (2006) *Principles of Anatomy and Physiology*, 11th edn. New York: John Wiley & Sons.

Ulfvarson J, Bardage C, Wredling R A-M, von Bahr C and Adami J (2007) Adherence to drug treatment in association with how the patient perceives care and information on drugs. *Journal of Clinical Nursing* **16**, 141-148.

Vermeire E, Hearnshaw H, Van Royen P and Denekens J (2001) Patient adherence to treatment: three decades of research: a comprehensive review. *Journal of Clinical Pharmacy and Therapeutics* **26**, 331-342.

Wainwright S P and Gould D (1997) Non-adherence with medication in organ transplant patients: a literature review. *Journal of Advanced Nursing* **26**, 968-977.

Walsh M (1997) *Watson's Clinical Nursing and Related Sciences*, 5th edn. London: Baillière Tindall.

Williams C (2002) Using medications appropriately in older adults. *American Family Physician* **66**, 1917-1924.

Xue Q-L, Fried L P, Gloss TA, Laftan A and Chaves P H M (2008) Life space constriction, development of frailty and the competing risk of mortality (The Women's Health and Aging Study 1). *American Journal of Epidemiology* **167**, 2, 240-248.

Yang J C, Tomlinson F and Nagle G (2001) Medication lists for elderly patients: clinic demand versus in-home inspection. *Journal of General Internal Medicine* **16**, 112-115.

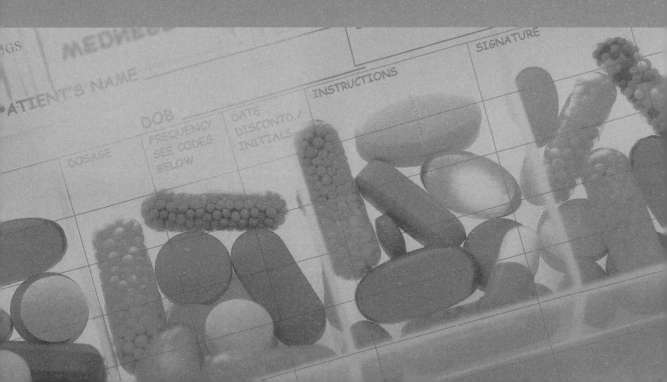

Part 4

Patient scenarios

Chapter 9

Rheumatoid arthritis:
a woman with long-standing rheumatoid arthritis who has also developed osteoporosis

Rheumatoid arthritis results in continual pain and discomfort and affects the person's mobility. This can have a major impact on the individual's life and lifestyle. Using the patient scenario of Mrs Ishbael Stewart, a woman with long-standing rheumatoid arthritis who has also developed osteoporosis, this chapter explores the medicines management issues that have presented in the treatment of these conditions, such as managing chronic pain and patient concordance. The chapter also considers the nursing implications and interventions that arise in relation to the medications that can be used to treat both of these conditions.

The medications that may be prescribed to improve the patient's symptoms are not without their side effects and risks. Helping to ensure the effective management of the chronic symptoms that people such as Mrs Stewart experience involves using both the art and the science of nursing.

Unpicking the issues presented in this scenario of Mrs Stewart's experiences demonstrates much of the underpinning knowledge base. It also emphasises the appropriate attitudes and understanding needed by nurses in order to help Mrs Stewart to manage her medication, so helping her to live more comfortably with her long-term condition.

✔ Learning outcomes

By the end of this chapter you should be able to:

✔ Give an overview of rheumatoid arthritis and osteoporosis

✔ Describe the potential impact of rheumatoid arthritis and osteoporosis on the individual

✔ Discuss pharmacological approaches to the management of the inflammatory process

✔ Discuss the actions and effects of aspirin and prednisolone related to the specific patient scenario

✔ Discuss the pharmacological approaches to the treatment of osteoporosis

✔ Identify the nursing knowledge needed to support this patient

✔ Identify the supporting nursing interventions for this patient.

Chapter at a glance

The nature of rheumatoid arthritis
Pharmacological treatments used to manage rheumatoid arthritis
The nature of osteoporosis
Pharmacological treatments used to manage osteoporosis
Quick reminder
References

Mrs Ishbael Stewart

Mrs Ishbael Stewart has had rheumatoid arthritis since she was 22; she is now 48 years old. Not only did the disease progress very rapidly during her mid-twenties but it was also extremely intractable (difficult to treat successfully) to many treatments. As for most people with rheumatoid arthritis, Ishbael's life, and that of her husband and family, has been greatly affected by her illness. However, she began taking inflix-imab about 4 months ago and after about 8 weeks she said that she felt as though she had finally 'got her life back'. She has much more flexibility in her joints now and is considerably more mobile; the pain, stiffness and swelling have almost disappeared too. She tells everyone that she feels 'like a new woman' and is relishing the experience of not having to rely on others for everyday personal care. Her family and friends are amazed by the difference they see in her.

Ishbael and her husband Ted have four children – two sons and two daughters.

THE NATURE OF RHEUMATOID ARTHRITIS

Rheumatoid arthritis (RA) is a disease of unknown aetiology. It is recognised by pain, stiffness (particularly in the early morning), and swelling in some of the body's joints, along with resulting immobility and joint deformity. It is unpredictable in nature, but the synovial joints (fingers, toes, wrists, knees, ankles and shoulders) are affected most commonly (Boon *et al.*, 2006; Panayi, 2006). However, it should be remembered that rheumatoid arthritis is a systemic condition and may also affect many of the organs. It affects about 1% of the population, and women are affected more commonly than men. People in the middle decades of life are most commonly affected (**www.arc.org.uk**). Rheumatoid arthritis is an autoimmune disease – that is, a disorder brought about by the immune system responding against the individual's own cells and tissues.

Essential terminology

Aetiology
Study of the causes of disease.

Systemic
Widespread throughout the body.

To enable patients to manage their condition successfully, it is important that nurses are able to differentiate between rheumatoid arthritis and osteoarthritis. Unfortunately, many people use use the term 'arthritis' rather than 'musculoskeletal disorder' to describe joint pain and disease in a general way. However, although osteoarthritis and rheumatoid arthritis do have some similar features, they also have some very marked differences (Table 9.1; Oliver and Ryan, 2004).

Table 9.1 Overview of the characteristics and symptoms of osteoarthritis and rheumatoid arthritis

Osteoarthritis	Rheumatoid arthritis
Primary (idopathic) or secondary, e.g. trauma, metabolic	Inflammatory arthritis – systemic autoimmune disease
Few or single joint involvement (occasionally more than three joints involved)	Symmetrical arthritis affects a number of joints
No extra-articular features	Extra-articular feature may be present, including organ involvement (lung, cardiac, renal) and rheumatoid nodules
Joints commonly affected: fingers, distal interphalangeal joints, proximal interphalangeal joints, first carpometacarpophalangeal joint (base of thumb), hips and knees, hallux valgus (bunion); cervical and lumbar spine can also be involved	Joints commonly affected (presentation is often bilateral): metacarpophalangeal joints, for example knuckles, and metatarsophalangeal joints, for example joints in the toes, wrists, shoulders, elbows, knees and ankles
Blood results generally normal but may show mildly raised inflammatory indices, especially with osteoarthritis of the hip	Blood results demonstrate inflammation, C-reactive protein, plasma viscosity and erythrocyte sedimentation rate; anaemia of chronic disease may also be present
On examination: tenderness on joint margins, coarse crepitus, firm swelling and signs of mild inflammation, e.g. cool effusion	On examination: joints feel hot, frequently swollen and tender on palpation; pain at rest
Pain: A strong feature of disease but generally exacerbated by: ● weight-bearing or movement; ● ascending or descending stairs; ● rising from low chairs; ● stiffness – after resting and inactivity Can be unremitting with severe disease	Pain: ● Chronic pain with flares of disease exacerbating pain ● Strong feature of the disease ● Pain can be experienced without exacerbating factors, e.g. pain at rest ● Joints are generally warm or hot when painful ● Additional chronic pain as a result of osteoarthritis secondary to rheumatoid arthritis
Functional decline attributed to: ● joint deformity (structural and mechanical failure of cartilage, osteophyte formation); ● loss of bone in severe cases; ● joint deformity, osteophyte formation and loss of bone in severe cases can result in joint instability; ● muscle weakness; ● stiffness – sometimes described as 'gelling'	Functional decline attributed to: ● multiple joint involvement; ● erosive disease; ● inflammatory component – joint damage and functional decline linked to increase in overall disease activity; ● early-morning stiffness increases with more active disease; ● secondary osteoarthritis; ● muscle weakness
Consequences of disease related to functional decline and pain	Pain, functional decline, fatigue, weight loss and anaemia

Nursing Standard **18**, 50, p. 44 www.nursing-standard.co.uk

Personal and professional development 9.1

Consider how it would feel to have constant joint pain and restricted mobility. How would it affect your life? How would you feel about having to take a number of medicines regularly?

Personal and professional development 9.2

Write short notes that you could use to help you explain the inflammatory response to Mrs Stewart. Think about how comfortable you would feel explaining the inflammatory response to her. If you think you would find this difficult, consider what further reading might assist you to develop your ability to do this.

Related knowledge Pathophysiology

Autoimmune disease is the consequence of a number of interrelated reactions that take place in the immune system. As a result of these responses, some of the T-cells (white blood cells that are specialised in aspects of immunity) become ineffective and others are deactivated. The affected organ or system is then unable to recognise itself and attempts to defend itself against attack. Almost every organ and system in the body can be affected by autoimmunity (Phillips *et al.*, 2001). A number of cytokines (proteins produced by lymph cells that influence the inflammatory process) are found in the joints of people with rheumatoid arthritis. One of these cytokines, produced by T-cells, is tumour necrosis factor α (TNF-α). TNF-α is responsible for stimulating the production of other cytokines that produce inflammation. Stopping the action of TNF-α seems to prevent the production of the other cytokines that stimulate the inflammatory process in the affected joints, which leads to rheumatoid arthritis (Luqmani *et al.*, 2006).

Unfortunately, as with many chronic diseases, there is no available cure for rheumatoid arthritis. However, there are a number of useful therapies and interventions that can help to reduce both the clinical features of the disease and the impact of the disease on the patient, thus aiding people such as Mrs Stewart to live more comfortably with the disease. A greater understanding of the inflammatory process, technological developments such as magnetic resonance imaging (MRI) and developments in haematological screening (investigations of blood and the tissues that produce blood cells) has led to a better understanding of the development of rheumatoid arthritis and the development of more effective treatments, such as the biological therapies (medicines based on agents that occur in the immune system).

Many of the treatments used in rheumatoid arthritis interfere with the normal inflammatory process, and so it is important that the nurse understands both the normal inflammatory response and how it is affected by treatment. Once you understand these processes, you can then transfer your understanding of these principles into caring for patients with other diseases caused by inflammation, where similar interventions may be used.

Related knowledge Pathophysiology

In most situations, inflammation is a protective response by the body to either trauma or infection. Inflammation is the first step in the sequence of healing, repair and recovery, which begins with an acute process aimed at scavenging the injury's cause and the remains of the cells in that area. If the acute process is not effective, it can become chronic. When an insult is made on the body, it sets off a chain reaction of physiological activity at the cellular level. A series of chemicals are produced in response to the trauma or infection; these chemicals produce the classic signs of inflammation that were first described in Western culture by Celsus, an ancient Roman physician - redness (rubor), swelling (tumour), heat (calor) and pain (dolor). Although this description summarises both what can be seen and felt on the skin's surface when inflammation occurs, it must be remembered that inflammation also takes place internally.

The inflammatory response is a complex set of reactions. It begins with the immediate release of histamine from the mast cells (Table 9.2), which results in vasodilation. If the vasodilation is on the skin's surface, the classic signs of inflammation can be seen: erythema (redness), swelling and heat (which can be remembered easily as a red, hot, painful swelling). If the inflammation is internal, the same process occurs but is not visible to the nurse. If inflammation is systemic (widespread), vasodilation may lead to hypotension and hypovolaemic shock. Following vasodilation, there is an increase in capillary permeability, causing the capillaries to leak serum; if this happens too quickly for the serum to be reabsorbed, some degree of swelling develops in the tissues.

Monocytes arrive at the site of the injury or trauma and begin the process of phagocytosis (engulfing and ingesting bacteria and tissue cell debris), aiming to inactivate any infective substance. If monocytes arrive in large numbers, they contribute to the size of the swelling and eventually are discharged as pus.

Any accompanying pain and itch are protective functions as a result of stimulation of the sensory receptors by histamine.

The chemicals in this process are known as inflammatory mediators. Some of these mediators, such as prothrombin, are always present in the bloodstream, as inactive precursor mediators. However, other mediators are produced from cells following tissue damage, as a result of injury or infection, such as serotonin.

▶

▶ *(continued)*

There follows a further series of reactions, which includes the fibrin, fibrinolytic and kinin cascades. Alongside these, damage to cell membranes causes the cell membrane phospholipids to release arachidonic acid. This stimulates the formation of two metabolic pathways, the cyclo-oxygenase and the lipoxygenase pathways. The nociceptors are stimulated by the prostaglandins that are produced in the cyclo-oxygenase pathway (Mera, 1997; Phillips *et al.*, 2001).

Table 9.2 Cells involved in inflammation

Cell type	Function and location	Product
Neutrophils	Phagocytic cell with membrane receptors for chemotactic messengers; normally comprise 60% of leucocytes. Engulf and ingest microorganisms and cells. Also have receptors on their cell membranes that recognise chemicals so that they can move towards or away from high concentrations of chemicals.	Enzymes and free radicals, which kill or digest microorganisms. Leukotrienes – chemical messengers found in a variety of tissue that influence state of blood vessels, airways and some white blood cells.
Monocytes/ macrophages	Blood monocytes migrate into the tissues and differentiate into macrophages. Possess membrane receptors for chemotactic messengers, cytokines and growth factors. Phagocytose small and large particles.	Free radicals, thromboxanes (found in platelets – stimulates blood clotting and constricts blood vessels) and leukotrienes.
Eosinophils	Involved in allergic responses. Normally comprise 2–4% of blood leucocytes.	Superoxide radical, leukotriene C_4.
Mast cells	Present in connective tissues (tissues that support the body, e.g. collagen) and mucous membranes (linings of body passages, e.g. airways that are moistened by mucus produced by their specialised cells).	Histamine (chemical that produces allergic reactions), heparin (prevents blood clotting, occurs naturally in the body and also is produced synthetically for medicinal use). Prostaglandins (influence smooth muscle contraction, blood pressure, body temperature and inflammation), leukotrienes, thromboxanes and chemotactic factors.

Leukotrienes, prostaglandins, prostacyclin and thromboxanes are the hormone-like chemicals (mediators) that facilitate the chain reaction in response to inflammation. These mediators come from the phospholipids in cell membranes. The first step in the process is the conversion of phospholipids into arachidonic acid by the phospholipase enzymes. The next stage involves the chemicals that are produced joining one of two production processes – the cyclo-oxygenase or the lipoxygenase pathway. If they go into the lipoxygenase pathway, they become leukotrienes; if they go into the cyclo-oxygenase pathway, they become prostaglandins, prostacyclin and thromboxanes. Platelets contain the enzyme thromboxane synthetase and can synthesise thromboxane. This enzyme is absent in vascular endothelium, which instead produces prostacyclin. Most other cells of the immune response contain the enzymes necessary to produce the other leukotriene and prostaglandin intermediates and end products.

Adapted from Mera (1997)

Mrs Ishbael Stewart

Over the years Mrs Stewart has used a range of treatments. Initially she hoped that she would be cured, but once she came to terms with having RA her aim was to be pain-free and as mobile as possible. She used enteric-coated aspirin initially, but as the disease progressed this medicine became ineffective at managing her symptoms. Her symptoms became increasingly intractable. The medicines she has used over the years include aspirin, ibuprofen and prednisolone; the latter seemed to her to be the most successful at controlling the disease. Consequently, she took large doses of prednisolone for many years. She always carried a steroid treatment card with her and impressed on her family its whereabouts. Mrs Stewart has also tried a variety of complementary and alternative therapies, including massage, chiropractic and the herbal medicine gamma-linolenic acid (GLA).

Mrs Stewart began smoking the occasional cigarette when she was 14 years old. When she started work, aged 16, she began to smoke more, until she admitted to regularly smoking at least 20 cigarettes a day. However, as her hands became increasingly deformed and disabled as a result of the rheumatoid arthritis, she found that she could no longer easily take a cigarette out of its packet, light it or hold it between her fingers. Consequently, she found that she smoked less and less over a period of time, until she stopped all together when she was 33 years old.

By this time, Mrs Stewart had had a variety of treatments for her RA, both medical and surgical. Over the years, Mrs Stewart has had arthroplasty, synovectomy and fusion to some of her finger joints, thumbs, wrists, knees and toe joints. She has also had hydrotherapy and splinting and tried a variety of aids, such as large-handled cutlery and insoles.

Mrs Stewart's ill-health began before rheumatology became the specialised service that it is today, and so Mrs Stewart has benefited from her local rheumatology service for only a relatively short period of time. Consequently, she would be managed in a very different way if she presented to her GP today with the same problems. Current recommendations are that the person is referred to the multidisciplinary rheumatology team as early as possible and given aggressive combination disease-modifying anti-rheumatic drug (DMARD) therapy (Luqmani et al., 2006). Many people that you care for will have had their ill-health for many years, and their treatments will probably have evolved over this time. Recognising when people should be referred for specialist advice is an important responsibility of healthcare professionals today. However, there still seem to be barriers to people getting quick and efficient access to early, effective treatment for rheumatoid arthritis; two of these barriers are an insufficient number of specialist healthcare practitioners, such as nurse specialists, and a lack of funding to enable patients to benefit from the biological therapies such as infliximab, as recommended by the NICE guidelines (Luqmani et al., 2006; NICE, 2007a).

PHARMACOLOGICAL TREATMENTS USED TO MANAGE RHEUMATOID ARTHRITIS

Non-steroidal anti-inflammatory drugs (NSAIDs)

The NSAIDs include some common drugs, such as aspirin and ibuprofen, as well as the newer cyclo-oxygenase (COX2)-selective inhibitors such as etoricoxib and alecoxib. If used regularly and in the prescribed dosage, all NSAIDs have both an anti-inflammatory effect and an analgesic effect, making them effective for 'continuous or regular pain associated with inflammation' (**www.bnf.org.uk**).

Although paracetamol is thought to have some cyclo-oxygenase-inhibiting properties (**www.bnf.org.uk**; Greenstein and Gould, 2004), it has little in the way of anti-inflammatory properties. Therefore, the use of paracetamol as an anti-inflammatory is limited; it is, however, a commonly used analgesic and antipyretic, with its biggest advantage being that it does not have the side effect of gastric irritation, dyspepsia and haemorrhage that aspirin has. Paracetamol is used by patients with rheumatoid arthritis to manage their joint pain.

Greenstein and Gould (2004) classify the NSAIDs into three categories: the older NSAIDs, such as indometacin; the non-selective COX-inhibiting NSAIDs, such as ibuprofen and naproxen; and the selective COX2-inhibiting NSAIDs, such as etoricoxib. However, there are other ways of classifying the NSAIDs; for example, Thompson and Dunne (2004) classify NSAIDs according to their half-life. However, for many nurses Greenstein and Gould's (2004) classification would seem to be the most useful.

> ## Personal and professional development 9.3
>
> Think about whether you understand the concept of half-life and what this may mean for the person taking the medicine.

The NSAIDs prevent the production of two isoenzymes (enzymes that are chemically different but work in the same way) – COX1 and COX2. These isoenzymes have slightly different functions in the body. Small quantities of COX1 are found in almost all tissues and seem to have two roles: regulation of platelet aggregation (sticking together) and protection of the mucous membranes lining the stomach, thus protecting the stomach from the corrosive effects of gastric acid. COX1 reduces the ability of the stomach's parietal cells to produce hydrochloric acid.

Conversely, the site of production of COX2 is the inflamed tissue itself, and its function seems be in maintaining the blood supply to the kidneys (Greenstein and Gould, 2004; Simonsen *et al.*, 2006).

Pharmacokinetics NSAIDs

Absorption: Most of the NSAIDs are absorbed fully from the gastrointestinal tract (**www.bnf.org.uk**; Greenstein and Gould, 2004).

Distribution: The NSAIDs are bound strongly to plasma proteins. Consequently, only a small percentage of the dose taken circulates freely in the blood and is available to bring about a pharmacological effect (McGavock, 2005; Rang *et al.*, 2003).

Metabolism: The NSAIDs are metabolised in the liver by enzymes (**www.bnf.org.uk**; Greenstein and Gould, 2004).

Elimination: The metabolites (end products of the metabolic process) of the NSAIDs are excreted via the urine (McGavock, 2005; Thompson and Dunne, 2004).

Pharmacodynamics NSAIDs

Under normal circumstances, following tissue damage as a result of trauma or infection, COX1 and COX2 convert arachidonic acid into prostaglandins and thromboxanes (Figure 9.1). Many of these prostaglandins stimulate central and peripheral nociceptors (pain receptors). These prostaglandins contribute to the acute inflammatory response by producing vasodilation, making the blood vessels more porous and reducing the ability of platelets to aggregate; the thromboxanes have the reverse effect. The non-selective NSAIDs (e.g. ibuprofen, naproxen) block both COX1 and COX2, while the selective COX2 inhibitors (e.g. eterocoxib) block only COX2. The selective NSAIDs spare the COX1 isoenzyme and its effect on the stomach.

Personal and professional development 9.4

From the information given previously, identify what the implications could have been for Mrs Stewart taking NSAIDs.

The effects of non-selective NSAIDs lead to an increase in acid secretion in the stomach, with the risk of gastritis and formation of gastric ulcers. The development of gastric ulcers frequently results from an infection with *Helicobacter pylori*, and this may make some people taking NSAIDs more vulnerable to gastric ulcers. The newer NSAIDs, such as etoricoxib, selectively inhibit the production of COX2 isoenzymes, therefore protecting the stomach. However, COX2 inhibitors seem to increase the risk

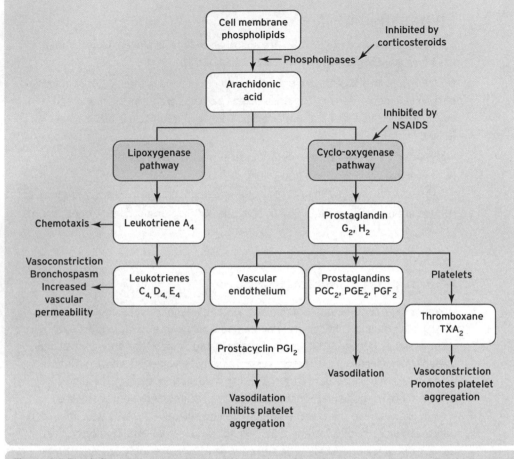

Figure 9.1 The inflammatory process and the action of corticosteroids and non-steroidal anti-inflammatory drugs (after Mera, 1997)

of the patient developing coronary heart disease and stroke, and some COX2 inhibitors have been withdrawn from use or are no longer prescribed for vulnerable people (**www.bnf.org.uk**; NICE, 2007a). Kearney and colleagues (2006) suggest the picture may be more complex than this: it could be that this risk is present with all NSAIDs, but the earlier medicines have simply not been subjected to the same scrutiny as the newer NSAIDs. It should also be remembered that rheumatoid arthritis is a significant risk factor for coronary heart disease (Goodson *et al.*, 2002).

A further effect of NSAIDs is the reduction in renal blood flow, and infrequently renal failure can be accelerated in people with heart failure, liver cirrhosis, existing renal disease, or in those people who take diuretics (**www.bnf.org.uk**). The blood clotting mechanism is affected by NSAIDs, increasing bleeding time.

Aspirin

Although aspirin is rarely prescribed for its analgesic properties nowadays, it has been used in the management of rheumatoid arthritis and a number of other inflammatory diseases for almost 100 years (**www.aspirin-foundation.com/what/100.html**). As well as its anti-inflammatory action, aspirin also has an antipyretic effect, although this is seen only in people with a raised body temperature; aspirin has little effect on normal body temperature (Greenstein and Gould, 2004). Aspirin has been available over the counter for many years, and consequently many people use it for the relief of mild to moderate pain. However, its popularity as an analgesic has been hindered by its side effects. Its chief side effect is gastrointestinal irritation, but it may also cause hyper-sensitivity reactions in some individuals and increases the time it takes for the blood to clot. In addition, if taken in high doses, aspirin can stimulate the middle ear via the VIII cranial nerve, producing tinnitus, deafness, dizziness and vomiting.

In children, aspirin can have devastating effects on the brain (Reye's syndrome); conse-quently, it is now recommended that it is not used in children under the age of 16 years (**www.bnf.org.uk**). Since October 2003, the MHRA (2003) suggests that products contain-ing aspirin should carry a caution alert on the label advising not to give aspirin to children under the age of 16 years, except on the advice of a doctor.

The BNF states that GP prescribing of aspirin is much less common than previously, with many GPs preferring to prescribe what are seen as safer alternatives – other NSAIDs.

Intrestingly, some of the disadvantages of aspirin are being used intentionally. The effect of aspirin on preventing the production of thromboxane, and thus inhibiting the clotting process, has changed the treatment and prevention of a number of diseases. Aspirin is now recommended and used routinely to both treat and prevent coronary heart disease and stroke (DH, 2000; NICE, 2001); in addition, research studies are begin-ning to suggest that aspirin may be effective in preventing such diverse problems as bowel cancer, fetal growth retardation, pre-eclampsia, dementia, and the retinopathy and nephropathy of diabetes mellitus (**www.aspirin-foundation.com/what/100.html**).

Despite being used for over 100 years, it was discovered only relatively recently that aspirin is an NSAID. It was also thought until relatively recently that the anti-inflamma-tory properties of the NSAIDs made them the ideal choice as a first-line treatment for the inflammation caused by rheumatoid arthritis. There was an understanding that rheumatoid arthritis was a progressive disease in which the inflammatory process slowly destroyed the synovial membranes of the affected joints. However, it has become evident that the process of inflammation causes most damage within the first few months of the first presentation of the disease. Consequently, the traditional approach of initially prescribing the least toxic drugs and proceeding to the most toxic has been turned on its head (Panayi, 2006).

Nursing implications

It is important to ensure that people on non-selective COX NSAIDs (e.g. naproxen, ibuprofen) take them with food or a glass of milk and take small, frequent meals in an attempt to protect the stomach from the risk of irritation and ulceration.

Corticosteroids

As we mentioned earlier, Mrs Stewart took large doses of prednisolone for a number of years. When she was taking this medicine, she felt that it managed her symptoms more successfully than any of the other medicines she had tried.

Prednisolone is a synthetic glucocorticoid. It belongs to a group of drugs classified as the corticosteroids. Prednisolone can be administered by a variety of routes to treat rheumatoid arthritis – orally, intravenously, intramuscularly, intra-articularly and injected directly into soft tissue; however, like most medicines that have to be taken on a long-term basis, most commonly prednisolone is administered orally. It is available in plain and enteric-coated forms.

Sometimes the corticosteroids are referred to as adrenocorticosteroids. This name is technically more accurate, as it refers to where these hormones are produced: they are secreted by the cortex of the adrenal glands. The term 'corticosteroids' is the collective name given to a group of naturally occurring hormones produced by the body to maintain homeostasis and to aid the body in times of stress.

In reality

In day-to-day practice, many clinicians and patients use the term 'steroids' to refer to these hormones.

Personal and professional development 9.6

Reflect on your knowledge and understanding of the adrenal glands. Do you need to develop your understanding of the anatomy and physiology of the adrenal glands in order to explain their position and function to Mrs Stewart?

As with all hormones, the body's output of corticosteroids varies. In order to maintain homeostasis, blood levels are monitored by the body and maintained at the appropriate level by adrenocorticotropic hormone (ACTH) produced by the anterior lobe of the pituitary gland. This in turn is controlled by ACTH-releasing factor produced in the hypothalamus.

Three types of corticosteroid hormone are secreted by the adrenal cortex:

- *Glucocorticoids*: These hormones, e.g. hydrocortisone, affect protein and carbohydrate metabolism. They act in response to the increased metabolic demand of the body as a result of stress or injury.
- *Mineralocorticoids*: These hormones, e.g. aldosterone, affect the body's ability to maintain fluid and electrolyte balance, thus safeguarding sodium homeostasis.
- *Androgens*: The male sex hormones, including testosterone, are produced in small amounts in both males and females.

The corticosteroids are used mainly to treat allergic and inflammatory conditions, such as asthma, but they can also be given as replacement therapy. A classic example is the use of hydrocortisone in the treatment of Addison's disease, in which the adrenal cortex is unable to secrete the hormones that the body needs. The effects of the corticosteroids on the immune system mean that corticosteroids are also used as part of the anti-rejection therapy given following organ transplantation.

The corticosteroids are available in synthetic form, for example, hydrocortisone, betamethasone, prednisolone and dexamethasone. They are available for oral use, for injection via various routes (for example, intravenous, intra-articular), for rectal use and for topical application.

Pharmacokinetics Corticosteroids

Absorption: Oral glucocorticoids are well absorbed. When given intramuscularly, glucocorticoids are completely absorbed (**www.bnf.org.uk**; Greenstein and Gould, 2004; McGavock, 2005; Rang *et al.*, 2003; Simonsen *et al.*, 2006).

Distribution: Corticosteroids are bound to the plasma proteins and are therefore distributed via the bloodstream.

▶

▶ *(continued)*

Metabolism: Corticosteroids are metabolised by the liver. If the liver is not working to its full potential, e.g. in older people and in people with liver failure, the blood levels of corticosteroids can be markedly increased. Conversely, corticosteroids will be less efficient if drugs that affect the production of liver enzymes (e.g. phenytoin) are taken at the same time (**www.bnf.org.uk**).

Elimination: The glucocorticoids are excreted by the kidneys.

Pharmacodynamics Corticosteroids

The corticosteroids have complex actions on the inflammatory response and the immune response. They prevent leucocytes (white blood cells) moving to the location of the inflammation and interfere with the function of leucocytes, fibroblasts and endothelial cells. Almost all body cells have numerous corticosteroid receptors. The corticosteroids bind to receptors. Prednisolone, a glucocorticoid ligand, attaches to receptors on the cell surface and moves through the cell into the cell's nucleus. Once in the cell's nucleus, prednisolone attaches to glucocorticoid receptors and blocks the production of arachidonic acid in the cell, therefore preventing the production of cytokines, and as a result, the production of prostaglandins and thromboxanes. Consequently, regardless of the route of administration of prednisolone, its effects are felt across the whole body, and it affects all of the organs and the metabolic pathways.

Prednisolone and the other glucocorticoids have anti-inflammatory, metabolic and immunosuppressant effects on the body (Table 9.3). At times of physical or emotional stress, the production of glucocorticoids increases in order to meet the increased demands of the body.

Essential terminology

Receptors

Sites found on all cells where chemicals can attach and affect the way the cell works.

Ligand

Chemical that attaches to a particular cell receptor site and alters the functioning of the cell.

Table 9.3 Metabolic and immunosuppressant effects of prednisolone

Metabolic effects	Immunosuppressant effects
Increase the rate at which proteins are broken down into amino acids, consequently increasing gluconeogenesis in the liver	Moderate the production of eosinophils (type of white blood cell)
Speed up fat breakdown and initiate the metabolism of fat before that of carbohydrate, leading to increased plasma glucose levels	Instigate the atrophy of lymphatic tissues
Redistribution of body fat as a result of increased lypolytic (fat breakdown) activity	Decrease the production of lymphocytes and plasma cells
Increase the breakdown of muscle tissue, leading to loss of muscle mass	Reduce the production of histamine by mast cells

Essential terminology

Gluconeogenesis
Production of glucose from non-carbohydrates, e.g. fats and amino acids. Occurs most commonly in the liver.

Personal and professional development 9.7 The nurse's role

Using this information, write short notes about the conclusions that can be drawn from the pharmacokinetics and pharmacodynamics information given above.

Like all drugs, prednisolone and the other glucocorticoids have benefits as well as undesirable, or adverse, effects. The benefits include increased wellbeing, increased appetite, and reduction of inflammation and associated problems. For Mrs Stewart, this meant that her joint pain and swelling was much improved, leading to a better quality of life; she was pain-free and more mobile.

Personal and professional development 9.8

The benefits of increased wellbeing and increased appetite have the potential to become a disadvantage for Mrs Stewart. Write short notes about why this might be and identify the nurse's role in this situation.

For Mrs Stewart, after many years of pain and fatigue, and the inability to care for herself fully or to fulfil her roles within her family, feeling well may lead to her enjoying her food more and taking more of an interest in food. She may have started to eat more than she normally did. Her increased appetite may have encouraged her to eat more to appease it. The result of this could be that Mrs Stewart quickly began to put on weight. If she were underweight, this would be an advantage, as it would enable her to reach a more healthy weight; but if her body mass index (weight in relation to height) rose so much that she became overweight, this would compromise her joints and her mobility (**www.food.gov.uk**).

Taking large doses of corticosteroids for many years can have disadvantages, some of which Mrs Stewart is seeing now. The adverse effects of prednisolone and the other glucocorticoids tend to be seen more commonly as a result of high doses taken over long periods of time, and can include:

- osteoporosis;
- atrophy of the adrenal cortex;
- Cushing's syndrome;
- diabetes;
- immunosuppression;
- peptic ulceration;
- impaired wound healing;
- mental instability;
- cataracts (**www.bnf.org.uk**; Rang *et al.*, 2003; Simonsen *et al.*, 2006).

Mrs Stewart took large doses of prednisolone for a long period of time and as a result could be experiencing some of the disadvantages of the prolonged use of corticosteroids. Corticosteroids can increase the physiological effects, which can produce effects linked to both the mineralocorticoid and the glucocorticoid activity.

One of the other, sometimes very distressing, side effects for patients such as Mrs Stewart is the possible development of features similar to those of Cushing's syndrome. This is recognised by a typical appearance of: 'moon' face, **striae**, **hirsutism**, muscle **atrophy**, bruising, oedema and acne. When the corticosteroids are stopped, these altered features usually resolve (**www.bnf.org**).

Essential terminology

Striae
Silvery marks on the abdomen and upper legs.

Hirsutism
Widespread hairiness.

Atrophy
Wasting away.

Personal and professional development 9.9

Write short notes to explain what you would be looking for to suggest that Mrs Stewart has experienced mineralocorticoid side effects from taking long-term prednisolone.

Nursing implications

As both the NSAIDs and the glucocorticoids bind to plasma proteins, it is imperative that Mrs Stewart has sufficient plasma proteins in the bloodstream; therefore, it is important to ensure that Mrs Stewart is not undernourished. If she is undernourished then it is likely that she has insufficient circulating plasma proteins. If Mrs Stewart is undernourished, the nurse needs to encourage her to eat a healthy high-protein diet in order to restore her blood levels to normal. This would be an opportunity to explore her diet more fully. The nurse would also consider whether Mrs Stewart needs to be referred to a dietitian.

Glucocorticoids mask the clinical features of infection, which may become serious before it is recognised. Therefore, whenever possible it is advisable for patients on these drugs to avoid situations where there may be exposure to infection. As a result, Mrs Stewart is advised to consider carefully the implications of being in poorly ventilated, overcrowded environments, or being exposed to children with infections. The nurse should also ensure that Mrs Stewart understands the importance of washing her hands regularly.

Personal and professional development 9.10

Write short notes to help you explain to Mrs Stewart why she should carry a steroid treatment card when she is taking large doses of corticosteroids.

Taking high-dosage, long-term corticosteroids leads to atrophy of the adrenal cortex, which may take a number of years to return to normal once the medication is stopped. The impact of this is that when the body needs an increased supply of corticosteroids, over and above that provided by the medication, the adrenal cortex is unable to comply. If during this time the patient has another major illness, suffers notable trauma or has to have surgery, this will put extra demand on the adrenal cortex to produce more hormones; the adrenal cortex will be unable to respond appropriately, and so the patient will need a temporary increase in the dosage of corticosteroid or if the patient has recently stopped medication, a temporary course of corticosteroid treatment (**www.bnf.org.uk**). Steroid treatments cards are available from the DH and should be carried by patients taking steroids for more than three weeks. The card identifies the steroid(s) that the patient is prescribed.

Pharmacological knowledge Disease-modifying anti-rheumatic drugs (DMARDs)

While the NSAIDs and glucocorticoids control the clinical features of rheumatoid arthritis, the disease-modifying anti-rheumatic drugs (DMARDs) affect the progression of the disease itself. DMARDs are very slow-acting and frequently take months to show any effect. DMARDs include gold, hydroxychloroquine, leflunomide, penicillamine, sulfasalazine and the immunosuppressants (e.g. methotrexate).

Infliximab

Infliximab, a monoclonal antibody, is a recently introduced anti-TNF drug. These drugs are also referred to as 'biologic therapies', as they have been developed from substances found in the human immune system. They are genetically engineered antibodies that recognise and lock onto specific cell proteins, thus triggering the body's immune system. They are used in the treatment of rheumatoid arthritis and other autoimmune inflammatory diseases (e.g. Crohn's disease) as they interfere with the inflammatory process. Monoclonal antibodies are also used in the treatment of cancer. They work by deactivating the cytokine TNF-α found in the joints of people with rheumatoid arthritis. TNF-α is a major element of the immune response, and consequently deactivation of it reduces the immune response. This can have positive benefits, as it has for Mrs Stewart, but it also means that the normal defence mechanism to infection is seriously reduced.

Infliximab is an antibody to TNF-α; it binds to TNF-α and consequently renders it inactive. It is therefore referred to as a TNF-α blocker. Infliximab is a protein; if taken orally, it would be digested in the stomach, and so it is given by injection. Mrs Stewart had intravenous injections, which were administered by a rheumatology nurse specialist, while she was a day patient at the local rheumatology unit. As infliximab is a relatively new drug, the long-term implications for Mrs Stewart are not yet fully known. The drug seems to have little effect on normal body cells other than reducing the number of antibodies, but it must be remembered that there is still little long-term evidence on the use of infliximab. The BNF states that early clinical trials have identified some of the adverse effects of the drug as rash and fever. This supports the evidence collated by Ledingham and Deighton (2005), which identifies the major risk of the TNF-α blockers as infection.

Personal and professional development 9.11

Think about how comfortable you would feel explaining to Mrs Stewart what a monoclonal antibody is. If you feel that you need to know more, John W Kimball's online biology textbook is a useful resource (**http://users.rcn.com/ jkimball.ma.ultranet/BiologyPages/M/Monoclonals.html**).

In reality

People who have rheumatoid arthritis and healthcare professionals may not always look for the same things when evaluating the effectiveness of treatment. Healthcare professionals tend to be focused on the physiological effects and the damage to the joints, while patients with the disease may focus on the impact of both the disease and the treatment on their life and relationships (Ledingham and Deighton, 2005). Perhaps, as Pearson (2006) suggests, this 'is because for centuries health care professionals have attempted to understand sickness and disease in order to prevent, cure or control it.' It could be argued that this reflects the subjective stance of the patient and the more objective stance of the healthcare professional. However, this indicates the importance of the practitioners listening carefully to the patient's comments about their pain, disability and fatigue in relation to their disease and treatment. Rheumatology services are beginning to recognise this, and guidelines now suggest that they do this in a more meaningful way than previously (Luqmani *et al.*, 2006). To do this needs a team of healthcare professionals and the patient to work together collaboratively to best manage the patient's treatment and care (Ledingham and Deighton, 2005).

Personal and professional development 9.12

Write a list of the members of the multidisciplinary team who may be involved in helping Mrs Stewart have a better quality of life.

Depending on the degree of disability and the social support available, a large number of healthcare professionals may be involved in the care and support of a person with rheumatoid arthritis. The multidisciplinary team could include the occupational therapist, physiotherapist, GP, rheumatologist, rheumatology specialist nurse, podiatrist, social worker, community psychiatric nurse and psychiatrist.

Complementary Medicinal Products

Mrs Stewart is not alone in using complementary and alternative therapies alongside conventional medicine. When chronic symptoms are not relieved and have a marked impact on the person's life, they may choose to explore other means of treatment than conventional medicine. Using complementary and alternative therapies gives the person easier access to treatments, restoring their sense of independence. However, the evidence for the efficacy of complementary medicinal products in the treatment of rheumatoid arthritis is rather limited.

Mrs Stewart has tried a variety of complementary and alternative therapies, including massage, aromatherapy and the herbal medicine gamma-linolenic acid (GLA). GLA can be bought over the counter. A Cochrane systematic review stated that it had 'some potential benefit although further studies are required to establish optimum dosage and duration of treatment' (Little and Parsons, 2006).

Mrs Ishbael Stewart

About 3 months ago, while walking to a taxi outside her son's front door, Mrs Stewart slipped and fell on some ice. As a result, she sustained a right Colles' fracture, fractured ribs and a fractured right temporal bone. At the time, there were concerns that Mrs Stewart may have extensive osteoporosis. Following dual-energy X-ray absorptiometry (DEXA) scans to measure the density of her bone structure, this was confirmed. Mrs Stewart is anxious about how this will further impact on her life. Her youngest son and his wife had their first child the day before her accident. Mrs Stewart is upset that she has been unable to be a 'proper grandmother' to Ami-Louise, her first grandchild. She had previously thought that, as her arthritic symptoms had improved and she felt so well, she may be able to help with the care of Ami-Louise, as she has never come to terms with doing so little hands-on parenting with her own children because of her disability, deformities, pain and fatigue. The fall has shaken her rather fragile self-confidence and self-esteem much more than she would care to admit. Mrs Stewart has now begun to take alendronic acid.

> ### Personal and professional development 9.13
>
> Consider what you know about osteoporosis, referring to the case study about Mrs Stewart. Write a list of the possible reasons that may have led to Mrs Stewart developing osteoporosis.

From Mrs Stewart's history, you can see that she has a number of risk factors that have led to her developing osteoporosis. One of the major risk factors for her has been having rheumatoid arthritis since she was a young woman. It is likely that this meant her activity levels have been low. Consequently, she has done little high-impact exercise, such as walking, to stimulate bone growth and ensure strong healthy bones into late adulthood (**www.nos.org.uk**; Phillips *et al.*, 2001). The other risk factors include taking long-term, high-dose corticosteroids, smoking and (at 48 years) being menopausal.

THE NATURE OF OSTEOPOROSIS

The word 'osteoporosis' means porous bones. Unfortunately, it is usually **asymptomatic** until either the patient fractures a bone or a kyphosis of the vertebral column develops. Healthy bone is hard and impermeable, but it is not an inert structure. Healthy bones actively accumulate calcium, which is then available for the body to use in a complex range of metabolic activities, such as blood clotting, conduction of nerve impulses and the contraction of muscle (Mera, 1997). In order to maintain these metabolic activities, the body needs a constant supply of calcium. If such a supply is not provided by dietary means, healthy bones can provide calcium. Thus, healthy bones act like a reservoir for calcium, storing it when blood levels are high and releasing it when blood levels are low. Specialised cells known as osteoblasts carry out bone synthesis, which is why they are often referred to as 'bone builders'. Bone resorption is the role of other cells called osteoclasts.

> **Essential terminology**
>
> **Asymptomatic**
> Without any symptoms; as a result, the affected person does not feel any different from normal.

Osteoporosis is the most common metabolic bone disease. It affects more women than men because of the lack of oestrogen production that occurs in postmenopausal women. Osteoporosis causes the normally hard bone to become spongy and weak.

Bone demineralisation increases as we age and is why many people lose height and become shorter as they get older. This loss of calcium and other minerals eventually leads to changes in the bone structure such that the bones become less dense (low density). Osteoporosis occurs when this demineralisation of the bones occurs more severely than would normally be expected. Consequently, the bones of the affected person become softer and spongy and are much more brittle than healthy bone. As a result, the bones fracture more easily. In osteoporosis, this demineralisation process affects all bones in the skeleton, but fractures are seen most commonly in the forearm, hip and spine.

> **Personal and professional development 9.14**
>
> Write short notes about three of the key points relating to the development of osteoporosis. You should feel comfortable using these notes to explain to Mrs Stewart why she has osteoporosis.

Helping Mrs Stewart understand why she has osteoporosis will help her to appreciate how she can try to prevent the problem getting worse. The health-promotion information that the nurse offers should include a discussion of long-term oral corticosteroids, smoking, low body weight, excess alcohol intake, lack of physical activity, family history of osteoporosis, early menopause, postmenopause and vitamin D deficiency.

Nursing knowledge Supporting strategies

Heath promotion for Mrs Stewart should include information about diet, exercise, rest, pacing, alcohol consumption and her current medication. However, it should be borne in mind that given the long-term impact of rheumatoid arthritis on Mrs Stewart's ability to take conventional weightbearing exercise to ensure healthy bones (**www.nos.org.uk**) she needs to be referred to a physiotherapist who can work closely with her in order to maximise her abilities.

PHARMACOLOGICAL TREATMENTS USED TO MANAGE OSTEOPOROSIS

Alendronic acid

Alendronic acid (alendronate) is one of the group of medicines known as bisphosphonates. They are available in tablet form and can be prescribed to be taken daily, weekly or monthly. Bisphosphonates are non-hormonal. They act by inhibiting the activity of osteoclasts (therefore preventing bone reabsorption) and stimulating osteoblasts to synthesise bone more swiftly (therefore slowing down the rate of bone loss). As a result, the bisphosphonates improve bone density and reduce the risk of further fractures (**www.bnf.org.uk**; Libermann et al., 1995; Lindsay et al., 1999; Simonsen et al., 2006).

The major side effect of the bisphosphonates is irritation of the oesophagus, leading to inflammation and ulceration. As a result, the treatment instructions regarding these medicines can appear extremely complicated; it has been suggested that this is one reason why many women with osteoporosis fail to comply with treatment (Cooper et al., 2006; NICE, 2007a). Alendronic acid is effective only if it is taken on an empty stomach; therefore, it has to be taken at least half an hour before the first food or drink of the day. The tablets must be swallowed whole with at least 200 ml of plain water. The individual must then stay upright for at least 30 minutes after taking the medication; the person may sit, walk or stand during this time, but not bend or lie down. Some forms of the medicine are taken only weekly, although this is be seen as a disadvantage by some patients as they forget to take it.

Personal and professional development 9.15

Consider your activities first thing in the morning. How easy would it be for you to not bend over in any way for at least 30 minutes and not to eat or drink for 30 minutes first thing in the morning? Identify some strategies that would help you do this.

Nursing knowledge Health promotion strategies

It is important when giving medication advice to Mrs Stewart that it is done in such a way that she understands the potential impact of having to stay upright when swallowing and for a minimum of 30 minutes after taking her medication. Helping her to think about how she and her family could reorganise her morning may help her to prevent potential side effects and continue to take her medication.

Pharmacological knowledge Other medication

Raloxifene belongs to the group of drugs known as selective oestrogen receptor modulators (SERMs). These are antagonists and block the action of oestrogen in a number of tissues, including breast tissue; they do not affect all tissue in the same way, however, as they are selective. Raloxifene acts as an anti-bone-resorptive agent and is usually well tolerated. It has some side effects, but these are usually mild and include leg cramps and swelling of the hands and feet. Because of the slightly increased risk of venous thromboembolism (blood clotting) with raloxifene, it is contraindicated (not to be given to) in women with a past history of venous thromboembolism (**www.bnf.org.uk**).

Hormone replacement therapy of oestrogen and (in women with an intact uterus) progesterone prevents postmenopausal bone loss, but its continued use is controversial as it has been implicated in increasing the risk of breast cancer and stroke (**www.bnf.org**; Rang *et al.*, 2003; Simonsen *et al.*, 2006).

Strontium ranelate, unlike the bisphosphates, is designed to be taken before bed. It suppresses osteoclasts and stimulates osteoblasts, thus replicating normal bone turnover more closely by increasing bone formation and decreasing bone reabsorption. This results in an increase in bone mass and bone mineral density. Adverse effects include nausea and diarrhoea, but these are usually mild and transient (**www.bnf.org.uk; www.emc-medicines.co.uk**).

Calcium and vitamin D supplements may also be used, although the evidence of their effectiveness is contentious (**www.bnf.org.uk**; Rang *et al.*, 2003).

The NICE (2007a) guidelines support the use of bisphosphonates as first-line treatment of osteoporosis in postmenopausal woman. However, this has proved to be controversial and an appeal has been heard against the latest technology appraisal guidance.

The Appeals Committee upheld only one part of this appeal – to provide guidance when alendronate is 'contraindicated, poorly tolerated or ineffective' (NICE, 2007b). The new technology appraisal advice and the new guidelines are still being developed as the book goes to press. Public perceptions of NICE guideline decisions are frequently represented in the media as 'penny-pinching' and are often seen as a means of rationing the service provided by the NHS. Being able to explain such decisions to patients and their families can be problematic for nurses and other healthcare professionals. Community prescribing is also 'rationed' by the local primary care trust, which can reinforce the perception that whether a medicine is prescribed for a particular condition or not is a 'postcode lottery'.

As we have seen, many of the treatments that have been prescribed for Mrs Stewart have had advantages as well as disadvantages. Persisting with any treatment is often difficult, and it may be more so for people with long-term conditions, as their medicines may have to be taken for many years. It is usually possible for most people to persevere for a relatively short period of time with some of the disadvantages of medicines, but it becomes more difficult to maintain concordance in the long term.

Quick reminder

✔ Rheumatoid arthritis is a disorder caused by inflammation of the joints and characterised by severe pain, general debility and some degree of limited mobility, which can have a major impact on the affected person's lifestyle.

✔ Rheumatoid arthritis affects approximately 1% of the UK population and affects more women than men.

✔ Treatments for the disease have changed considerably relatively recently; for example, activity is now encouraged for affected people.

✔ Recommendations include that the affected person is referred to a specialist rheumatology service (rather than be treated by their GP), where a variety of specialists and contemporary interventions can be accessed.

✔ Many people with rheumatoid arthritis have been, or continue to be, treated with aspirin, other non-steroidal anti-inflammatory drugs (NSAIDs), corticosteroids and disease-modifying anti-rheumatic drugs (DMARDs). A number of people are still maintained on these traditional medicine regimes prescribed by their GP.

✔ Contemporary treatment for rheumatoid arthritis reverses this pattern and focuses first on using combination DMARD prescribing and biologic therapies to resolve the acute inflammatory process.

✔ Osteoporosis, another musculoskeletal disorder, changes the structure of the bones, making them brittle and more easily fractured. It affects both men and women but is more common in postmenopausal women. It can be prevented.

✔ Osteoporosis develops gradually and has no obvious symptoms, and so it is easily missed by both the patient and healthcare professionals.

✔ Prescribing and treatment frameworks, e.g. NICE guidelines, can be controversial and lead to demands for changes. Primary care trust prescribing budgets and spending are increasingly being challenged by patients and patient groups.

✔ Nurses at the 'front line' can be caught up in such challenges and so must be prepared for presenting professional and informed, rather than personal, opinions.

REFERENCES

Boon N A, Colledge N R, Walker B R and Hunter J A A (2006) *Davidson's Principles and Practice of Medicine*, 20th edn. Edinburgh: Churchill Livingstone Elsevier.

Cooper A, Drake J and Brankin E (2006) Treatment persistence with once monthly ibandronate and patient support vs. once weekly alendronate: results from the PERSIST study. *International Journal of Clinical Practice* **60**, 896–905.

Department of Health (DH) (2000) *Coronary Health Disease: National Service Framework for Coronary Heart Disease – Modern Standards and Service Models*. London: The Stationery Office.

Greenstein B and Gould D (2004) *Trounce's Clinical Pharmacology for Nurses*. Edinburgh: Churchill Livingstone.

Goodson N J, Wiles N J, Lun M, Barret E M, Silman A J and Symmons D P M (2002) Mortality in early inflammatory polyarthritis: cardiovascular mortality is increased in seropositive patients. *Arthritis Rheumatology* **46**, 2010–2019.

Kearney P M, Baigent C, Godwin J, Halls H, Emberson J R and Patrono C (2006) Do selective cyclo-oxygenase 2 inhibitors and traditional non-steroidal anti-inflammatory drugs increase the risk of atherothrombosis? Meta-analysis of randomised trials. *British Medical Journal* **332**, 1302–1308.

Ledingham J and Deighton C (2005) Update on the British Society for Rheumatology guidelines for prescribing TNF alpha blockers in adults with rheumatoid arthritis (update of previous guidelines of April 2001). *Rheumatology* **44**, 157–163.

Libermann U, Weiss S, Broll J, *et al.* (1995) Effects of alendronate on bone mineral density and the incidence of fractures in postmenopausal osteoporosis. The Alendronate Phase III Osteoporosis Treatment Study Group. *New England Journal of Medicine* **333**, 1437–1443.

Lindsay R, Cosman F, Lobo R A, Walsh B W, Harris S T, Reagan J E, Liss C L, Melton M E and Byrnes C A (1999) Addition of alendronate to ongoing hormone replacement therapy in the treatment of osteoporosis: a randomized, controlled clincial trial. *Journal of Clinical Endocrinology and Metabolism* **84**, 3076–3081.

Little C V and Parsons T (2006) Herbal therapy for treating rheumatoid arthritis. *Cochrane Database Systematic Review* (1), 2948.

Luqmani R, Hennell S, Estrach C, *et al.* (2006) British Society for Rheumatology and British health professionals in rheumatology guideline for the management of rheumatoid arthritis (the first two years). *Rheumatology* **45**, 1167–1169.

McGavock H (2005) *How Drugs Work: Basic Pharmacology for Healthcare Professionals*, 2nd edn. Oxford: Radcliffe Publishing.

Medical and Healthcare Products Regulatory Agency (MHRA) (2003) *Aspirin and Reye's Syndrome in the Under 16 Years*. London: Medical and Healthcare Products Regulatory Agency.

Mera S (1997) *Understanding Disease: Pathology and Prevention*. Cheltenham: Stanley Thornes.

National Institute for Health and Clinical Excellence (NICE) (2001) *Guidance on the Use of Cyclo-oxygenase (COX) 2 Selective Inhibitors Celecoxib, Rofecoxib, Meloxicam and Etolold for Osteoarthritis and Rheumatoid Arthritis*. London: National Institute for Health and Clinical Excellence.

National Institute for Health and Clinical Excellence (NICE) (2007) *Adalimumab, etanercept and infliximals for the treatment of rheumatoid arthritis*. Technology Appraisal 130. London: National Institute for Health and Clinical Excellence.

National Institute for Health and Clinical Excellence (NICE) (2007a) *Biphosphonates (Alendronate, Etidronate, Risedronate), Selective Oestrogen Receptor Modulators (Raloxifene) and Parathyroid Hormone (Teriparatide) for the Secondary Prevention of Osteoporotic Fragility Fractures in Postmenopausal Women*. Technology appraisal 87. London: National Institute for Health and Clinical Excellence.

National Institute for Health and Clinical Excellence (NICE) (2007b) *Osteoporosis: Secondary Prevention - Appeal Panel Letter*. London: National Institute for Health and Clinical Excellence.

Oliver S and Ryan S (2004) Effective pain management for patients with arthritis. *Nursing Standard* **18**, 43–52.

Panayi G (2006) *What is RA?* www.rheumatoid.org.uk/article.php?article_id=224&printer_friendly.

Pearson A (2006) Understanding the illness experience. *International Journal of Nursing Practice* **12**, 177.

Phillips J, Murray P and Kirk P (2001) *The Biology of Disease*, 2nd edn. Oxford: Blackwell Science.

Rang H P, Dale M M, Ritter J M and Moore P K (2003) *Pharmacology*, 5th edn. Edinburgh: Churchill Livingstone.

Simonsen T, Aarbakke J, Kay I, Coleman I, Sinnott P and Lysaa R (2006) *Illustrated Pharmacology for Nurses*. London: Hodder Arnold.

Thompson P W and Dunne C (2004) *Non-Steroidal Anti-Inflammatory Drugs: Use and Abuse*. Chesterfield: Arthritis Research Campaign.

Chapter 10

Coronary heart disease:
an adult male with hyperlipidaemia, who has an acute myocardial infarction and develops heart failure

Coronary heart disease (CHD) is a condition of the coronary blood vessels that supply the heart. It is the most common form of heart disease (**http://coronary heartdisease.org**). It is caused by a narrowing of the coronary arteries as a consequence of atheroma (fatty plaques) development. Much research has been, and is still being, undertaken to try to understand the causes of CHD. We are able to identify risk factors such as smoking and obesity (factors relating to lifestyle) and the presence of other conditions such as high blood pressure (hypertension). It is thought that many deaths related to CHD could be prevented by lifestyle changes.

This chapter introduces John Edmonds, a patient with CHD. The chapter discusses the key groups of medicines used to manage this condition. The specific medicines identified for the patient and the implications of this treatment for the patient will be discussed. The chapter provides some information to contextualise the treatment given to this patient.

✔ Learning outcomes

By the end of this chapter you should be able to:

✔ Give an overview of coronary heart disease

✔ Discuss the potential impact of coronary heart disease on an individual

✔ Identify pharmacological approaches used to manage coronary heart disease

✔ Discuss the actions and effects of statins, oxygen, diamorphine, aspirin, thrombolytics, metclopropamide, diuretics, ACE inhibitors and beta-blockers related to the specific patient scenario

✔ Identify nursing knowledge needed to manage this patient and his coronary heart disease

✔ Identify supporting nursing interventions for this patient.

Chapter at a glance

The nature of coronary heart disease
Pharmacological interventions used to manage hyperlipidaemia
The nature of myocardial infarction
Pharmacological interventions used to manage myocardial infarction
The nature of left ventricular failure and pulmonary oedema
Pharmacological interventions used to manage heart failure and
    pulmonary oedema
Discharge advice in relation to medication
Professional guidance
Compliance/adherence
Family involvement
Quick reminder
References

Mr John Edmonds

John Edmonds is a 44-year-old man employed as a drug company representative. He met his wife Tracy, a doctor's receptionist, during one of his visits to a local GP surgery.

He has a family history of coronary heart disease, and his GP wants to treat his raised cholesterol level with simvastatin 10 mg daily (at night) initially, to be reviewed in 4 weeks, in line with NICE guidelines.

John and Tracy have no children and have a busy social life. They both enjoy eating and drinking with friends, taking it in turns to play host at their houses. They see this as a much-needed stress reliever at the end of a busy working week.

John is reluctant to take his medication. He doesn't believe in thinking too much about the future, and he would rather live life to the full. With his insider knowledge, he is worried about experiencing ill-effects from the treatment.

THE NATURE OF CORONARY HEART DISEASE

The reduction of CHD is a major government priority. CHD is the single most common cause of premature death in the UK (DH, 2000):

It is a condition that makes a significant impact on every aspect of an individual's life including their quality of life, future employment and personal relationships as well as increasing their risk of dying early. Much can be done to reduce the suffering caused by CHD and to stop it developing in the first place.
(DH, 2000)

CHD is also referred to as coronary artery disease and ischaemic heart disease, both of which are useful descriptive terms to help us understand the disease. CHD is a disease that affects the coronary circulation, and as a consequence there is reduced blood flow to the heart, resulting in ischaemia.

Coronary heart disease describes the situation in which there is a build-up of **atheroma** within the coronary blood vessels. This atheroma is laid down within the lining of the arteries and results in plaque formation (Figure 10.1).

> ## Personal and professional development 10.1
> ### Related physiology
>
> You may wish to remind yourself of the functions of the heart and revise the pulmonary, systemic and coronary circulations in order to understand the implications of CHD for the patient.

Essential terminology

Atheroma
Fatty deposits in the walls of the arteries.

Hyperlipidaemia
Hyper – high; *lipid* – from the Greek word for 'fat'; *aemia* – 'in the blood'.

Hyperlipidaemia

Hyperlipidaemia is a continuously high concentration of lipids such as cholesterol in the bloodstream. Hyperlipidaemia produces atherosclerotic changes. This process can be triggered by the presence of conditions such as diabetes mellitus or by behaviour such as smoking, which over a period of time can cause damage to coronary blood vessels.

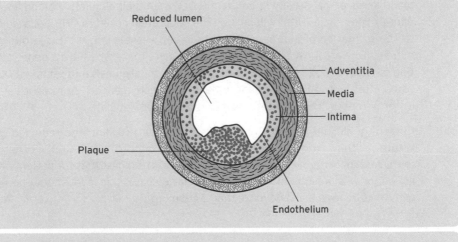

Figure 10.1 Atheroma

The first stage is the infiltration of lipids into the lining of the coronary arteries to form fatty streaks. This progresses into a thick fibrous plaque (atheroma), which hardens with time due to the presence of calcium (Phillipe and Whittaker, 2004). The impact upon the patient depends upon how much of the artery is occluded (narrowed); the patient may be unaware, be suffering from angina or develop a myocardial infarction (MI), which may be fatal, depending upon the extent of the damage to the heart muscle.

Cholesterol

A raised level of cholesterol in the bloodstream is a risk factor for the development of CHD. Treatment is directed towards reducing the intake of cholesterol in the diet and, where dietary change is not enough, the use of medication such as statins, which reduce the production of cholesterol in the body.

Cholesterol and triglycerides are fat-like substances (lipids) used by the body. Cholesterol is used to form cell membranes, some hormones and bile acids. Triglycerides are the body's main energy store. Although cholesterol is taken into the body in the diet (contained in animal fat, also referred to as saturated fat), it is also produced by the liver (biosynthesis). The liver uses an enzyme called 3-hydroxy-3-methylglutaryl coenzyme (HMG-CoA reductase) to synthesise (manufacture) cholesterol.

Cholesterol travels in the bloodstream using protein carriers; the combination of cholesterol and protein is called a lipoprotein. There are two main types of lipoprotein – low-density and high-density, which are 'in balance'. If an individual has high circulating blood levels of low-density lipoprotein (LDL), then their circulating blood levels of high-density lipoprotein (HDL) will be low. The lipoprotein linked to CHD because it can lead to the formation of plaques within the blood vessels is LDL. It is thought that the patients who are most at risk of heart disease are those who have a genetic predisposition to developing hyperlipidaemia – these people are unable to remove LDL from the blood effectively. HDL is thought to have a protective action – it removes surplus cholesterol from the cells and returns it to the liver for elimination.

Current guidelines (DH, 2000; Foxton *et al.*, 2004) recommend reducing cholesterol levels within the bloodstream to 5.0 mmol/l, although other sources (**www.lesscholesterol.co.uk**; Williams *et al.*, 2004) suggest that for patients with established, or with a high risk of, cardiovascular disease, this level should be 4.0 mmol/l, with the LDL level being no more than 2.0 mmol/l.

PHARMACOLOGICAL INTERVENTIONS USED TO MANAGE HYPERLIPIDAEMIA

Statins

Statins are recommended by the National Service Framework (NSF) for Coronary Heart Disease (DH, 2000) as the medication of choice to reduce circulating blood levels of LDL. Statins act by inhibiting the enzyme HMG-CoA reductase, used by the liver to produce cholesterol; this results in an increased clearance of LDL from the bloodstream, and therefore a reduction in LDL levels. Statins can reduce LDL by up to 60% (McTaggart, 2003). However, they do not 'cure' – that is, rectify the underlying cause of – lipidaemia and so statins and dietary modification need to be continued for an indefinite period. The choice of statin used is related to the individual patient's risk profile. One of the factors to be considered is the desired LDL level.

Mr Edmonds has been prescribed simvastatin 10 mg daily, to be taken at night. In this situation, the medicine has been prescribed to reduce Mr Edmonds' raised cholesterol and to prevent the further development of CHD.

Pharmacological knowledge Availability of drugs and medicines

The UK government has stated its aim to reduce CHD. Strategies include education targeted at people identified as at risk – that is, having a family history of the disease (DH, 2000). In tandem with this, the Medicines and Healthcare Products Regulatory Agency (MHRA) has approved an initiative for simvastatin 10 mg to be supplied by pharmacists, so this medicine is now available (in this small dose) over the counter. The MHRA is 'the goverment agency ... responsible for ensuring that medicines and medical devices work and are acceptably safe' (**www.mhra-gov.uk**).

Adverse effects of statins include gastrointestinal disturbance, tiredness, rashes and effects on the muscles, such as myalgia, muscle weakness, myositis (inflammation of the muscle) and rhabdomyolysis (severe myositis, which can lead to muscle break-down); effects such as rhabdomyolysis are extremely rare (**www.bnf.org**). The adverse effects of statins are frequently related to the dose given. It is important, given the role of the liver in cholesterol synthesis, that liver function tests (LFTs) are undertaken before treatment, and at intervals following the introduction of statins. Statins are contraindicated in patients with liver disease.

It is recommended that statins are given at night because this is when cholesterol synthesis predominantly takes place; however, newer statins, such as rosuvastatin, can be given at any time, as they have a longer half-life (Foxton *et al.*, 2004).

Greenstein and Gould (2004) suggest that statins are the most valuable of the lipid-lowering medicines; other medicines include:

- *Bile acid-binding resins*: These medicines combine with bile acids and cholesterol, inhibiting absorption of cholesterol and promoting the conversion of cholesterol to bile acids. This results in an increase in the excretion of bile acids via the faecal route. This further results in the conversion of cholesterol to bile acids in the liver, ultimately leading to reduced cholesterol levels.
- *Fibrates*: These medicines increase the number of LDL receptors in the liver, altering the metabolism of lipoproteins, which results in lower LDL and triglycerides in the bloodstream.
- *Nicotinic acid*: This medicine inhibits fatty acid release from fat cells in the body, reducing the production and levels of LDL and raising levels of HDL (Foxton *et al.*, 2004; **www.bnf.org**)

In reality

Until recently, it was thought that statins could not reverse atheroma, but could prevent further build-up and therefore limit progression of the disease. However, a recent report (**http://newsbbc.co.uk**) has stated that 'intensive' treatment with statins could reverse the development of atheroma. If you wish to read more about this, see Nissen *et al.* (2004).

Nursing knowledge Patient education

Mr Edmonds is reluctant to alter his lifestyle and worries about the side effects of medicines. He should be given the following information to help him get the maximum benefit from his treatment with simvastatin:

- He should be advised to follow a cholesterol-lowering diet.
- It is important for him to take the treatment because of his family history.
- Alcohol is not recommended.
- Regular blood tests are required so that the doctor can monitor the effectiveness of the treatment.
- Simvastatin has relatively few side effects; the most common are flatulence, headache and muscle ache.
- Any muscle pain should be reported immediately to the doctor.
- Grapefruit juice should be avoided, as it alters the metabolism of simvastatin.
- The tablets can be taken with or without food.

Pharmacokinetics Simvastatin

Absorption: Well absorbed; it undergoes extensive first pass effect. Maximum plasma concentration of the active drug is reached approximately 1–2 hours after administration. Food does not affect absorption.

Distribution: 95% protein-bound.

Metabolism: The half-life of the drug is approximately 2 hours.

Elimination: Excreted mainly via the faeces.

Essential terminology

Atherosclerosis
Thickening and hardening of the coronary arteries associated with patchy deposits of fat.

Unfortunately, many people are unaware that they have coronary heart disease until they suffer from its consequences. Coronary heart disease can result in atherosclerosis, angina pectoris, myocardial infarction and sudden death.

Mr John Edmonds

Mr Edmonds is admitted at 2 a.m. to the coronary care unit. He awoke with severe central chest pain and was very distressed. Tracy immediately called an ambulance, which took him to the local accident and emergency department. He was assessed quickly and given diamorphine 5 mg intravenously (for pain relief) with metclopropamide 10 mg, which has made him more comfortable.

After being seen by the doctor, and a provisional diagnosis of MI being made, he is given another dose of diamorphine 2.5 mg intravenously and assessed for thrombolysis using the thrombolysis algorithm. It is decided that Mr Edmonds is a suitable candidate for thrombolysis. He is given a dose of dispersable aspirin 300 mg, followed by reteplase intravenously.

THE NATURE OF MYOCARDIAL INFARCTION

NICE (2002) claims that about 240 000 people in England and Wales suffer an MI each year and that 50% of these die as a consequence within 30 days.

Myocardial infarction is defined by Alexander *et al.* (2006) as 'the death or necrosis of a portion of myocardium as a result of reduction, interruption or cessation of blood flow'. They state that most acute MIs are the result of 'total occlusion of a coronary artery by a thrombus'. The thrombus (stationary clot) occurs as a consequence of a series of events. First, platelets break up as they pass over a damaged area in the lining of a blood vessel (in this case, usually as a result of plaque rupture), releasing platelet factors. One result of this is that the platelets start to adhere to the damaged area. The increasing local number of platelets causes the increased platelet factors to combine with prothrombin and other substances such as calcium, resulting in the formation of thrombin. Thrombin reacts with fibrinogen and becomes fibrin (a thread-like structure/web) (Thibodeau, 2003).

The classic picture of a person suffering an MI is the experience of severe and sudden central chest pain, usually when the patient is at rest (caused by the myocardial ischaemia), associated with fear, shock, dyspnoea, cyanosis and nausea.

Depending upon the size and position of the damaged myocardial tissue, the patient may experience a cardiac arrest, unstable heart rhythm or heart failure, or go on to have a further MI. Consequently, early assessment and treatment are vital. To confirm his diagnosis, Mr Edmonds' history will be recorded; to establish the characteristics of the chest pain, an electrocardiograph (ECG) will be recorded (damage to the myocardium, depending upon the site, may be visible on the ECG, such as changes to the ST segment and T waves); and blood samples will be taken in order to identify the presence of cardiac enzymes such as troponin.

Personal and professional development 10.2
Related physiology

Remind yourself of the cardiac cycle and how this is represented as the QRST complex on an ECG recording.

Related knowledge Diagnostic tests

Cardiac enzymes

Troponin is the cardiac enzyme most commonly used to confirm diagnosis of MI because it can be identified early (i.e. within 4-6 hours) (Leahy, 2006).

Troponins are a family of proteins found in skeletal and heart muscle, which, following damage, are released into the bloodstream. Troponin I is specific to heart muscle.

PHARMACOLOGICAL INTERVENTIONS USED TO MANAGE MYOCARDIAL INFARCTION

The aims of nursing interventions and treatment following MI are to:

- reduce mortality;
- limit the extent of the MI;
- reperfuse the myocardium in order to limit morbidity;
- provide support.

This is managed pharmacologically by the administration of oxygen, analgesia and thrombolytics.

Supportive treatments

In MI, the heart muscle is deprived of its circulation and, therefore, oxygen. This results in the oxygen reserves within the myocardium being depleted quickly. The consequences of this are that the contractility of the heart is affected, reducing cardiac function, and electrolyte imbalances may occur.

Oxygen

The DH (2000) recommends the administration of oxygen. There are three key reasons for this.

- *To reduce the work of the heart*: Cardiac contraction is affected by the availability of oxygen treating the hypoxia will decrease the effort of breathing and stress on the myocardium.
- *To relieve tissue hypoxia*: Reducing the ischaemia of the myocardium lowers the irritability of the myocardium, thus reducing the risk of arrhythmias (irregular, usually fast heart rate).
- *To relieve pain*: Cardiac ischaemia results in cardiac pain; giving the patient oxygen reduces this pain by reducing tissue hypoxia (Rang *et al.*, 2003).

Oxygen used in healthcare is described as a medical gas and, as such, requires a prescription. Wherever possible, the patient is assessed for lung function using the patient's history, X-ray and arterial blood gas analysis. Oxygen is given in a concentration higher than that found inspired air (21%). The concentration to be given and the means (mask, nasal cannula) are prescribed. Patients with impaired lung function should be prescribed only small doses of oxygen.

Personal and professional development 10.3
Applying information

The hypoxic drive is a form of respiratory drive in which the body uses oxygen chemoreceptors (cells or specialised sensory nerve endings that are able to respond to chemical stimuli such as oxygen levels in the blood) instead of carbon dioxide receptors to regulate the respiratory cycle. Normal inspiration is driven mostly by high levels of carbon dioxide in the bloodstream rather than low oxygen levels. An increase in carbon dioxide causes chemoreceptor reflexes to trigger an increase in respirations. However, where there are chronically high carbon dioxide levels in the blood, such as in patients with chronic chest disease, the body begins to rely more on the oxygen receptors and less on the carbon dioxide receptors. In this case, if there is an increase in oxygen levels (such as following prescribed oxygen therapy), the body decreases the respirations. This is why patients using the hypoxic drive should receive oxygen only in low concentrations and be monitored carefully. Nurses should observe the patient's respiratory rate and characteristics (e.g. shallow or laboured) and pulse oximetry (non-invasive way of measuring oxygen saturation).

In this situation, because Mr Edmonds has no history of pulmonary problems or disease, he can be given higher concentrations of oxygen (Worster, 2000).

Analgesia

Diamorphine

One of the priorities in the treatment of Mr Edmonds is to relieve his chest pain. The pain, particularly in this situation, is associated with anxiety, which, if not treated effectively, can increase myocardial demand and therefore make the situation worse. Diamorphine is the analgesia of choice (Alexander *et al.*, 2006).

Diamorphine is classified as an opioid analgesic. It is derived from morphine and acts in a similar way. It acts more rapidly and has a shorter duration of action than morphine (Greenstein and Gould, 2004).

Essential terminology

Agonist
Chemical substance/drug that produces an effect.

Antagonist
Chemical substance/drug that prevents an action from occurring.
An overview of agonists and antagonists is given in Chapter 4.

The nervous system produces endorphins and encephalins in response to pain. Their action is to inhibit the transmission and perception of pain by acting on opioid receptors within the central nervous system. The term 'opioid analgesics' is used to describe those medicines used for pain relief that produce morphine-like effects. It is thought that opioids exert their effects by binding with the body's opioid receptors. The opioids bind to many different types of receptor, hence their wide range of effects, including analgesia, sedation and pupillary constriction. Opioids with an agonist action at one type of receptor may also act as antagonists at other receptors and are blocked by antagonists such as naloxone (Rang *et al.*, 2003).

Opioid receptors are found mainly within the brain and spinal cord, but there is evidence to suggest that they are also are found in other areas of the body, such as peripheral nerves. The exact action of opioids is still not clearly understood. They are prescribed for acute and chronic pain and achieve their analgesic effects by exerting an anti-nociceptive action; that is, they interfere with the transmission of nociceptive impulses. Opioid analgesia is also discussed in other chapters, e.g. Chapter 7.

Nursing knowledge Pain

The classic definition of pain used in nursing is that offered by McCaffrey and Beebe (1994): 'Pain is whatever the experiencing person says it is and existing wherever he says it does'. This implies that pain is subjective. The International Association for the Study of Pain (Merskey and Bogduk, 1994) define pain as 'an unpleasant sensory and emotional experience associated with actual or potential tissue damage, or described in terms of such damage'.

Pain is thought to be transmitted by pain receptors in cutaneous and visceral tissues, referred to as nociceptors. Nociceptors respond to any type of stimulus that is strong enough to cause damage and are associated with acute pain.

Another reason why diamorphine is the medicine of choice for a patient with MI is related to its effect on the limbic system within the brain, which results in euphoria. Thus, the patient receiving diamorphine experiences pain relief associated with a sense of wellbeing. This effect should not be underestimated, as pain, particularly that associated with MI, provokes anxiety. The anxiety activates the sympathetic nervous system and has the potential to alter clotting, reduce the immune response and increase the heart rate (Frazier *et al.*, 2002). This in turn can make the pain perception worse, and so a vicious circle is set up. Like the pain experience, the euphoric effects of opioids vary, depending upon individual circumstances. There is also the possibility of sedation with opioids.

Adverse effects of opioids include respiratory depression, suppression of the cough reflex, nausea and vomiting, pupillary constriction, tolerance and dependence. It would be unusual for these effects to occur in Mr Edmonds' case, however, as they are more long-term effects and he is likely to require only one or two doses as he recovers from his MI. However, the patient may be concerned about the effect of diamorphine on the gastrointestinal tract: opioids often cause nausea, which is the reason for administering a concomitant dose of metoclopramide.

Nursing knowledge Quick reminder

Tolerance and dependence

Tolerance is used to describe the situation that occurs when increasing doses are required to produce an effect. This is often because the liver becomes more efficient at metabolising the medicine, so that the amount of medicine that survives its first pass through the liver is less.

Tolerance can be explained partly by downregulation (a decrease in the number of receptors to bind to the medicine). In relation to opioids, it is thought that the receptors become desensitised (Wickens, 2005).

Dependence may be physical or psychological dependence, such that withdrawal of the medicine results in physical symptoms or psychological craving, respectively.

Neither of these mechanisms is well understood. Tolerance does not automatically result in dependence, but there is a link between the two.

Nursing knowledge Nursing interventions

Because of the known side effects of opioids, we can anticipate the impact of these medicines and provide the patient with the following supportive measures;

- Provide information and support.
- Assess the patient's pain, and evaluate the effects of the analgesia.
- Observe for unwanted effects.
- Administer prescribed anti-emetics to combat the effects of nausea and vomiting.
- If the patient is going to have repeated doses, a stool softener and advice regarding diet and fluids are necessary.

Because John Edmonds is in severe acute pain, associated with anxiety, diamorphine is a good choice of analgesic. It is likely that his pain relief will be given by injection, preferably intravenously. The rationale for this is that he needs his pain relief quickly, and he will probably have some accompanying shock (see below), which will slow down absorption if the drug is given by the intramuscular route. The usual dose of diamorphine in MI is 5 mg followed by a further 2.5–5 mg if necessary by slow intravenous injection (1 mg/minute) (**www.bnf.org**).

Nursing knowledge Quick reminder – pathophysiology

Shock can be caused by many different situations, such as severe allergic reaction (anaphylactic shock), severe infection (septic shock), blood loss (hypovolaemic shock) and following MI because of reduced blood flow to the heart (cardiogenic shock). In all of these cases, the common feature is a reduction of blood supply and therefore a reduction of the supply of oxygen and nutrients to the vital organs, such as the brain, heart and kidneys, which may be damaged as a consequence. The body tries to maintain the circulation to these important organs and, as a consequence, other peripheral organs, such as the skin, show signs of reduced blood flow, for example pallor and being cool to the touch. There are degrees of shock, but early recognition and treatment are important in order to prevent it becoming a serious situation (Collins, 2000; Harrison and Daly, 2001).

Pharmacodynamics Diamorphine

Diamorphine is a narcotic analgesic obtained from opium. It acts upon the central nervous system, where it has a depressant effect, and on smooth muscle. It has some stimulatory action, which results in nausea and vomiting.

Pharmacokinetics Diamorphine

Absorption: Absorbed rapidly and completely, even when taken orally, although absorption from the gastrointestinal tract may be erratic.

Distribution: Diamorphine metabolites rapidly cross the blood-brain barrier.

Metabolism: Half-life of 2-3 minutes.

Elimination: Up to 80% of the dose is excreted in the urine within 24 hours (http://emc.medicines.org.uk).

Anti-emetics

Anti-emetic medicines are used to prevent or reduce nausea and vomiting. A wide range of anti-emetic medicines are available, and the choice of medicine is determined by the cause of the vomiting. Metoclopramide is prescribed for migraine. In the case of Mr Edmonds, metoclopramide is prescribed to counteract the effect of other medicines, such as diamorphine. Metoclopramide is also given with cytotoxic medicines. It is important that Mr Edmonds is given an anti-emetic to 'cover' the diamorphine, as he may be experiencing nausea and vomiting as a consequence of his MI (Hand, 2001a).

Metoclopramide

Metoclopramide is a dopamine receptor antagonist. Dopamine is a neurotransmitter found within the central nervous system and involved in the control of gastric motility. Dopamine receptor antagonists increase peristalsis. Metoclopramide has both local and central effects. It causes the stomach to empty more quickly but also acts on the vomiting centre. The drug improves the muscle tone in the intestinal tract, it exerts its effects by increasing the release of acetylcholine locally within the intestinal tract, increasing the tone in the lower osophagus. This improves gastric and duodenal emptying by increasing gastrointestinal motility. The gastro-oesophageal reflux is also reduced.

Metoclopramide may cause drowsiness, restlessness and diarrhoea. It can be administered by intramuscular or intravenous injection (slow, 1-2 minutes) up to three times daily.

Pharmacodynamics Metoclopramide

The action is associated closely with parasympathetic nervous control of the upper gastrointestinal tract and encourages normal peristaltic action.

Pharmacokinetics Metoclopramide

Metabolism: Metabolised by the liver

Elimination: Eliminated by the kidneys; patients with reduced renal function should start with a reduced dose.

Pharmacological knowledge Other anti-emetic medicines

Other groups of anti-emetics are classified as follows:

- Acetylcholine receptor antagonists (e.g. hyoscine) block the action of acetylcholine on the vomiting centre in the brain; used for motion sickness.
- Antihistamines (e.g. cyclizine) block the action of histamine on its receptors; used in pregnancy and motion sickness.
- 5-HT3 antagonists (e.g. ondansetron) prevent vomiting associated with cytotoxic therapies and vertigo.
- Phenothiazines (e.g. prochlorperazine, chlorpromazine) act on the central nervous system; they are also antipsychotics. They block the effects of chemoreceptor trigger zones. In small doses, they control nausea and vomiting, particularly when occurring as adverse effects of other treatments.

Reperfusion/limiting myocardial damage

One of the aims of medication for the patient experiencing an MI is to limit the size of the infarction, thereby reducing the risks to the patient of a traumatised myocardium and further complications (Simonsen *et al.*, 2006). The range of medicines used includes antiplatelets, thrombolytics and anticoagulants.

Related knowledge Quick reminder – pathophysiology

A thrombus (clot) is made up of red and white blood cells, platelets and fibrin (threads). The clot is referred to as a thrombus only when it stays where it was produced; a clot that travels is termed an 'embolus'.

Aspirin

Aspirin is a salicylate; it is also known as acetylsalicylic acid. Aspirin is used to inhibit the production of prostaglandins. Aspirin in this situation is being given for its antiplatelet effect – it prevents platelets (thrombocytes) from binding together and to the atheromatous plaques. Simonsen *et al.* (2006) describe aspirin as the 'most important platelet inhibitor'. Its antiplatelet action can be achieved by using small doses.

Aspirin has been demonstrated to reduce mortality after MI. It works by inhibiting the production of the prostaglandin thromboxane A2, which is responsible for platelet **aggregation**. Specifically, aspirin blocks the production of the enzyme cyclo-oxygenase, which interferes with the conversion of arachidonic acid to thromboxane A2, and therefore blocks this pathway of platelet aggregation.

It is recommended that a dose of 300 mg aspirin is given as soon as possible; this makes best use of its effect on platelet inhibition. This is followed by a daily dose of 75 mg to maintain this effect, continued for a minimum of 4 weeks to prevent further infarction (DH, 2000; Worster, 2000).

Unfortunately, aspirin can irritate the lining of the stomach, thought to be due to the absence of the protective prostaglandins, although this is not such a problem with the low maintenance dose that Mr Edmonds is prescribed. He could be advised to take the aspirin with food or be prescribed soluble aspirin to overcome the problem, but he will probably be prescribed gastro-resistant aspirin 75 mg.

Pharmacodynamics Aspirin

Aspirin inhibits platelet adhesion and aggregation by its inhibitory effect on cyclo-oxygenase in thrombocytes.

Pharmacokinetics Aspirin

Absorption: Aspirin is absorbed well from the stomach and small intestine, unless gastro-resistant to slow its absorption. Food in the stomach slows absorption. Aspirin is converted into the active metabolite salicylate.

Distribution: Aspirin is distributed widely through body tissues and fluids. In high doses, aspirin can bind to plasma proteins, resulting in a chemical change to the protein. The body may then recognise this different acetylated protein as foreign and produce antibodies, resulting in an allergic reaction next time the aspirin is taken (Greenstein and Gould, 2004).

Metabolism: Aspirin is metabolised by the liver, but approximately 25% is unchanged.

Elimination: Aspirin is excreted by kidneys, which is enhanced when the urine is alkaline (**www.bnf.org**; **www.emc.medicnes.org.uk**).

Related knowledge Dealing with inadvertent or intentional overdose

When a patient presents with aspirin overdose, the treatment involves making the urine more alkaline in order to enhance excretion; this entails administering large volumes of intravenous fluids – forced alkaline diuresis (**www.bnf.org**).

Nursing knowledge Health education related to medicines

Mr Edmonds should be informed about the actions, side effects and interactions of aspirin and how to store it, as he will be taking it for some time after discharge. He should be advised to take the aspirin as directed by the doctor, but what general advice could be given?

Answers can be found at the back of the book.

Thrombolysis

The aim of thrombolysis is to break down clots in the coronary arteries (hence the term 'clot buster') in order to re-establish blood flow. Thrombolytic therapy targets the fibrin (mesh) within the clot and therefore involves the use of fibrinolytic medicines. Fibrinolytic medicines such as streptokinase and recombinant tissue plasminogen activator (rt-PA) are used during and after an acute MI to achieve patency of the infarcted artery, thus reducing the size of the infarct and reducing mortality (death). Fibrinolytics can reduce mortality from 11.5% to 9.6% after MI within the first 30 days (Navuluri, 2001). Figure 10.2a demonstrates the action of thrombolytic drugs.

The NSF (DH, 2002) has established a 'call to needle time', which refers to the time between the first call for help and the administration of the prescribed thrombolytic therapy. The DH suggests that this should be no more than 1 hour and that 'door to needle time' (time between reaching hospital to administration of therapy) should be no more than 20 minutes.

The major side effect of thrombolytic therapy is haemorrhage, and so such medicines are contraindicated in patients who have anything in their history that may put them at risk of haemorrhage. Most NHS trusts have policies/algorithms in place to assess the risks to the individual patient.

(a)

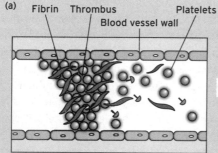
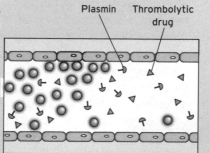

Before drug
When platelets accumulate in a blood vessel and are reinforced by strands of fibrin, the resultant blood clot, called a thrombus, cannot be dissolved by either antiplatelet drugs or anticoagulant drugs.

After drug
Thrombolytic drugs boost the action of plasmin, an enzyme in the blood that breaks up the strands of fibrin that bind the clot together. This allows the accumulated platelets to disperse, and restores normal blood flow.

(b)

Anticoagulants block the action of certain blood clotting factors that convert fibrinogen into fibrin, the protein that binds platelets into blood clots.

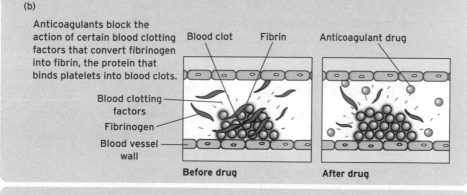

Figure 10.2 Action of (a) thrombolytics and (b) anticoagulants (after BMA, 1992)

Personal and professional development 10.4
Using medicines information

Can you identify three conditions that would render the patient unable to have thrombolytic therapy?

Answers can be found at the back of the book.

Williams (2002a) suggests that the thrombolytics available are equally effective, but issues such as cost, and route of administration contribute to the choice of the medicine to be used. The thrombolytics in current use are streptokinase, alteplase (rt-PA) and reteplase (Hand, 2001a).

Streptokinase

Streptokinase is the 'clot buster' that has been in use for the longest time, and therefore we have accrued a lot of information about it. It is also the cheapest of the thrombolytics. It is a protein/enzyme derived from the bacterium streptococcus, which combines with plasminogen to form plasmin. Plasmin disintegrates fibrin and therefore breaks up the thrombus. This produces a 'systemic lytic state', which means that the medicine's effect is upon the whole body and renders the body unable to produce clots in response to injury for up to 2 hours. For this reason, a careful medical history has to be taken. Because the source of streptokinase is a bacterial protein, it can cause allergic reactions; also, patients develop anti-streptococcal antibodies and so the medicine cannot be given again in the short term (the advice varies from 2–4 years). It is given intravenously, in a dose of 1 500 000 units in 100 ml of dextrose over 60 minutes (**www.bnf.org**; Hand, 2001a).

Pharmacodynamics Streptokinase

Streptokinase activates the endogenous fibrinolytic system. It binds to plasminogen, which accelerates the transformation of plasminogen into proteolytic and fibrinolytic plasmin.

Pharmacokinetics Streptokinase

Distribution: Peak activity in the bloodstream within 20 minutes.

Metabolism: There is a rapid reaction between streptokinase and antibodies, which results in small quantities being eliminated from the blood with a half-life of 18 minutes; otherwise, the half-life is 80 minutes.

Elimination: By the kidneys (**www.bnf.org**; **www.emc.medicines.org**).

Alteplase

Alteplase (rt-PA) is a naturally occurring substance (human protease) that is responsible for breaking down clots as part of the healing process. Although alteplase is more expensive than streptokinase, it is less problematic for the patient in that its action targets the clot, it can be used again and it is less likely to cause an allergic reaction. The BNF offers the following guidance for dosing: '15 mg by intravenous injection (bolus), followed by intravenous infusion of 50 mg over 30 minutes, then 35 mg over 60 minutes (total dose 100 mg over 90 minutes); lower doses in patients less than 65 kg' (www.bnf.org). Alteplase is given intravenously because it has a short half-life (Rang *et al.*, 2003).

Although alteplase occurs naturally, it is now produced within a laboratory using **genetic engineering** (recombinant DNA technology), hence its high cost. The term 'recombinant' refers to the joining of genetic material from two different sources, the primary source being DNA obtained from human tissue cultures; often the second source is viral.

Pharmacodynamics Alteplase

Alteplase is a glycoprotein that activates plasminogen directly into plasmin. Once alteplase is bound to fibrin, the fibrin is activated. The conversion of plasminogen to plasmin leads to the dissolution of the fibrin clot.

Pharmacokinetics Alteplase

Distribution: Cleared rapidly from circulating blood.

Metabolism: Metabolised mainly by the liver. Plasma half-life is 4–5 minutes (www.bnf.org; www.emc.medicines.org.uk).

Reteplase

Mr Edmonds has been prescribed reteplase, which is a new generation plasminogen activator, available since 1997. Alexander *et al.* (2006) claim that reteplase is as effective as streptokinase but does not produce antigens. Reteplase should be given within 12 hours of the onset of symptoms and administered as two intravenous 10-unit bolus injections 30 minutes apart (NICE, 2002). Each bolus should be given slowly, over 2 minutes (**www.bnf.org**). Reteplase should be followed by heparin – a bolus injection of 5000 units followed by a 1000 unit/hour infusion (Hand, 2001a).

Pharmacodynamics Reteplase

Generates plasmin from endogenous plasminogen. Plasmin degrades fibrin.

Pharmacokinetics Reteplase

Distribution: Given intravenously, reteplase is distributed immediately throughout the circulation.

Elimination: Exact data on the main elimination routes are not available.

Contraindications

Contraindications for thrombolytic therapy include a previous history of haemorrhagic stroke, any internal bleeding (e.g. following recent trauma or surgery), gastrointestinal bleeding, suspected aortic dissection, uncontrolled hypertension, cerebrovascular problems, cerebral tumours, pregnancy and other medicines such as anticoagulant therapy.

Personal and professional development 10.5

If you are unfamiliar with any of the conditions mentioned above, any nursing textbook should be able to supply you with explanations.

Navuluri (2001) suggests that a single thrombolytic medicine on its own is not effective because of the features of the thrombus and the medicine's action. Patient outcomes are improved when using a combination of fibrinolytic and antiplatelet medicines because of their synergistic activity. It is recommended by NICE (2002) that heparin is given with all thrombolytic therapy, with the exception of streptokinase; heparin would therefore be indicated for Mr Edmonds.

Anticoagulants

Heparin

Heparin is an anticoagulant. It does not have a fibrinolytic action but it prevents the formation of new thrombi and the extension of existing thrombi. It promotes the action of anti-thrombin III (anticlotting factor), which inhibits factors X, 1X and X1 (clotting factors). The outcome is inhibition of the conversion of prothrombin to thrombin, which prevents the conversion of fibrinogen to fibrin and thus prolongs clotting time. Normal blood flow depends upon clotting and anti-clotting factors being in balance. Figure 10.2b demonstrates the action of anticoagulants, while Figure 10.3 shows the various clotting factors.

Heparin administration is advised if the patient is unable to receive thrombolytic therapy and is used as an adjuvant to alteplase. Heparin in this situation is administered by injection; usually, a continuous intravenous infusion of standard heparin, which acts immediately on most clotting factors, is used. When heparin used prophylactically to prevent clotting during periods of immobility, such as before and after surgery, low-molecular weight (LMW) heparins are administered by subcutaneous injection from

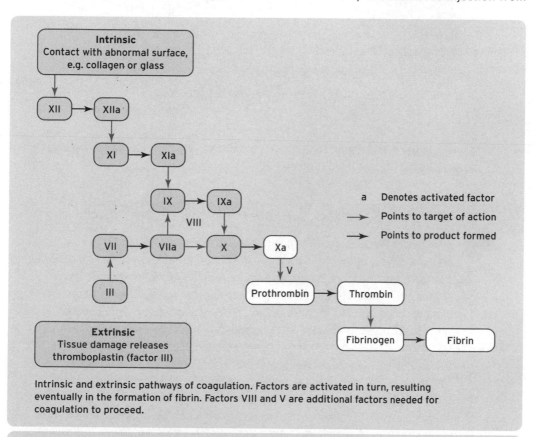

Intrinsic and extrinsic pathways of coagulation. Factors are activated in turn, resulting eventually in the formation of fibrin. Factors VIII and V are additional factors needed for coagulation to proceed.

Figure 10.3 Clotting factors (after Kindlen, 2003)

prefilled syringes. When used as an adjuvant to alteplase, heparin should be commenced 4 hours after the alteplase; a 5000-unit bolus is given, followed by 1000 units
per hour by infusion (Hand, 2001a; **www.bnf.org**).

Pharmacodynamics Heparin

Heparin is a naturally occurring anticoagulant that prevents the coagulation of
blood *in vivo* and *in vitro*. It potentiates the inhibition of several activated
coagulation factors, including thrombin and factor X.

Pharmacokinetics Heparin

Absorption: Heparin is not absorbed well from the gastrointestinal tract, and so
it is given by injection (intravenously in this situation). The onset of action is
amost immediate.

Distribution: Peak concentration levels occur within minutes.

Metabolism: Metabolised in the liver by the enzyme heparinase. Half-life is dose-
related (approximately 1–1.5 hours).

Elimination: Mainly by the kidneys (Rang *et al.*, 2003).

Aspirin is used as an adjuvant for streptokinase; aspririn increases survival when
accompanying thrombolytic therapy.

Related knowledge Other treatment approaches

There is growing evidence to suggest that primary **angioplasty** is more effective
than thrombolysis for reperfusing the myocardium. Keeley *et al.* (2003) reviewed
23 randomised trials that compared primary angioplasty with thrombolysis for
patients presenting with an acute MI who displayed a raised ST segment on ECG
(ST elevation MI: STEMI). In these studies, primary angioplasty 'demonstrated a
significant reduction in mortality'. This procedure is also recommended by the
GUSTO (Global Use of Strategies to Open Occluded Coronary Arteries in Acute
Coronary Syndromes) Trial Investigators (1997).

Primary angioplasty also limits the risk of reinfarction and haemorrhage
(Keeley *et al.*, 2003).

Angioplasty is a technique used to reconstruct damaged blood vessels. It is
referred to as 'primary' when it is the first-line treatment for patients with MI.

It involves a technique to open a blocked coronary artery. A balloon-tipped catheter is inserted into the arterial system via the groin and fed up to the affected coronary artery. The position of the catheter is confirmed by X-ray. Once in place, the balloon is inflated and the atheroma is compressed. The catheter usually carries a metal stent (latticed metal tube), which remains in place when the balloon is deflated to maintain the patency of the artery (Leahy, 2006). This technique requires a specialist team.

Pharmacological knowledge Other potential treatments

The National Service Framework for Coronary Heart Disease, DH (2000) suggests that, as well as the treatments identified above, the patient with an MI should receive beta-blockers and ACE inhibitors. The rationale for this is that these medicines reduce the work of the heart. Rang *et al.* (2003) suggest that there is only a small beneficial effect associated with beta-blocker use in acute MI but that ACE inhibitors are proven to improve survival. Both of these medicines are discussed below in relation to a change in Mr Edmonds' condition.

Mr John Edmonds

It is 48 hours since Mr Edmonds' admission. He has made an uneventful recovery and so has been transferred to the medical ward until his discharge. He awakes at 2 a.m. feeling frightened and dyspnoeic. He has developed a cough and is producing large amounts of frothy sputum. The doctor confirms a diagnosis of pulmonary oedema and prescribes furosemide 20 mg, ramipril 2.5 mg (an ACE inhibitor) and metoprolol 50 mg (a beta-blocker).

Mr Edmonds has developed pulmonary oedema, a feature of left ventricular failure, which is one of the complications of MI.

THE NATURE OF LEFT VENTRICULAR FAILURE AND PULMONARY OEDEMA

In heart failure, the heart is unable to maintain an adequate cardiac output (the volume of blood ejected by the ventricle per minute) to fulfil the body's metabolic requirements (Hand, 2001b). If the left ventricle has been damaged by MI and is unable to maintain an effective cardiac output, some blood remains within the ventricle, causing a build-up of pressure within the heart and ultimately within the pulmonary circulation (Figure 10.4). This is a problem of backward pressure: imagine the consequence of breaking down in your car at traffic lights and the pressure on the traffic behind you.

Increased pressure in the pulmonary circulation forces fluid into the alveoli (air sacs). The alveoli allow the transfer of gases, so that oxygen from inspired air can be transported to, and carbon dioxide excreted from, the tissues. In heart failure, because of the single-cell walls of the alveoli, fluid is also transferred, resulting in the production of large quantities of frothy, blood-tinged (pink) sputum - literally 'fluid on the lungs', or pulmonary oedema.

If cardiac output falls, the circulation of the kidneys is reduced, leading to diminished urinary output and retention of salt (sodium) and water. This results in the activation of the renin-angiotensin mechanism, which results in further sodium retention and oedema.

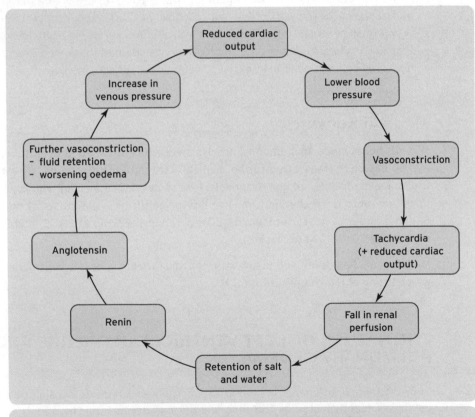

Figure 10.4 Heart failure (after Downie, Mackenzie and Williams, 2003)

PHARMACOLOGICAL INTERVENTIONS USED TO MANAGE HEART FAILURE AND PULMONARY OEDEMA

The aim of treatment for heart failure is to reduce the fluid overload by the use of **diuretics** and ACE inhibitors (Hand, 2001a, b). Diamorphine, in a dose of 2.5–5 mg, may also be given to the patient with acute pulmonary oedema. Diamorphine relaxes the patient and reduces the congestion in the lungs by dilating the veins (Prosser *et al.*, 2000). Other medicines prescribed for this condition are beta-blockers (**www.emc.medicines.org.uk**).

Nursing knowledge Nursing interventions

This acute situation would also require supportive nursing interventions, as the patient is distressed and dyspnoeic:

- Give oxygen as prescribed, to improve myocardial contractility.
- Provide reassurance and information to the patient.
- Promote rest.

Diuretics

The diuretics used in left ventricular failure are usually loop diuretics, such as furosemide and bumetanide (**www.bnf.org**) because of their fast action. Loop diuretics are so called because they act upon the loop of Henle in the nephron. They inhibit reabsorption of sodium and chloride from the ascending loop of Henle back into the bloodstream, resulting in an increased excretion of sodium and water (and chloride) from the body (Prosser *et al.*, 2000). Unfortunately, other substances and electrolytes such as potassium are lost. Hypokalaemia (reduced potassium) is therefore a potential adverse effect, which can cause arrhythmias. Loop diuretics are often prescribed with potassium supplements or potassium-sparing diuretics such as amiloride. Hypokalaemia can be assessed by taking blood samples to identify the levels of electrolytes such as potassium in the patient's bloodstream.

Increasing the urinary output helps to clear the oedema, but furosemide also has a vasodilator effect on the pulmonary veins, which further helps to relieve the pulmonary oedema.

Pharmacodynamics Furosemide

Furosemide is a potent loop diuretic that inhibits sodium and chloride reabsorption at the loop of Henle. Furosemide causes an increased loss of potassium in the urine and also increases the excretion of ammonia by the kidney.

Pharmacokinetics Furosemide

Absorption: Absorbed well.

Distribution: Distributed rapidly. Intravenous administration relieves breathlessness and can provide rapid relief. Loop diuretics are potent and short-lasting. Furosemide achieves a peak effect within 30 minutes; duration of action is 3–6 hours.

Metabolism: Metabolised by the liver.

Elimination: Eliminated primarily unchanged by the kidneys; some faecal excretion (**www.bnf.org**; **www.emc.medicines.org.uk**).

Pharmacological knowledge Other groups of diuretics

Other groups of diuretic that can be used include thiazide diuretics and potassium-sparing diuretics.

Thiazide diuretics (e.g. bendroflumethiazide) act by inhibiting sodium and chloride reabsorption in the distal tubule of the kidney, which increases sodium and therefore water secretion. These may cause hypokalaemia, hypotension, headaches and dizziness.

Potassium-sparing diuretics (e.g. spironolactone) increase sodium and chloride excretion in the distal tubule and cause retention of potassium. They may cause hyperkalaemia, dehydration, gastrointestinal disturbances and hypotension.

Figure 10.5 shows the action of various types of diuretic.

Spironolactone

The NSF (DH, 2000) recommends adding spironolactone in a low dose (e.g. 25 mg daily) to the other prescribed treatments as it has been demonstrated to reduce mortality and morbidity. Spironolactone is a potassium-sparing diuretic. It is an antagonist of aldosterone, a hormone that retains sodium. Spironolactone promotes the excretion of sodium; sodium is then lost from the bloodstream, with fluid, and is replaced by potassium (Downie et al., 2003). Spironolactone it is considered to be of minimal benefit on its own, but when given with furosemide the overall diuretic effect is enhanced and potassium replacement is unnecessary; therefore, the medicine regime is simpler. Another advantage is that both spironolactone and furosemide can be taken daily, whereas most potassium supplements are taken in multiple doses throughout the day, depending upon the medicine chosen.

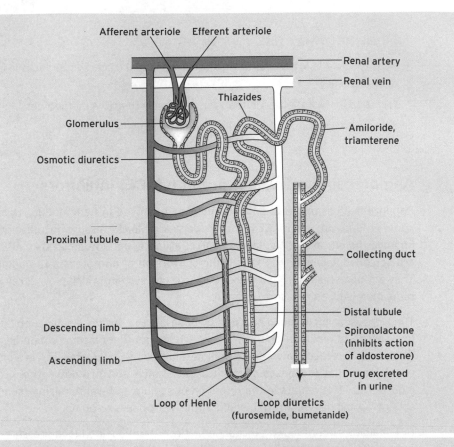

Figure 10.5 Action of diuretics (after Downie, Mackenzie and Williams, 2003)

Pharmacodynamics Spironolactone

Spironolactone is a competitive aldosterone antagonist. It increases sodium excretion whilst reducing potassium loss at the distal renal tubule. It has a gradual and prolonged action.

Pharmacokinetics Spironolactone

Absorption: Absorbed well in the gastrointenstinal tract. Spironolactone is only available orally.

Metabolism: Metabolised in the liver, principally to active metabolites.

Elimination: Eliminated primarily in urine and bile.

Angiotensin-converting enzyme (ACE) inhibitors

Ramipril is an example of an ACE inhibitor. It is used in heart failure to reduce the strain on a failing heart. ACE inhibitors decrease blood pressure, increase diuresis and improve the efficacy of the failing heart (Gallimore and Jordan, 2004). ACE inhibitors are so-called because they inhibit the conversion of angiotensin I to angiotensin II. They act upon the renin–angiotensin–aldosterone system, which plays a key role in the regulation of blood pressure.

The kidneys maintain blood pressure by releasing the hormone renin. Renin is released in response to reduced renal perfusion, acting upon the plasma protein angiotensin I. Angiotensin I is then converted to angiotensin II by ACE. Angiotensin II is a potent vaso-constrictor that increases peripheral resistance and promotes the secretion of aldosterone. This results in the retention of sodium and water, raising blood pressure and increasing the volume of blood that the heart needs to pump.

ACE inhibitors interfere with this action, effectively reducing blood pressure. They also reduce the pressure in the ventricle. Dilation of the arterioles reduces the load on the heart, therefore improving heart function. The results are a reduction in dyspnoea and an increase in exercise ability (heart failure is associated with fatigue). Figure 10.6 shows the action of ACE inhibitors.

ACE inhibitors are used in heart failure, usually in combination with a diuretic. They can reduce the patient's symptoms and improve mortality.

ACE inhibitors interact with many other medicines. They should be used with caution when patients are receiving diuretics (when used with potassium-sparing diuretics such as spironolactone) or potassium supplements, because hyperkalaemia may occur; and so serum potassium levels should be monitored. If the patient is already taking loop diuretics (e.g. furosemide), ACE inhibitors can cause first-dose hypotension; therefore, the patient should remain on bed-rest for at least 3 hours following the first dose and the patient's blood pressure checked. Because of this, the first dose is usually given at bedtime or in small starting doses for the first few days. The patient may experience postural hypotension (a fall in blood pressure associated with a change in posture, e.g. standing up from a lying or sitting position) (Gallimore and Jordan, 2004). Temporary

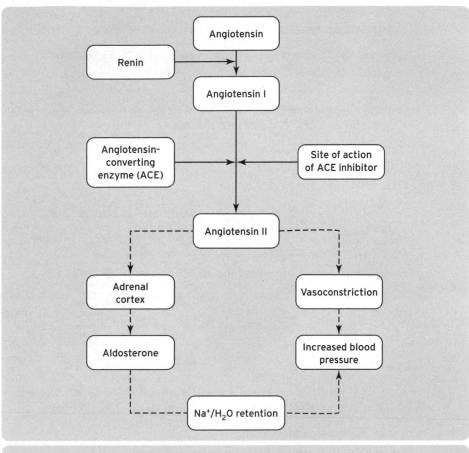

Figure 10.6 Action of ACE inhibitors (after Downie, Mackenzie and Williams, 2003)

withdrawal of ACE inhibitors can reduce the risk of postural hypotension but may result in severe rebound pulmonary oedema. ACE inhibitors also interact with beta-blockers.

Other adverse effects of ACE inhibitors are renal impairment, persistent dry cough, headache and fatigue.

Ramipril

Administration of ramipril causes an increase in plasma renin activity and a decrease in plasma concentrations of angiotensin II and aldosterone. The beneficial haemodynamic effects resulting from ACE inhibition are a consequence of the reduction in angiotensin II, causing dilation of peripheral vessels and a reduction in vascular resistance.

Pharmacodynamics Ramipril

Ramipril is a prodrug. It is hydrolysed in the liver to form the active angiotensin-converting hormone inhibitor ramiprilat. Ramipril is potent and long-lasting. It causes an increase in plasma renin activity and a decrease in plasma concentrations of angiotensin II and aldosterone, causing dilation of peripheral vessels and a reduction in vascular resistance.

Pharmacokinetics Ramipril

Absorption: Absorbed from the gastrointestinal tract and distributed to most body tissues.

Distribution: Peak concentrations are reached within 1 hour.

Metabolism: Almost completely metabolised.

Elimination: Metabolites excreted mainly by the kidneys; also excreted in the faeces.

Beta-blockers

This group of medicines exerts a protective effect on the heart, offering protection from the effects of stress, fright and excitement. They achieve this by:

- preventing increased heart rate;
- preventing increased cardiac output and workload;
- preventing increase in the oxygen expenditure of the heart.

Beta-blockers are used in hypertension, angina, MI, heart arrhythmias, anxiety and heart failure (Jordan and Knight, 2004). The risk of MI or cardiovascular death has been proven to be decreased by the use of beta-blockers (Conway and Fuat, 2007).

Adrenaline (epinephrine) and noradrenaline (norepinephrine) are naturally occurring catecholamines (stimulants) that exert their effects via alpha- and beta-adrenoceptors at sympathetic nerve endings. By occupying beta-receptor sites in the sympathetic nervous system, beta-adrenergic blockers (beta-blockers) compete with these stimulants, preventing them from occupying their natural target sites (the beta-adrenergic receptors) and therefore from exerting their stimulatory effects (Conway and Fuat, 2007). Beta-adrenoceptors are distributed widely within the heart, bronchi and blood vessels: β_1 receptors are found predominantly in the heart, while β_2 receptors are found mainly in the bronchi and blood vessels.

Stimulation of beta-adrenoceptors in the heart and coronary arteries results in an increase in heart rate, conduction and force of contraction (Conway and Fuat, 2007). By blocking these actions, beta-adrenergic blockers increase vascular resistance, decrease blood pressure and decrease the force of the heart's contractions. Oxygen consumption by the heart is then decreased, the impulse is slowed and cardiac output is decreased. In a patient newly diagnosed with heart failure, beta-blockers should be started slowly.

Beta-blockers are usually administered in tandem with diuretics.

Metoprolol

Metoprolol is a selective beta-blocker. It blocks the catecholamine action at β_1 receptors at a dose smaller than that required to block β_2 receptors, and so it can be described as cardioselective but not cardiospecific.

Pharmacodynamics Metoprolol

Metoprolol is a competitive beta-adrenoceptor antagonist. It inhibits beta-adrenoceptors. It has some cardioselectivity, and thus cardiac output and systolic blood pressure decrease rapidly following administration.

Pharmacokinetics Metoprolol

Absorption: Absorbed rapidly and well from the gastrointestinal tract. Food may enhance its absorption.

Distribution: Some protein binding, crosses the placenta and found in breast milk.

Metabolism: Metabolised extensively in the liver. There is variation in the rate of metabolism, and the dose should be adjusted to the individual patient.

Elimination: Mainly by hepatic metabolism.

DISCHARGE ADVICE IN RELATION TO MEDICATION

Hainsworth (2006) suggests that following MI, patients should be discharged on a combination of medications: statins, an antiplatelet such as aspirin, a beta-blocker and an ACE inhibitor.

Mr Edmonds will need appropriate advice to manage this complex cocktail of medicines. Mr Edmonds would be discharged on simvastatin, but recent evidence suggests that the dose should be 20–40 mg (Pottle, 2005) rather than the 10 mg he was originally prescribed. The advice given when it was initially prescribed should be reiterated and reinforced.

Furosemide should be taken in the morning. Taking the dose later in the day can lead to the patient getting up repeatedly through the night to go to the toilet; this effect may make the patient reluctant to take the medicine.

The ACE inhibitor should be continued for 5-6 weeks (www.bnf.org). Mr Edmonds should:

- avoid activities such as driving until it is established that the risk of dizziness and fainting (potential side effects) have passed;
- avoid activities such as drinking excess alcohol, as this can increase the risk of hypotension;
- be advised that the medicine should not be stopped without first seeking medical advice;
- be advised that a sudden change of posture (e.g. standing from sitting) may cause postural hypotension.

Nursing implications Pain management

The pain experienced by patients suffering an MI has a classic description: crushing central chest pain that radiates into the neck and jaw and down the left arm. The pain is associated with anxiety (some patients believe that they are going to die), nausea, vomiting and dyspnoea. It is important to note that not all patients present with this history; older patients often just have a sense of feeling unwell. Mr Edmonds has presented with the classic experience of chest pain. One of the priorities in the care of a patient with MI is to relieve the pain. Alexander *et al*. (2006) suggest that pain is a sign of 'ongoing myocardial ischaemia' and pain relief should be a nursing priority. The patient's pain should be assessed using an assessment tool. There are several chest pain assessment tools available to assess the character of the pain, such as the site, intensity and radiation (McAvoy, 2000). Monitoring and evaluating the pain response is of equal importance, and the patient should be informed about the need to report pain promptly.

On discharge, patients often express anxiety about experiencing further episodes of chest pain. It is important for nurses to be reassuring and to offer concrete advice about what to do if the pain reoccurs. It is likely that the patient will experience angina pain (Alexander *et al.*, 2006); the aim of the advice is to enable the patient to feel confident about how to manage the pain, how to identify the source of the pain, how to use appropriate pain-relieving strategies and how to access healthcare.

Nursing implications Reassurance

As the nurse looking after Mr Edmonds, what strategies can you employ to reassure him in this situation?

PROFESSIONAL GUIDANCE

National Institute for Health and Clinical Excellence

NICE offers guidance for health professionals regarding appropriateness of treatments after considering 'best' evidence in relation to medicines and treatments for specific conditions and diseases. NICE states clearly that what it provides is *guidance* and that ultimately treatment decisions should be made in relation to the patient's individual circumstances and with the patient and/or carer. NICE identifies the indicators for thrombolysis, offers an analysis of the effectiveness of each medicine, and calls for clear local guidelines so that risks and benefits to the individual can be assessed. NICE claims that thrombolysis is currently underused.

National Service Framework for Coronary Heart Disease

The National Service Framework (DH, 2000) is the government blueprint for combating CHD. It sets out a series of standards outlining the treatment and care related to the diagnosis, prevention and treatment of CHD. Part of Mr Edmonds' treatment will involve rehabilitation and **health promotion**. The World Health Organization (WHO) (1993) defines cardiac rehabilitation as:

> ... the sum of activities required to influence favourably the underlying cause of the disease, as well as the best possible physical, social and mental conditions, so that people might by their own efforts preserve or resume when lost, as normal a place as possible in the community. Rehabilitation cannot be regarded as an isolated form or stage of therapy but must be integrated within secondary prevention service of which it forms only one facet.

The NSF (DH, 2000) suggests four discrete phases of rehabilitation:

- *Phase 1*: This begins before discharge and involves an assessment of the patient's lifestyle, followed by advice to minimise risks.
- *Phase 2*: Health promotion that continues after discharge and includes a more comprehensive risk assessment and regular review.
- *Phase 3*: A cardiac rehabilitation course is recommended for some patients; this covers a broad range of approaches, such as exercise, relaxation and psychological support.
- *Phase 4*: Long-term maintenance offered by the primary care team.

Essential terminology

Health promotion
Advice and information to maintain a patient's health status; preventive.

Health education
Advice and information given to promote health; may occur before or after an illness/condition develops. The two terms are often used interchangeably.

Health education and promotion in relation to lifestyle

Although we are still not clear what causes coronary heart disease, we can identify risk factors within an individual's lifestyle that, if identified and minimised, can prevent further problems for the individual. Therefore, an important aspect of the care for Mr Edmonds is to provide him with information and advice about modifying these risk factors.

Related knowledge Risk factors

Risk factors related to coronary heart disease can be related to the individual's medical history, family history/characteristics and lifestyle.

- *Medical history*:
  - Diabetes mellitus
  - Hypertension
  - Hyperlipidaemia
  - Medicines such as oral contraceptives.
- *Family history/characteristics*:
  - Genetic predisposition
  - Age
  - Gender
  - Race/ethnicity.
- *Lifestyle factors*:
  - Smoking
  - Obesity
  - Physical inactivity
  - Alcohol intake
  - Salt intake
  - Diet high in saturated fats
  - Stress.

Personal and professional development 10.6

Access any relevant resource of your choice and, looking at Mr Edmonds' history, identify the information and advice you could give him about altering the factors within his lifestyle that could lead to a further MI. A useful resource is Foxton *et al.* (2004).

Answers can be found at the back of the book.

Mr Edmonds is being discharged on a complex therapeutic regime and there is the possibility that he might find this difficult to manage, and thus he might fail to take his medication as prescribed.

COMPLIANCE/ADHERENCE

The definition of compliance still used frequently is that of Haynes *et al.* (1979):

> ... the extent to which the patient's behaviour (in terms of taking medications, following diets or executing lifestyle changes) coincides with medical or health care advice.

There is a suggestion that this definition implies that the patient should do what the health professional wants them to do. In other words, the doctor is in control and the role of the patient is to comply. Fawcett (1995) identifies that the term has been changed to 'adherence', but this still implies that patients are required to accept the best advice of professionals. It is suggested that in order to encourage patients to participate actively in decisions about their own care, there should be effective communication between professional and patient and appropriate information needs to be given that takes account of the beliefs and expectations of the patient (Playle and Keeley, 1998).

It is important that Mr Edmonds is involved in his treatment decisions. He has a family history of CHD, he has raised cholesterol levels and he has suffered an MI. He has demonstrated non-adherence with previous treatment and is taking risks in relation to his diet.

There are differing levels of adherence, relating to the patient's individual circumstances. The onset of an acute illness such as MI can make patients feel helpless. They may feel that they have lost their independence, finding themselves suddenly 'dependent upon strangers for their survival' (Gillespie and Melby, 2003). This might be a useful time to reinforce the importance of lifestyle changes to reduce CHD risk. Events such as this can cause patients to rethink their approaches to healthcare, but clearly this needs to be approached sensitively, due to the vulnerability of the patient.

Patients should be actively involved in their own care. Hainsworth (2006) suggests that one way of achieving this is to promote the use of risk factor charts to reinforce the benefits of lifestyle changes.

Nursing knowledge Patient education

There is a growing belief that there is a link between coronary heart disease and erectile dysfunction (ED). Indeed, erectile dysfunction may be the first indicator of CHD in men. Kirby (2007) states that 'the patient with ED and no cardiac symptoms is a cardiac patient until proven otherwise' and that 'ED and CHD share many risk factors'.

Nurses need to be aware of this. Kirby (2007) suggests that sexual function is so important for men that they are likely to take risks, such as failing to take medication that they believe will worsen their ED.

FAMILY INVOLVEMENT

It is important to involve Mr Edmonds' wife in his health education. They have no children, and we do not know what other family support is available. Their shared interests and social life seem to centre around seeing friends for meals and drinks, and so any change to his lifestyle will impact on hers. It will create a much more supportive situation if both Mr and Mrs Edmonds follow the same kind of meal plans. Nuttall (2002) suggests that whether people have coronary heart disease or not, they can still benefit from advice about their lifestyle; this is a compelling reason to include Mrs Edmonds when discussing advised changes.

Quick reminder

✔ Coronary heart disease is responsible for 110 000 deaths per year in the UK (DH, 2000). The main features are related to the development of atheroma, which can predispose to an acute situation such as myocardial infarction.

✔ Statins are one of the newer treatments for the reduction of circulating blood cholesterol levels. They interfere with the production of cholesterol by the liver.

✔ Treatments are directed at reperfusing the damaged coronary artery and thus limiting cardiac damage (aspirin and thrombolysis) and at treating ongoing problems, such as heart failure (diuretics, ACE inhibitors and beta-blockers).

✔ The treatment of MI is also directed at supportive interventions, such as the administration of oxygen and diamorphine to reduce the work of the heart and to reduce pain and anxiety.

✔ Heart failure (left ventricular failure) is a complication of MI that results in pulmonary oedema. Treatments include diuretics, ACE inhibitors and beta-blockers.

✔ Patients with coronary heart disease benefit from lifestyle advice and support to encourage involvement in treatment, including taking their medicines appropriately.

REFERENCES

Alexander MF, Fawcett J N and Runciman P J (2006) *Nursing Practice: Hospital and Home – the Adult,* 3rd edn. Edinburgh: Churchill Livingstone.

Collins T (2000) Understanding shock. *Nursing Standard* **14**, 35–43.

Conway B and Fuat A (2007) Recent advances in angina management: implications for nurses. *Nursing Standard* **21**, 49–56.

Department of Health (DH) (2000) *National Service Framework for Coronary Heart Disease.* London: The Stationery Office.

Downie G, Mackenzie J and Williams A (2003) *Pharmacology and Medicines Management for Nurses,* 3rd edn. Edinburgh: Churchill Livingstone.

Fawcett J (1995) Compliance: definitions and key issues. *Journal of Clinical Psychiatry* **56** (Suppl. 1), 4–8.

Foxton J, Nuttall M and Riley J (2004) Coronary heart disease: risk factor management. *Nursing Standard* **19**, 47–54.

Frazier S K, Moser D K, O'Brien J L, Garvin B J, An K and Macko M (2002) Management of anxiety after acute myocardial infarction. *Heart and Lung* **31**, 411-420.

Gallimore D and Jordan S (2004) Prescription drugs uses and effects: ACE inhibitors. *Nursing Standard* **18**, 4.

Gillespie M and Melby V (2003) Assessing acute myocardial infarction. *Emergency Nurse* **11**, 26-29.

Greenstein B and Gould D (2004) *Trounce's Clinical Pharmacology for Nurses*. Edinburgh: Churchill Livingstone.

GUSTO Trial Investigators (1997) A clinical trial comparing primary coronary angioplasty with tissue plasminogen activator for acute myocardial infarction. The Global Use of Strategies to Open Occluded Coronary Arteries in Acute Coronary Syndromes (GUSTO IIb) Angioplasty Substudy Investigators. *New England Journal of Medicine* **336**, 1621-1628.

Hainsworth T (2006) Improving the prevention of cardiovascular disease. *Nursing Times* **102**, 23-24.

Hand H (2001a) Myocardial infarction: part 1. *Nursing Standard* **15**, 45-55.

Hand H (2001b) Myocardial infarction: part 2. *Nursing Standard* **15**, 45-53.

Harrison R and Daly L (2001) *Acute Medical Emergencies: A Nursing Guide*. Edinburgh: Churchill Livingstone.

Haynes R B, Sackett D L and Taylor D W (1979) *Compliance in Health Care*. Baltimore, MD: Johns Hopkins Press.

Jordan S and Knight J (2004) Prescription drugs uses and effects: beta blockers. *Nursing Standard* **18**, 49.

Keeley E C, Boura J A and Grines C L (2003) Primary angioplasty versus intravenous thrombolytic therapy for acute myocardial infarction: a quantitive review of 23 randomised trials. *Lancet* **361**, 13-20.

Kindlen, S (ed) (2003) *Physiology for Health Care and Nursing*. Edinburgh: Churchill Livingstone.

Kirby M (2007) Helping the failing heart and penis. *International Journal of Clinical Practice* **61**, 716-718.

Leahy M (2006) Primary angioplasty for acute ST-elevation myocardial infarction. *Nursing Standard* **21**, 48-56.

McAvoy J A (2000) Cardiac pain: discover. *Nursing* **30**, 34-39.

McCaffrey M and Beebe A (1994) *Pain: A Clinical Manual of Nursing Practice*. London: Mosby.

McTaggart F (2003) Comparative pharmacology of rosuvastatin. *Atheroscerosis Supplements* **4**, 9-14.

Merskey H and Bogduk N (1994) *Classification of Chronic Pain*, 2nd edn. Seattle, WA: International Association for the Study of Pain Press.

National Institute for Health and Clinical Excellence (NICE) (2002) *Guidance on the Use of Drugs for Early Thrombolysis in the Treatment of Acute Myocardial Infarction*. London: National Institute for Health and Clinical Excellence.

Navuluri R (2001) Antiplatelet and fibrinolytic therapy: part two of a four-part series on antithrombic therapies. *American Journal of Nursing* **101**, 24A-24D.

Nissen S E, Tuzco E M, Schoenhagen P *et al.* (2004) Effect of intensive compared with moderate lipid-lowering therapy on progression of coronary atherosclerosis. *Journal of the American Medical Association* **291**, 1071-1080.

Nuttall M (2002) Primary care strategies to reduce the risk of coronary heart disease. *Professional Nurse* **17**, 680-681.

Phillipe M and Whittaker N (2004) Coronary heart disease. In Whittaker N (ed.) *Disorders and Interventions*. Basingstoke: Palgrave Macmillan.

Playle J and Keeley P (1998) Non-compliance and professional power. *Journal of Advanced Nursing* **27**, 304-311.

Pottle A (2005) Familial hypercholesterolemia: clinical features and management. *Nursing Standard* **20**, 14-16, 55-65.

Prosser S, Worster B, MacGregor J, Dewar K, Runyard P and Fegan J (2000) *Applied Pharmacology: An Introduction to Pathophysiology and Drug Management for Nurses and Healthcare Professionals*. London: Mosby.

Rang H P, Dale M M, Ritter J M and Moore P K (2003) *Pharmacology*, 5th edn. Edinburgh: Elsevier.

Simonsen T, Aarbakke J, Kay I, Coleman A, Sinnot P and Lysaa R (2006) *Illustrated Pharmacology for Nurses*. London: Hodder Arnold.

Thibodeau G A (2003) *Anatomy and Physiology*, 5th edn. St Louis, IL: Mosby.

Wickens A (2005) Foundations of Biopsychology. Harlow: Pearson Education.

Williams B, Pouter N R, Brown M J, *et al*. (2004) British Hypertension Society Guidelines. Guidelines for management of hypertension: report of the fourth working party of the British Hypertension Society. *Journal of Human Hypertension* **18**, 139–185.

Williams H (2002a) Acute coronary syndromes. *Pharmaceutical Journal* **269**, 747–749.

World Health Organization (WHO) (1993) *Needs and Action Priorities in Cardiac Rehabilitation and Secondary Prevention in Patients with CHD*. Geneva: World Health Organization.

Worster B (2000) Drugs and cardiovascular disease. In Prosser S, Worster B, MacGregor J, Dewar K, Runyard P and Fegan J (eds) *Applied Pharmacology: An Introduction to Pathophysiology and Drug Management for Nurses and Healthcare Professionals*. London: Mosby.

Chapter 11

A man with acute intestinal obstruction

I n this chapter, we consider the pharmacological interventions relating to a patient with acute abdominal pain admitted to an accident and emergency unit and his consequent surgery and recovery. We use the patient scenario of Mr Giancarlo Rossi, a 54-year-old man. Mr Rossi's experience of this acute condition provides a number of opportunities to examine a variety of pharmacological treatments. These treatments include acute pain management in the pre- and postoperative phases, managing nausea and vomiting and reducing the risks of major gastrointestinal surgery; we also examine the implications that having an ileostomy may have on medications. This chapter also considers the supportive nursing interventions that arise in relation to the medications used in the treatment and management of acute intestinal obstruction.

More controversially, this chapter highlights not only the possible influence of nursing's urban myths about opioids but also how the values and beliefs of some healthcare professionals may result in poor pain control for some patients. We also see how society's values in relation to drugs may affect patient concordance with their prescriptions.

✔ Learning outcomes

At the end of this chapter you should be able to:

✔ Give an overview of acute intestinal obstruction

✔ Explain the relevant anatomy and physiology of the gastrointestinal tract

✔ Discuss the potential impact of acute intestinal obstruction on an individual

✔ Identify supporting pharmacological approaches to the management of acute intestinal obstruction

✔ Discuss the actions and effects of the medicines identified in this patient scenario, namely morphine sulphate, tinzaparin, metoclopramide, cefuroxime and metronidazole

✔ Discuss the nursing knowledge needed related to medicines management for this patient

✔ Identify supporting nursing interventions for this patient

✔ Identify the non-pharmacological approaches that can be used to help manage pre- and postoperative pain

Chapter at a glance

Overview of 'acute abdomen'
The nature of acute intestinal obstruction
The nature of acute abdominal pain
Preoperative pain management of acute abdominal pain – changing schools of thought
Pharmacological interventions used to manage acute abdominal pain
Preoperative medication
The nature of anaesthetics
Reducing the risks of surgery
The nature of postoperative nausea and vomiting
Postoperative pain management
Factors affecting patient education about medicines
Quick reminder
References

Mr Giancarlo Rossi

Mr Giancarlo Rossi has been admitted to the accident and emergency unit complaining of severe abdominal pain, nausea and vomiting and constipation, a syndrome frequently referred to as acute abdomen. He is a 54-year-old man who came to live in the UK after meeting Natasha, the woman who was later to become his wife of 28 years. He works for a local landowner, as head gardener, on a large estate, where he and his family live in a tied cottage (i.e. the cottage is part of his wages). Following examination and investigations, Mr Rossi was diagnosed as having an acute intestinal obstruction, which seemed to be as a result of a tumour of the large bowel (colon). This was explained to Mr Rossi by the surgeon, who then gained consent for immediate surgery to relieve the obstruction. Following this, Mr Rossi was prescribed intravenous morphine sulphate 15 mg and tinzaparin 3500 units preoperatively and once daily for the following 7 days. Along with the drugs used for the induction of general anaesthesia, he was also given intravenous cefuroxime 1500 mg and intravenous metronidazole 500 mg. He was also prescribed a further two doses of intravenous cefuroxime 750 mg and intravenous metronidazole 500 mg, both 8-hourly.

OVERVIEW OF 'ACUTE ABDOMEN'

Many people who use the NHS in an emergency have pain as one of their clinical features. Pain may be the only symptom in a patient or it may be accompanied by other symptoms. Pain may be acute or chronic; however, in an emergency situation, pain is more likely to be acute. Lyon and Clark (2006) define acute abdominal pain as 'pain of less than one week's duration'. It is likely that Mr Rossi's set of symptoms were described using the all-encompassing provisional diagnosis of acute abdomen. The term 'acute abdomen' is used frequently to represent a set of symptoms, or syndrome, in which the patient experiences acute pain, nausea and vomiting, and some change in their bowel habit (Boon et al., 2006). As with many diseases and disorders, in the early stages the immediate cause of these symptoms is not always clear, and further investigation is necessary. In order to establish a diagnosis for a patient with an acute abdomen, investigations include a thorough physical examination, abdominal examination, X-rays, ultrasound, computed tomography (CT) scanning, measurement of vital signs and blood screening (a variety of blood tests, including urea and electrolytes (U&Es), full blood count, liver function tests and serum amylase – an enzyme found in serum that is raised in pancreatitis (Nunes and Lobo, 2005).

The information in the opening scenario picks up the care of a patient who presented to the accident and emergency department with acute abdomen. Following examination and investigation, a diagnosis of acute intestinal obstruction was made.

THE NATURE OF ACUTE INTESTINAL OBSTRUCTION

Disorders that cause abdominal pain can affect any of the organs that lie in the abdominal cavity. These organs in the upper gastrointestinal system are – stomach, duodenum, jejunum and ileum (small intestine) – and in the lower gastrointestinal system – ascending, transverse and descending colon (large intestine). The gastrointestinal system also includes the adjacent organs of the liver, gall bladder, pancreas, spleen and kidneys. The remainder of the organs of the gastrointestinal system – appendix, caecum, sigmoid colon, rectum, as well as the urinary bladder and (in females) uterus, fallopian tubes and ovaries – lie within the pelvis.

The contents of the duodenum, jejunum and ileuma are liquid, chyme, and it is here that carbohydrate, fat and protein are broken down into forms that are absorbable by the villi, which are mostly at the distal end of the ileum. Here, carbohydrates and proteins are transported into the capillaries through the epithelial cells that line the capillary walls, while fats are moved into the lacteals (lymphatic capillaries) in the villi.

Once these liquid contents pass through the ileocaecal valve into the ascending colon, water begins to be absorbed. By the time they reach the rectum, the contents are fairly solid. The bowel contents are propelled through the gastro-intestinal tract by a movement called peristalsis: a small portion of the muscular wall of the gut constricts, narrowing the diameter of that piece of gut. This constriction and narrowing action then moves slowly down the gut in a rhythmic action, propelling the bowel contents further through the gut. Peristalsis results from the stimulation of the gastrocolic reflex; this reflex is in response to ingesting (swallowing) food or fluid (Clancy *et al.*, 2002; Marieb, 2005).

Intestinal obstruction is a disorder in which something blocks the flow of faecal contents through part of the intestinal system, either the colon or the ileum.

Mr Giancarlo Rossi

On examination and during his surgery, it became apparent that Mr Rossi has colon cancer with some secondary spread into his liver.

Many people with colorectal cancer have few symptoms in the early days. Even when they do have some symptoms, the embarrassing nature of both the problem and the treatment often means that many people put off having investigations. As a result, when they do eventually present, they do so at a late stage of the disease, making it more difficult to treat the patient successfully. The symptoms may be many and mostly non-specific, such as fatigue, weight loss or altered bowel habit. The WHO (2006) states that the mortality of colorectal cancer is 19 per 100 000, which, given the population of the UK, estimated in 2008 to be just over 60 million (National Statistics Online, 2008), means that more than 11 000 people die as a result of this disease every year in the UK. Colorectal cancer is increasingly common after the age of 50 years. Risk factors for colorectal cancer are both genetic and environmental (influenced by diet and lifestyle) (Boon *et al.*, 2006).

The causes of intestinal obstruction include the following:

- Adhesions
- Tumours
- Hernia
- Intussusception
- Volvulus
- Impacted faeces
- Paralytic ileus
- Strictures resulting from inflammatory bowel disease (Boon *et al.*, 2006).

Personal and professional development 11.2

Write short notes about the way the gastrointestinal system works. Consider how comfortable you would feel about explaining this to Mr Rossi. If after doing this activity you feel you need to understand more fully how this system works, then identify in your portfolio three strategies that you will use to help you do this. Then write short notes in your portfolio exploring what you have learnt.

Related knowledge Pathophysiology

The obstruction in the bowel will be accompanied by inflammation. The inflammatory response will depend upon the severity of the obstruction and how long it has been there, the patient's age and any comorbidities. The inflammatory response is the same, regardless of which organ or body part is involved.

SEE CHAPTER 9

▶ *(continued)*

Inflammation leads to tissue stretching and some degree of distortion. Clinically, this typically produces pyrexia (raised body temperature), tachycardia (increased pulse rate) and a raised white blood cell count. There may be accompanying peritonitis (inflammation of the peritoneum).

The process of obstruction leads to the smooth muscle in the bowel wall contracting forcefully in an attempt to push the obstruction along the bowel. This reflex contraction is known as colic. If this continues and the obstruction is not relieved, the pressure in the lumen of the bowel increases and the bowel proximal to the obstruction becomes dilated. The patient's symptoms depend on the position and the severity of the obstruction and whether the blockage of the bowel is partial or complete. If the obstruction is partial, the obstruction may allow some passage of chyme or faeces through the bowel; the patient is therefore able to pass small amounts of faeces and flatus (wind/gas). If the obstruction is complete, then no chyme or faeces are able to flow past the obstruction; as a result, gas and faeces build up proximal (before) to the blockage. In this situation, the patient is unable to pass any faeces or flatus once the rectum is empty: absolute constipation. The resulting build-up of fluid, faeces (or chyme, if in the ileum) and flatus causes the bowel to distend (swell) as it becomes fuller and fuller, until the bowel wall becomes thinner and thinner. If this is not rectified, the bowel ruptures. At best, the bowel contents leak into the abdominal cavity, with resulting infection; at worst, this is accompanied by haemorrhage, as blood vessels in the bowel wall are ruptured. Both of these situations may be life-threatening. The exterior of the internal organs and the abdominal cavity are usually sterile. In health, the colon relies on a number of bacteria inhabiting the bowel. In the colon these anaerobic bacteria, such as enterococci, clostridia and enterobacteriacae, enhance the activity of the body's inflammatory response. These bacteria produce vitamin K, necessary for blood clotting and for converting indigestible substances such as cellulose (insoluble fibre) and partially digested saccharides (sugars) such as lactose into a more readily absorbable form (short-chain fatty acids). The bacteria also create the more 'antisocial' by-products of digestion – the gases methane and carbon dioxide.

Personal and professional development 11.3

On the diagram below, label the various parts of the gastrointestinal system and write short notes about the actions of each part of the system. Check your knowledge and understanding at the end of the chapter.

Answers can be found at the back of the book.

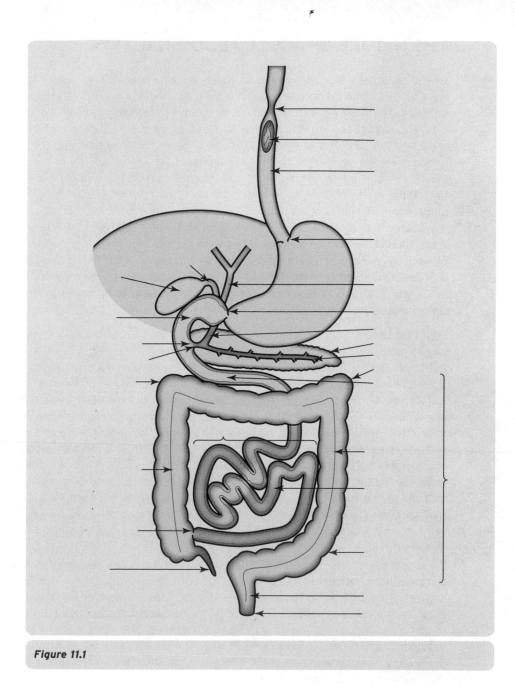

Figure 11.1

THE NATURE OF ACUTE ABDOMINAL PAIN

One of Mr Rossi's main complaints has been what he describes as severe cramp-like pain, or colic. This colicky pain results from the pathological process of obstruction. Constant pain made worse by movement, coughing or laughter is indicative of inflammation, especially seen in peritonitis. If Mr Rossi is lying very still so that he doesn't stimulate this pain, this suggests peritonitis. The character of pain and the way that humans feel pain are both subjective and multifaceted. The complexity of the nature of pain is too large a topic to cover in its entirety in this book. Consequently, we consider here some key points for you to understand in order to develop your insight into the pharmacotherapeutics of acute pain. The need for a comprehensive approach to pain management is identified in this section; this chapter also highlights the non-pharmacological approaches that may be used to treat pain, although these are not discussed in great detail. Aspects of pain management are addressed in a number of chapters in Part 4 of this book, in order to highlight its complexity; acute pain management is discussed in Chapters 10 and 11, while chronic pain management is explored in Chapter 9. Unfortunately, there is no 'one size fits all' model for pain relief.

Pain that occurs from nociception (arising from a noxious or harmful stimulus that causes pain) may be felt differently, depending on where it comes from. The type of pain felt by Mr Rossi is a result of disease in the bowel; such pain is known as visceral pain (from the internal organs), is rather widespread and dull, and can be referred to a more distant site. On the other hand, somatic pain is usually sharp, clearly defined, localised and limited. The visceral pain that Mr Rossi is experiencing comes from the distended (stretched) section of affected bowel, which is slowly becoming more and more distended. Think about how your skin feels when you stretch it; it can be stretched quite considerably before it begins to hurt. On the other hand, a burn is felt as painful almost instantly; indeed, even if you just get close to a heat source, your body lets you know that the action could be dangerous and you pull away from the heat. Pain can signal that something is wrong with the body (pathological) or it can be a warning signal (preventive). Pain is one of the normal functions of the nervous system, designed to protect us from threats of all kind, such as injury, infection and disease. Noxious stimuli irritate the sensory receptors (nociceptors) that abound in the skin and to a lesser extent in the viscera. These nociceptors are the final parts of the myelinated A-δ nerve fibres and unmyelinated C fibres. At the same time, any local insult, whether small or large, for example trauma or infection, results in the inflammatory process being brought into play. This causes the release of a number of chemical mediators, such as histamine, bradykinin and COX-2. These chemicals alter the polarity (electrical differences), so moving the message along the nerve to the dorsal horn of the spinal cord. In the spinal cord, various neuropeptides (chemicals that allow messages to be transmitted by nerves and nerve cells) help to pass the message upwards, to the brain. Magnetic resonance imaging (MRI) scans have demonstrated consistently that pain is perceived in the brain, as many areas of the brain 'glow' on the scan simultaneously, suggesting that the neurotransmitters are taking the pain message to many areas of the brain at the same time. Thus, it seems that at various points in the brain, meaning is added to the message: the limbic system adds emotions and feelings, whereas the frontal lobes are thought to use our memories and experiences in order to interpret the message.

Descartes (1662) was in some ways correct – pain is felt in the brain – but pain is much more complicated than he imagined. It is thought that the A-δ nerve fibres transmit messages straight to the brain when there is a sudden acute type of pain, for example when you burn yourself or trap your fingers in a door (Melzack and Wall, 1965, 1983). However, this sudden acute pain is soon replaced by a different feeling, frequently described as dull, throbbing, aching or burning pain. This is thought to be due to the more slowly reacting C fibres, which travel via a central part of the spinal cord called the dorsal horn. This is where Melzack and Wall's (1965, 1983) 'gate' is thought to lie: when the C fibres are stimulated by pain, they 'open' the gate, allowing pain sensations to be passed up the spinal cord to the brain and messages to be transmitted back down the spinal cord. This two-way traffic of stimulation of C fibres seems to result in pain being felt either more strongly or more weakly and engenders both the response to and the perception of pain in the individual.

In reality

The pain that results from diseased abdominal organs may not always be felt in the abdomen. For example, a patient with a perforated gastric ulcer may complain of severe acute pain at the tip of the shoulder; this is because the fluid and gas that have escaped from the stomach collect under the diaphragm and irritate the vagus nerve. This type of pain is known as 'referred pain' because it tracks along an associated nerve and the pain is perceived by the person to be at some distance to the true site of the pain.

Related knowledge Sociocultural factors

It is important to recognise that social, cultural and physical factors influence not only how people experience pain but also how they cope and deal with it. Consider the response of a soldier injured on a battlefield. The soldier has an expectation of injury. How does this compare with a person injured suddenly in an accident on their way to work?

It is particularly important that, as healthcare professionals, we each have an understanding of our personal and professional values and beliefs (philosophies). Having some insight into our personal philosophies enables us to develop professionally (Carper, 1978). Before you begin to be involved in managing a patient's pain, it is imperative to identify how you feel about pain and contrast this with how you should feel as a healthcare professional. The following exercise will help you to do this.

Personal and professional development 11.4

Here are some questions to ask yourself to help you understand the values and beliefs that you hold about important aspects of pain and pain management. Use this opportunity to explore your values and beliefs as honestly as you can. This is not always an easy thing to do, so this exercise may take you some time. You could record this learning in your professional portfolio.

	Yes	No
I believe that all patients who say they have pain do have pain.	☐	☐
I believe that it's possible to treat all pain with medicines.	☐	☐
As a nurse, I believe that I should ensure that all patients are pain-free.	☐	☐
I believe that patients who are prescribed opioids for pain easily become addicted to them.	☐	☐
I believe that respiratory depression is very common in patients who are given opioids for pain relief.	☐	☐
I believe that when no medical condition can be found in a patient with pain, they don't have any thing wrong with them.	☐	☐

After you have read this chapter, and you have cared for a number of patients in pain, it would be useful to reflect on whether your philosophy in relation to pain management has been challenged or has changed.

It may seem a rather contentious statement to make, but the initial focus of care in the management of pain is not pain relief. This is the case regardless of whether the pain is acute or chronic. The first priority of any healthcare professional when confronted by a person in pain is to seek the cause of the pain and then treat it. Before any pain-relieving strategies are suggested, it is important that the cause of the pain is found. Unfortunately, sometimes this first principle of pain management is ignored by healthcare professionals. For example, many people who are in the end stages of life complain of abdominal pain, but frequently the cause of the pain is not sought. It is thought that, even today, many people die in great distress because the cause of their pain is never looked for, and assumptions are made that the increasing pain is a result of either the process of dying or the patient becoming dependent on opioids. If the patient is taking opioid analgesia, a common response is often to increase the dosage of the opioid instead of looking for a cause of pain first. Frequently, however, for many of these patients the cause of their acute abdominal pain is constipation, usually as a result of a number of factors, including inactivity, insufficient intake of fluid and the use of medicines such as opioids that influence the action of the bowel. Establishing constipation as the cause of pain would save much suffering and distress.

Pain is an indication that something is wrong with the body. It has a variety of causes. Damage to the tissues, regardless of the cause, sets in motion a complex set of responses in the nervous system that the individual perceives as pain. The sensory nerve pathways help the body to identify the intensity, position and type of pain, and at the same time the emotional/affective pathways encourage the body to avoid the pain. The events that happen in response to a noxious stimulus occur at various points in the nervous system, with the activation of the ascending pain pathways in the spinal cord to the brain.

PREOPERATIVE PAIN MANAGEMENT OF ACUTE ABDOMINAL PAIN – CHANGING SCHOOLS OF THOUGHT

Traditionally, analgesia has been withheld from people with acute abdominal pain until a diagnosis has been made and an appropriate treatment regime prescribed. This common strategy is thought to have stemmed from a warning by a Dr Cope in 1921 (Gallagher *et al.*, 2006). Dr Cope's concern, and that of most general surgeons in the Western world since, seems to be that administering opiates before reaching a diagnosis would mask any symptoms and make it difficult for the surgeon to reach an accurate diagnosis. Gallagher and colleagues (2006), among others, argue that there are a number of reasons for surgeons to question the appropriateness of this much-used strategy. These reasons include the following:

- Much more reliable and sophisticated aids to diagnosis are now readily available, such as ultrasound and CT scans.
- Opioid antagonists (e.g. naloxone) that can reverse the effect of opioids have been developed.
- Antibacterials and antibiotics are now widely available, unlike in Dr Cope's day (Gallagher *et al.*, 2006).

Related knowledge Influences of the historical development of knowledge

The understanding since Descartes (1662) was that the focus of pain rested at the source of the pain and that pain was purely a mechanical response to injury. This belief led to the understanding within medicine that there are two types of pain, real pain and imaginary pain. The separation of mind and body that was the basis of Cartesian philosophy led to the commonly held assumption that when there was no obvious cause for the pain being complained of, then it must be 'psychological' in nature. This pain was referred to as 'psychogenic pain' and frequently compared disapprovingly with real pain and consequently viewed as

▶ *(continued)*

questionable. As a result, in difficult-to-manage pain situations, such as a person with intractable pain with no obvious cause (e.g. phantom limb pain, severe back pain) and that did not respond to analgesics, patients were often described as 'lead-swingers' (pretending to be ill in order to avoid having to work) or were considered mentally unstable. This Cartesian view of pain physiology was a widely held perceived wisdom in both medicine and nursing until the gate theory of pain was proposed by Melzack and Wall in 1983. Following the latter's work, much research has been undertaken that recognises the complexity of the pain process at a biochemical level. The first of the opioid receptors was identified in 1973, but, pharmacotherapeutics has not been able to capitalise on this and yet there is still no analgesic available that is as efficient as morphine but that does not have its adverse effects. Since then, healthcare professionals have increasingly questioned the Cartesian view of pain and based their understanding of pain and their practice of pain management on more recent pain theories.

PHARMACOLOGICAL INTERVENTIONS USED TO MANAGE ACUTE ABDOMINAL PAIN

Opioids

Many people are reluctant to take prescribed opioids such as morphine, even for severe pain. This seems to be because many people are concerned that they will develop an addiction to opioids and that they will experience unwanted effects. Many people think that morphine and other opioids come only in two forms: a liquid for injection (usually intravenous) and a powder that is inhaled. Many people are wary of having injections; injections are frequently perceived to be painful and some people have unpleasant childhood memories of mass vaccination (Drayer *et al.*, 1999).

Essential terminology

Narcotic

Any substance that brings about drowsiness, sleep or unconsciousness. The term 'hypnotic' is sometimes used instead of narcotic. The word 'narcotic' seems to be used most commonly in relation to the opioid group of drugs.

Morphine sulphate

Morphine is a powerful narcotic analgesic derived from opium. McGavock (2005) succinctly describes the nature of these, the most effective analgesics known, by saying that they 'are still unsurpassed in making bearable the unbearable'. Morphine acts centrally in the brain. The first of the opiate receptors in humans was identified in 1973 (Pert and Snyder) and a further two have been identified; these receptors are now classified by the Greek letters μ (mu), δ (delta) and κ (kappa). Discovery of the opioid receptors supported the long-held theory that the human body has naturally occuring (endogenous) opioid peptides and suggested that the Cartesian view of the body was extremely limited (Jackson, 2003; Pert, 1999). These endongenous opioid peptides were initially named enkephalins. This term is still used sometimes, but they are now more commonly known as endorphins.

Pharmacokinetics Morphine sulphate

Absorption: is administered directly into the general circulation. Oral morphine is poorly absorbed (**www.emc.medicines.org.uk**).

Distribution: Distributed widely across the body. Morphine crosses the placenta and is found in breast milk and sweat. Just over a third is bound to plasma proteins (**www.emc.medicines.org.uk**).

Metabolism: Morphine (and other opioids) is metabolised in the liver and is broken down into two main water-soluble metabolites. Mr Rossi's age should be considered in relation to the effects of any medicines he takes. Liver function becomes less efficient with ageing, and as a result drugs may not be metabolised (broken down) very well, so the toxic metabolites (breakdown products) build up in the bloodstream. MacIntyre and colleagues (2003) suggest that in some older people, this may lead to organ failure.

Elimination: The water-soluble metabolites of morphine and the other opioids are excreted by the kidneys (Greenstein and Gould, 2004; Rang *et al.*, 2003, Simonsen *et al.*, 2006). Oral morphine is excreted more slowly than IV morphine (**www.emc.medicines.org.uk**).

Nursing knowledge Nursing interventions

People with long-standing disorders of the gastrointestinal system are likely to have reduced quantities of circulating plasma proteins. This is usually because of symptoms such as anorexia, nausea and vomiting and diarrhoea, and the resulting malnutrition. This may lead to increased availability of morphine and other opioids, as more of the drug is available unbound in the plasma. The nurse therefore needs to monitor carefully the patient's response to the opioid in order to ensure that the dose is not too large.

Pharmacodynamics Morphine sulphate

Morphine sulphate is derived from opium. It is a powerful analgesic and narcotic. Its mode of action is not fully understood, but it is thought to act on the central nervous system and smooth muscle. This action means that it can cause a number of adverse effects. As it works centrally in the nervous system (in the brain), it can slow down respiration and cause respiratory depression, particularly in people who have not had opioids before (opiate naïve) and in individuals with obstructive airways disease. Morphine also acts on the vomiting centre in the brain and can make the individual feel nauseated; it can induce vomiting in susceptible people. Consequently, an anti-emetic (anti-sickness) medicine is often administered concurrently with morphine.

The influence of morphine on smooth muscle is seen most frequently in its effect on the bowel. Morphine makes peristalsis less efficient, leading to the slower passage of the bowel contents and resulting in constipation (**www.bnf.org**; **www.emc.medicines.org.uk**).

Interactions

Morphine and the other opioid analgesics interact with many other drugs, including those used socially. These interactions mostly potentiate (increase) the action of the other drug. Drugs that interact with morphine and other opioids are mostly those that have their mode of action in the brain and include alcohol, tricylic antidepressants, anxiolytics (reduce anxiety), hypnotics and antipsychotics (**www.bnf.org**). The BNF gives a long list of the drugs that interact with the opioids and the effects of these interactions in Appendix 1.

Nursing knowledge Nursing interventions

The majority of patients who are taking morphine therapeutically are likely to have some restriction of mobility levels and may not be drinking adequate amounts of fluid. As a result, they are at increased risk of constipation. Patients who are able to should be encouraged to increase their mobility and drink increased amounts of fluids to attempt to overcome this often debilitating side effect. For Mr Rossi, this will not be possible in the immediate postoperative period. There are many other situations when this is not possible, and so other means of preventing constipation may have to be considered.

Communicating professionally – what's in a name?

A number of anxieties and concerns have led to misconceptions about the use of opioids, particularly morphine and diamorphine. These misconceptions may influence patients' and healthcare professionals' behaviour in acute and chronic pain management. These concerns are thought to be a result of the stigma attached to the historical use of opioids (Ballantyne, 2007). UK regulation of opioids first began in 1920 under the Drug Enforcement Act. Before this, opioids were widely available from chemists shops, doctors' surgeries and opium dens, and choosing whether to use opioids was entirely up to the individual. However, this presented major problems for society, which led to legal restrictions. The stigma surrounding the use of opioids increased after the legal regulations were introduced, when the possession of opioids other than on prescription became a criminal offence. Many people believe that opioid dependence easily results from its use and that people adopt criminal behaviours to pay for their habit (Ballantyne 2007; Sykes, 2007), One of the concerns of healthcare professionals is that opioids cause respiratory depression; however, this is seen only rarely and usually only in opioid-naive patients. Titrated doses are recommended in such patients; this means beginning with the smallest possible effective dose in the range.

Nursing knowledge Patient education

As we mentioned earlier, many people are extremely reluctant to take prescribed opioids for pain (Ballantyne, 2007; Sykes, 2007). Some people are concerned that they will become addicted to opioids, that they will experience severe adverse effects and that they will have to have injections. Chumbley and colleagues (2002) and Dihle and colleagues (2001) suggest that a number of strategies help to lower patients' concerns about opioid analgesics and consequently can lead to increased use of this type of analgesia in severe pain. Such strategies include giving information about:

- the low incidence of dependence (addiction);
- the adverse effects of the opioids, and how these will be managed;
- the various non-injection routes available, such as oral dosing and transdermal patches.

If possible, the patient should be encouraged to collaborate with the prescriber to choose their preferred route of administration.

PREOPERATIVE MEDICATION

Premedication

The drugs that are given to prepare a patient for a general anaesthetic are usually referred to as premedication (or premed). A number of medications may be prescribed for a patient going to theatre for surgery. Medications that are commonly administered as premedication are given to aid the surgeon and to keep the patient safe. Premedication may include various groups of medicines to produce some or all of the following effects: anxiolysis (reduction of anxiety), analgesia, amnesia and anti-emesis. The anaesthetist is responsible for the safe delivery of a general anaesthetic, but they are also responsible for assessing the patient's fitness for anaesthesia and for prescribing any necessary premedication. Premedication used to be given routinely to all patients before general anaesthetic. However, with the improvement in the drugs that are available, particularly those used to induce inhalation anaesthesia, there is often little need today to administer medicines that reduce bronchial secretions.

A number of factors influence the anaesthetist's prescribing decisions. Such factors will include the following:

- Whether the operation that is to take place is an emergency or is planned. This may affect not only whether the patient has a premedication but also the type of premedication.
- The patient may have some degree of anxiety before surgery. Factors that can influence anxiety levels in such situations include the patient's personality and coping strategies, their medical condition, the type of surgery they are going to have, how well they understand the information given to them and previous surgical experiences (Vingoe, 1994). Patients who are anxious may be prescribed an **anxiolytic** (a drug that reduces anxiety) if the anaesthetist assesses that it would be appropriate.

Related knowledge Legal issue

One of the key roles of all the healthcare professionals involved is to ensure that the patient understands why they are having surgery and that their written consent to have the operation has been given. Informed consent is both a legal requirement and a moral imperative. Patients should understand not only what they have consented to but also what they are likely to experience postoperatively (DfCA, 2005).

Informed consent is a legal requirement, but it has also been shown to be crucial to successful postoperative recovery (Boore, 1978; Hayward, 1975). Although informed consent provides an explanation and reassurance for the patient, the anaesthetist may judge that the patient requires some form of medication to allay the patient's anxieties – an anxiolytic. For planned surgery, the anxiolytic is usually one of the benzodiazepines, such as lorazepam. The benzodiazepines have to be used with caution, as with medium- to long-term use they lead to reliance and dependence; therefore, they are best used as a short-term measure to manage anxiety (McGavock, 2005).

Continuing previous medication

The anaesthetist will consider whether Mr Rossi is taking medicines for diseases and disorders unrelated to the proposed surgery. Although many medicines can (and will) be stopped suddenly before an operation, some cannot. One of the most common examples of this is a patient who takes an oral hypoglycaemic (a blood-sugar-lowering medicine) for type 2 diabetes mellitus and is going for planned surgery. The patient is asked not to take the oral hypoglycaemic (or, if they are in hospital, the nurse does not administer the medicine) on the day of surgery. This is for two reasons: first, there will be an increased metabolic demand as a result of the surgery, which the oral hypogly-caemic will be unable to meet; second, the patient will be advised not to eat or drink before surgery, which makes the absorption of oral medicines unreliable; the anaes-thetist will therefore prescribe an intravenous infusion of insulin, which will enable the patient's blood sugar to be controlled more accurately both during and after surgery.

THE NATURE OF ANAESTHETICS

Mr Rossi will have a general anaesthetic so that the surgeon can operate on him safely. Anaesthetists use a variety of medicines to induce and maintain anaesthesia. Many laypeople consider anaesthesia as 'being put to sleep'. Although in some ways this is true, it does not recognise fully the complexities of anaesthesia itself or of the drugs used to facilitate it. Anaesthetics is a medical speciality in its own right. To date, there are no nurse anaesthetists in the UK, although this practice is common in some European countries and the USA. We therefore explore only a limited aspect of the medicines used in anaesthesia.

To facilitate the management of a particular patient, the anaesthetist may use addi-tional medicines other than anaesthetics. For example, in order to use surgical techniques in deep structures and tissue, such as the bowel resection that Mr Rossi will have, the anaesthetist will administer a muscle relaxant along with the anaesthetic. The muscle relaxant affects the muscles of respiration (intercostals and diaphragm), and as a result the patient will be unable to breathe spontaneously. Therefore, Mr Rossi will be artificially ventilated during surgery. The anaesthetist will take care to ensure that spontaneous breathing returns as the surgery finishes.

Over the years, as anaesthetists have refined and developed their role in response to a greater understanding of how the body works and the large variety of drugs and improved technology, the word 'anaesthetic' has lost some of its true meaning. The word is derived from the Greek *aisthesis*, which means sensation. Placing 'an' in front of the word changes its meaning to without sensation. The primary focus of the main medicines used to pro-mote anaesthesia is the induction of a loss of sensation to all or part of the body.

There are three main types of anaesthesia:

● *General*: The effect applies to the whole body.

- *Local*: The effects apply within a clearly defined area of the body. For example, you may have had a local anaesthetic if a dentist has carried out work on your teeth. Following injection of the anaesthetic, a certain area around the jaw and mouth has no sensation. As the effects of the medicine wear off, you can feel sensation returning to the area in the form of tingling. If you eat while the jaw area is anaethetised, you can easily chew your cheek as well as the food.
- *Topical*: This is a direct limited application to intact skin or mucous membranes, such as the eye. The effects are in the superficial tissue rather than being felt throughout the whole depth of tissue, as occurs in local anaesthesia.

General anaesthesia

The anaesthetics used to produce generalised loss of sensation to the whole body have traditionally been classified into two groups. This classification system is based on the route by which they are delivered to the patient, namely inhalation and intravenous.

Pharmacokinetics Inhalation anaesthetics

Absorption: The inhaled gases (anaesthetic gas mixed with oxygen) enter the alveoli in the lungs. Each alveolus is closely wrapped in blood vessels. Generally, gas passes from an area of high tension, or partial pressure, to an area of low partial pressure. The alveolar air will have more anaesthetic gas in it than is in the bloodstream surrounding the alveoli. The inhaled gases therefore move from the alveolar air (higher partial pressure) into the bloodstream (lower partial pressure) in an attempt to equal the partial pressure between the two environments.

Distribution: These gases dissolve very readily in the plasma. Consequently, the organs that have the highest blood flow, such as the brain, liver, heart and kidneys, feel the effects quickly.

Metabolism: Some of these gases are metabolised by the liver.

Elimination: The lungs primarily eliminate most of the anaesthetic gases, but some metabolites are excreted in urine.

Pharmacodynamics Inhalation anaesthetics

The anaesthetic gases affect the central nervous system and produce a widespread loss of sensation to some degree. The result is some level of unconsciousness, analgesia, muscle relaxation and the loss of reflexes such as those involved in swallowing, vomiting and blinking.

The extent of the effects on the body will depend on the concentration of the gas mix administered – that is, anaesthetic gas (or gases) mixed with oxygen. By altering this mix, and also by using injectable muscle relaxants and analgesics, a varying and sophisticated degree of anaesthesia can be achieved. This means that the anaesthetist can have fine control over the rate and depth of the anaesthesia; this is particularly valuable for surgical techniques that are lengthy, extensive, painful and/or complex.

Mr Rossi will have an intravenous injection to induce anaesthesia. The intravenous anaesthetics are usually used in procedures that require a shorter period of time, before inhaled gases are used, for induction of anaesthesia or to enhance the effects of inhaled anaesthetics. Commonly used intravenous anaesthetics include drugs from the following groups of medicines: barbiturates, benzodiazepines, hypnotics and opiates.

Pharmacokinetics Intravenous anaesthetics

Distribution: Generally distributed well throughout the body. Most intravenous anaesthetics are lipid soluble.

Metabolism: These drugs are metabolised in the liver.

Excretion: Excreted by the kidneys.

Pharmacodynamics Intravenous anaesthetics

Each group of these drugs has slightly different effects on the central nervous system by preventing some aspect of neurotransmission and interfering in some way with the neurotransmitters, such as acetylcholine (Simonsen *et al*., 2006; **www.bnf.org**).

In reality

In other clinical situations that are different from that of Mr Rossi, some of the medicines prescribed may be different. Other medicines may be prescribed to deal with a patient's pre-existing specific disorder; for example, a patient with atrial fibrillation may be prescribed digoxin to be administered before to surgery.

Mr Giancarlo Rossi

Before surgery, Mr Rossi was prescribed subcutaneous tinzaparin 3500 units preoperatively and once daily for 7 days, and intraveneous cefuroxime 1500 mg and intravenous metronidazole 500 mg on induction, with a further two doses of intravenous cefuroxime 750 mg and intravenous metronidazole 500 mg, both 8-hourly. He was also asked to wear anti-embolic (thrombo-embolic disease, TED) stockings.

REDUCING THE RISKS OF SURGERY

One of the major risks of prolonged immobility is deep vein thrombosis (DVT) and pulmonary embolus, which is potentially life-threatening. With major surgery, there is prolonged immobility during and immediately following the operation. Vincent (2006) suggests that 'DVT occurs after approximately 20% of all major surgical procedures and over 50% of orthopaedic procedures'. Colorectal surgery seems to carry a higher risk of venous thromboembolic episodes than other general surgery. The reasons for this increased risk are unclear, but it is thought that either the positioning of the patient during surgery or the use of pelvic dissection could be possible factors, either individually or jointly (Wille-Jørgensen et al., 2004). The Agency for Healthcare Research and Quality states that prophylaxis to prevent both venous thromboembolism and postoperative infection in patients at risk are two of the 11 practices that they highlight that have robust evidence demonstrating their value (Shojania et al., 2001). Although this is a systematic review from the USA, the practice of medicine there is comparable to that in the UK and Western Europe, and concerns about patient safety within all Western healthcare systems are similar (Vincent, 2006).

The pharmacological treatment that aims to prevent or reduce the incidence of venous thromboembolism uses the group of medicines known as anticoagulants. Anticoagulants interfere with the coagulation (clotting) process of blood, by decreasing its capability to coagulate (clot). They are used in both the prevention and the treatment of venous thromboembolic disorders, such as DVT and pulmonary embolism.

Pharmacological knowledge Other groups of medicines

Once a thrombus has formed, two groups of drugs may be used to liquefy it: platelet inhibitors and fibrinolytics. The platelet inhibitors reduce the ability of platelets to aggregate (stick together) and to trigger further coagulation. The fibrinolytics stimulate the process of fibrinolysis, which means they increase the breakdown of fibrin and fibrinogen, thus liquefying arterial and venous thrombi (**www.bnf.org**; Greenstein and Gould, 2004; Simonsen *et al.*, 2006). For a more detailed explanation of both platelet inhibitors and fibrinolytics, please see Chapter 10.

There are two groups of anticoagulants, the heparins and vitamin K antagonists. Each group works in a different way, and so they are used for different disorders.

Low-molecular-weight heparin

The prophylactic use of low-dose subcutaneous heparin before general surgery is recommended by the BNF for patients who are at high risk of thromboembolic disorders. Patients considered to be at high risk include 'those with obesity, malignant disease, history of deep vein thrombosis or pulmonary embolism, patients over 40 years, or those with an established thrombophilic disorder or who are undergoing large or complicated surgical procedures' (**www.bnf.org**). Following a systematic review of the research studies that have evaluated a combination of interventions used in the prophylaxis (prevention) of deep vein thrombosis and pulmonary embolus, Wille-Jørgensen *et al.*, (2004) recommend that a combination of the heparins and graduated compression stockings offer the best protection for people undergoing colorectal surgery. Their review also raises the question of whether aspirin may be a possible prophylactic because of its antiplatelet effect. However, there are no studies comparing the heparins with aspirin for preoperative prophylaxis (Wille-Jørgensen *et al.*, 2004).

Nursing knowledge Nursing interventions

Wille-Jørgensen *et al.* recommmend that all patients undergoing colorectal surgery should have graduated compression TED stockings applied. Patients should wear the correct length and size and so must be measured for these stockings.

The anticoagulant tinzaparin is one of a number of low-molecular-weight forms of heparin available for the prophylaxis and treatment of venous thromboembolic events. Heparin is a naturally occurring substance in the body and is a very powerful anticoagulant (Greenstein and Gould, 2004). It is a large molecule with a complicated structure; it is possible to break up each molecule into a number of smaller fragments. Only some of these smaller fragments have anticoagulant abilities; the low-molecular-weight heparins such as tinzaparin are made up of only these fragments (fractions). In order to avoid confusion, the whole molecule of heparin is known as unfractionated heparin (Greenstein and Gould, 2004).

Pharmacokinetics Tinzaparin

Absorption: Tinzaparin, like all heparins, cannot be absorbed if taken orally. Therefore, it is given subcutaneously. (Unfractionated heparin can also be given intravenously.) The absorption half-life is 200 minutes.

Distribution: Peak plasma activity is seen 4-6 hours after injection, which is the maximum effect seen.

Metabolism: After being injected subcutaneously, bioavailability is about 90%, and so much of the tinzaparin is available for use.

Elimination: The reticulo-endothelial system (the collection of phagocyctic cells found mostly in the liver, spleen and bone marrow) removes heparin from the circulation (Simonsen *et al.*, 2006; **www.emc.medicines.org.uk**).

Nursing knowledge Nursing interventions

Tinzaparin is injected subcutaneously into the abdominal wall. About 25 mm of skin should be pinched together and the needle inserted at right-angles to the skin.

Pharmacodynamics Tinzaparin

Tinzaparin is described as an anti-thrombotic, because it interferes with the complex cycle of blood clotting. It inhibits a number of the clotting or coagulation factors, particularly factor Xa (**www.emc.medicines.org.uk**). It attaches to anti-thrombin 111 and as a result slows down the conversion of thrombin to fibrin (Simonsen *et al.*, 2006).

Surgical site infection prophylaxis

Infection is another significant risk for Mr Rossi. All surgery causes some kind of break to the skin, the body's major defence against infection. Therefore, all surgery runs a risk of infection, although some types of surgery are riskier than others. Mr Rossi is at greater risk of infection because he is having gastrointestinal tract surgery. During the operation, the surgeon will make incisions into the bowel, and even if it appears that none of the bowel content is spilled into the abdominal/peritoneal cavity, some aerosol spread is inevitable. The normal flora of the bowel includes many naturally occurring microorganisms; in addition, the normal skin flora include staphylococci and streptococci. A type of *Staphylococcus aureus* is well known because of its resistance to methicillin and the majority of other antibiotics available today; this bacterium is known as methicillin-resistant staphylococci aureus (MRSA).

In Mr Rossi's case, the risk of him developing a surgical site infection (SSI) is extremely high. In order to reduce the risk of this happening, it has been almost standard practice for a number of years to give the patient some antibiotic cover that is administered, usually intravenously, close to the beginning of the surgery and then continued for 48 hours. This is particularly important in a situation such as Mr Rossi's, when there is no opportunity to prepare the bowel for surgery. If there is to be an elective operation to the ileum, colon or rectum, the patient is starved for about 4 hours before their anaesthetic and usually has extensive bowel preparation in order to ensure that the bowel is empty. This reduces the risk of contamination of the operation site and also leaves a much clearer site, thus aiding the surgical team to visualise properly the area in which they are working.

Surgical site infections can be local or systemic and cause much pain, misery and mortality. Any surgery on the bowel carries a high risk of infection because of spillage or aerosol contamination of the site. However, not everyone exposed to a particular pathogen will become infected. A number of factors seem to be important in defining whether an individual develops an infection after exposure to a pathogen, including nutritional status, age (e.g. an immune system that is immature or one that is wearing out) and genetic variations. The efficiency of an individual's immune system is crucial in determining whether a pathogen will successfully colonise that individual (Phillips *et al.*, 2001).

Pharmacodynamics Cefuroxime

The cephalosporins are active against Gram-positive organisms such as staphylococci and streptococci and so are used to treat a variety of infections. Cephalosporins are also used to prevent infection following surgery where it is known that the risks of developing an infection are increased. The types of surgery where prophylaxis with cefuroxime are recommended are abdominal, pelvic, orthopaedic, cardiac, pulmonary, oesophageal and vascular surgery (www.emc.medicines.org.uk).

Pharmacokinetics Cefuroxime

Absorption: Like most of the cephalosporins, cefuroxime is absorbed poorly from the gastro-intestinal tract and consequently is given parenterally (Simonsen et al., 2006; www.bnf.org.uk). Plasma half-life is 70 minutes and up to half is bound to plasma proteins (www.emc.medicines.org.uk).
Distribution: Widespread throughout the body. Crosses the blood/brain barrier and the placenta as well as being found in breast milk (www.emc.medicines.org.uk).
Elimination: Most is excreted unchanged by the kidneys with some being excreted in bile (www.emc.medicines.org.uk)

Cefuroxime

Mr Rossi was prescribed cefuroxime, which is one of a group of antibacterials known as cephalosporins.

The cephalosporins are related to the penicillins; therefore, there is a risk of **hypersensitivity** in a small number of patients. Hypersensitivity reactions that have been reported include urticaria, pruritis, maculopapular rash and arthralgia. It is recommended that cephalosporins should be given only with caution to people who have had a severe hypersensitivity reaction (anaphylaxis) (**www.emc.medicines.org.uk**).

As cefuroxime is one of the cephalosporins, it acts on the cell wall of the microorganism (Rang *et al.*, 2003; Simonsen *et al.*, 2006). The choice of cefuroxime as prophylaxis for Mr Rossi is based on the types of organism that are likely to be found at the site of his surgery. Cefuroxime is bactericidal (kills bacteria).

Metronidazole

Mr Rossi was also prescribed metronidazole, which is one of a group of antibacterials prescribed for the prevention and treatment of infection caused by anaerobic bacteria. This group of medicines has a broad spectrum of activity, which means that they are active against a variety of types of bacteria. These medicines are prescribed and administered in situations where it is likely that any infection will be caused by anaerobes and when culture and sensitivity will not be available initially. For surgical prophylaxis, metronidazole is prescribed, with an initial bolus given immediately before surgery and then 8-hourly.

Pharmacokinetics Metronidazole

Distribution: Given intravenously it spreads extensively throughout the body. It also passes across the placenta to the fetus and is found in breast milk. Only 10% of the dosage binds to plasma proteins.

Metabolism: Metabolised in the liver.

Elimination: Excreted by the kidneys (**www.emc.medicines.org.uk**). Metronidazole has a number of adverse effects, most commonly as a result of prolonged therapy. It diffuses across the placenta and is also found in breast milk. These adverse effects include peripheral neuropathy and disturbances of the gastrointestinal tract (from the mouth to the rectum) (**www.bnf.org; www.emc.medicines.org.uk**).

> ### Pharmacokinetics Metronidazole
>
> Metronidazole does not react with cefuroxime or heparin, but it does interact with alcohol, phenobarbitone and 5-fluorouracil (**www.bnf.org**; **www.emc.medicines.org.uk**). The actions of metronidazole are both antibacterial and anti-protozoal. It is effective against anaerobic bacteria (Rang *et al.*, 2003; **www.emc.medicines.org.uk**).

THE NATURE OF POSTOPERATIVE NAUSEA AND VOMITING

Nausea and vomiting are caused by stimulation of the chemoreceptor trigger zone (CTZ) in the brain. The CTZ lies near the medulla, where the vomiting centre is located. Nausea and vomiting at any time is a distressing set of feelings and events, but to have nausea and vomiting after an operation only adds to the distress of the surgery. Postoperative nausea and vomiting (PONV) is thought to be one of the most important areas of apprehension in patients who are about to have a general anaesthetic (Carlisle, 2006; Macario *et al.*, 2006). Indeed, Sweeney (2007) cites Kapur (1991) as describing PONV as the 'big, little problem'. Lachaine (2006) suggests that PONV affects some 30–80% of patients in the first 24 hours after their operation, although Wallenborn (2006) suggest that the figure is actually 20–30%. This is a considerable number of people who are affected by a very distressing problem. It is thought that some people are more at risk of PONV than others, although the physiological mechanism for this is not understood (Carlisle, 2006). The mechanism responsible for nausea and vomiting as a side effect of medicines, such as those used in chemotherapy, is better understood (**www.emc-medicines.org.uk**).

Lachaine (2006) states that previous studies have suggested a number of risk factors, including being female, non-smoking, a history of previous postoperative nausea and vomiting or motion sickness, and opioid use. Consequently, some treatment guidelines are available to help to prevent and manage PONV, and many NHS trusts have such guidelines. Lachaine (2006) confirms the need for sound preoperative assessment of the patient to identify their risk factors. She also suggests that the patient's prescription should be tailored appropriately, beginning in theatre.

Metoclopramide

Traditionally in the UK and Europe, metoclopramide has been the drug of choice to reduce PONV. However, some studies seem to suggest that metoclopramide is ineffective for many people (Lachaine, 2006; Wallenborn *et al.*, 2006), perhaps because the dosage prescribed was too small and not tailored to the individual patient. The standard dose prescribed of metoclopramide is 10 mg, but Wallenborn *et al.* (2006), Lachaine (2006) and the BNF suggest that this dose is too small: Wallenborn and colleagues

(2006) and Lachaine (2006) propose that some individuals need a larger dose or should be given metoclopramide combined with another anti-emetic medicine.

Metoclopramide is described by the BNF as 'an effective anti-emetic'. It is used to treat nausea and vomiting caused by a number of different conditions, including PONV, migraine and cytotoxic drugs (chemotherapy).

Mr Rossi has been given intravenous injections of metoclopramide.

Pharmacokinetics Metoclopramide

Elimination: Mainly via the kidneys (**www.emc.medicines.org.uk**).

Nursing knowledge Nursing implications

The ageing process means that older people are often less able to metabolise and/or excrete metoclopramide, as the liver and kidneys become less efficient with age.

Pharmacodynamics Metoclopramide

The action of metoclopramide is very similar to the way in which the parasympathetic nervous system controls the upper gastrointestinal tract. Metoclopramide is thought to encourage normal peristaltic action (Greenstein and Gould, 2004; Rang *et al.*, 2003; Simonsen *et al.*, 2006).

Pharmacological knowledge Anti-emetics

Another group of anti-emetic medicines that are commonly prescribed is the serotonin 5-HT$_3$ receptor antagonists, such as ondansetron and granisetron. These medicines are highly selective receptor antagonists and block the serotonin 5-HT$_3$ receptors on the cells in the chemoreceptor trigger zone (CTZ) in the brain. Their exact mechanism of action in PONV is not known (**www.emc.medicines.org.uk**). For people identified as being at high risk of PONV, a dose of one of these medicines may be administered intravenously on induction of general anaesthesia. However, there may be some impact on the large bowel, and so these medicines are used with caution. For a fuller discussion of this group of medicines, please see Chapter 7.

POSTOPERATIVE PAIN MANAGEMENT

Overview

Pain is a very common experience for most people. Given that pain is such a common experience and that pain relief has been known about since ancient times, it would seem safe to presume that in our sophisticated society no one would have to suffer pain for long. Sadly, however, this is not always the case. Not all pain is managed in the best way that it could be, and there is evidence that many healthcare professionals have a long way to go in their understanding of pain and its management (Coulling, 2005; Edwards *et al.*, 2001; Prowse, 2006; Schafheutle *et al.*, 2001; Tcherny-Lessenor *et al.*, 2003). Since the Audit Commission (1997) reported that large numbers of hospitalised people experienced 'unacceptable levels of post-operative pain', similar views have been expressed by a variety of studies.

Over the past couple of decades, there have been advances in pharmacological and pharmacotherapeutic understanding and provision. This has resulted in a number of guidelines and the development of acute pain teams led by anaesthetists in most large NHS hospitals in the UK (RCA and Pain Society, 2003; RCS and RCA, 1990).

Related knowledge User viewpoint

In a study carried out on patients following major surgery, Zalon (2004) identified three main factors that were expressed by patients as being imperative to their recovery:

- Pain
- Depression
- Fatigue.

Kirkevold and colleagues (1996) and Moore (1999) recognise that most people undergoing or recovering from major surgery are apprehensive about whether they will recover their full independence.

If postoperative pain is not managed well, this can have implications for some patients. In long-term comparisons between patients with severe pain and patients with mild pain, the risk of developing chronic pain increases in patients who have complained of severe pain for a week following their surgery (Callesen *et al.*, 1999; Caplan *et al.*, 1999; Carr *et al.*, 2005; Wright *et al.*, 2002).

Although the majority of prescribing of analgesia for post-operative pain in NHS hospitals is still carried out by medical staff, much of the pain management undertaken in wards is carried out by nurses (Prowse, 2006; Schaufheutle *et al.*, 2001). In order to do this successfully, nurses need sound assessment skills and must be able to administer and evaluate the effects of the prescribed pharmacological and non-pharmacological strategies used. Underlying these skills are sound theoretical knowledge and understanding and the ability to apply this understanding appropriately in clinical situations (Bird and Wallis, 2002; Higgins *et al.*, 2004). There are a variety of pain assessment tools that can be used, varying from the numerical pain scale (where the patient describes their pain on a scale of 0 to 10, with 0 being no pain and 10 being the worst possible pain) to the complex McGill assessment scale.

Nursing knowledge Nursing interventions

Interventions for pain relief may include any or all of the following:

- Immobilisation of an affected part e.g as in a fracture
- Positioning the patient comfortably
- Local application of heat or cold
- Empathy
- Reassurance
- Giving information
- Complementary therapies, such as relaxation and guided imagery.

Mr Giancarlo Rossi

During surgery, it was confirmed that a carcinoma, a tumour of the epithelial tissue, was the cause of Mr Rossi's obstructed ascending colon. The tumour, which was removed, involved part of the ileocaecal junction (where the ileum joins the caecum, the first part of the colon), and so an ileostomy was formed in order to relieve the obstruction. Mr Rossi made an uneventful immediate recovery from the anaesthetic. He was transferred from recovery to the ward with patient-controlled analgesia (PCA).

Following major surgery, any pain is best managed by the patient, using a syringe driver that the patient controls by pressing a switch when they require pain relief (patient controlled analgesia – PCA). A Cochrane review of 55 randomised controlled trials confirmed that patient-controlled analgesia 'provided better pain control and greater patient satisfaction than parenteral as needed analgesia' (Hudcova *et al.*, 2006). These authors did identify, however, that patients who used higher amounts of opioids complained more often of the adverse effect of pruritis (itchy skin).

Nursing's urban myths about opioid analgesia

McCaffrey and Pasero (1999) identified a number of wrongly held beliefs – 'myths' – about opioid analgesia and pain relief. In this section, we refer to these beliefs as 'nursing's urban myths', as they are still commonly held by some people on the ward floor. Sadly, these urban myths represent a lack of understanding in relation to the action and risk of opioids, and some healthcare professionals withhold medication in order to, as they perceive it, best manage the care of their patients. Here we highlight three of the myths that McCaffrey and Pasero (1999) identify:

> **Urban myth number one – respiratory depression is fairly common in patients who receive opioids for severe pain.**
>
> **The risk of respiratory depression is less than 1%.**
> (McCaffrey and Pasero, 1999, pp 267-270).

The opioids do cause some degree of respiratory depression. Although this is rare, it is life-threatening and we are unable to identify clearly in advance the people who it will affect. Consequently, it is important that postoperatively a careful watch is kept on the patient's respiratory character, depth and rate, while they are recovering from a general anaesthetic and receiving opioids.

> **Urban myth number two – people taking opioids for pain relief easily become physically dependent.**
>
> **Less than 1% do.**
> (McCaffrey and Pasero, 1999, pp 50, 173-174).

McCaffrey and Pasero's discussion recognised that all of the studies reviewed identified physical tolerance in more patients than dependence, but dependence was very rare, at less than 1%. If a patient seems to need more analgesia than the nurse deems appropriate for a particular type of surgery, there is no reason to withhold analgesia. Successful pain management is highly unlikely to lead to dependence, particularly in people who are opioid-naive (have not had opioids before). This is one of the main reasons given by nurses (Schafheutle *et al*., 2001) for withholding analgesia from patients, resulting in poor pain management for the individual. Recognising that pre-emptive analgesia provides a much more satisfactory experience for the patient is the mark of an expert nurse.

> **Urban myth number three – patients who gain relief from a placebo do not have pain.**
>
> **Many patients who have physical cause for their pain obtain temporary relief from a placebo.**
> (McCaffrey and Pasero, 1999, pp 54-56).

Although the science of placebos is not yet clearly understood, it is thought that they produce their effects by releasing the body's natural endorphins (opioids). It has been suggested that all medicines have some placebo effect and that this is due partly to the communication skills of the healthcare professional, which encourages trust. McCaffrey and Pasero (1999) highlight that all of the evidence to date identifies that a placebo effect does not last for very long.

> ## Personal and professional development 11.5
>
> Choose two nursing activities that may be used for Mr Rossi to help him cope with his postoperative pain. Write short notes about each of these activities to justify your choice.

Schafheutle *et al.* (2001) suggest that there are a number of issues surrounding the mismanagement of pain control for some postoperative patients. They propose that the following factors have a major influence on effective pain management after surgery:

- The appropriateness of carrying out pain assessments during the medicine round. Interruptions to the nurse carrying out the medicine round have been highlighted as a major risk factor for medication errors, and patients do not have pain only when medicines are due.

- Nurses often use their 'judgement' about whether a patient is in pain or not. The decision-making process may be rather arbitrary and subjective. For example, nurses may use the patient's behaviour and other non-verbal cues rather than asking the patients.

- Regular prescriptions should be written rather than using PRNs ('when required'). Using PRN medication is an unreliable method as it is more difficult to use pre-emptive analgesia, it relies on patient self-reporting, timing is unpredictable, and nurses' decisions rest on their personal philosophies and ritualistic practice.

- Patient self-administration is a more suitable means of ensuring adequate analgesia. However, some patients are unable to self-adminster, and therefore assessment of the patient's abilities is important before the patient can be deemed capable.

FACTORS AFFECTING PATIENT EDUCATION ABOUT MEDICINES

We have been told that Mr Rossi came to the UK as a young adult. It is important that we do not assume that a person who speaks good English can also read English well. For many people in the UK, English is a second language; many of these people have a good command of spoken English but cannot read or write in English. Other patients may have other difficulties with reading such as dyslexia, learning disability or sight problems.

A study of almost 400 patients explored patients' understanding of the labels on the medication that they used (Schillinger 2006). This study demonstrated clearly that a third of people misunderstood their medication instructions, often because they had difficulty in reading the label. Having multiple prescriptions compounded the problem. Therefore, any written information that is supplied to a patient must be easy to understand and provided in an accessible and appropriate form.

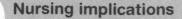

Nursing implications

Mr Rossi has had an ileostomy (part of the ileum brought to the skin's surface) in order to help to manage his bowel obstruction. This may have implications for Mr Rossi in the future in relation to the medicines he may have to take. As highlighted in Chapter 4, medicines that are taken orally are absorbed via the gastrointestinal tract, most in the distal portion of the ileum; sustained-release and enteric-coated medicine forms are designed to be absorbed here. Depending on where the ileostomy is sited, it is likely that some of these medicine forms will be passed out through the stoma unaltered, before they have been absorbed. Such medicine forms should therefore be avoided in individuals with an ileostomy. Some medication may also influence the gastrointestinal tract musculature and innervation, either speeding up or slowing down the rate at which the bowel contents travel. The consistency of the faecal output of the stoma (the portion of bowel that opens on to the skin's surface) may be affected by medicines that alter the amount of water in the gastrointestinal tract; for example, penicillins and iron supplements may cause it to be more fluid (diarrhoea), while codeine, iron supplements and tricylic antidepressants may make it less fluid (constipation). This information should be part of the patient's education about their ileostomy management as well as their medicines management.

Quick reminder

✔ Acute intestinal obstruction is a fairly common general surgical emergency. It has a number of causes, including cancer. It has the potential to be life-threatening.

✔ Effective pain management both before and after surgery is paramount, as is the relief of other symptoms such as nausea and vomiting. The opioids are still the mainstay of providing effective pain relief, both pre- and postoperatively. Delivery of opioid analgesia following surgery is best managed by the patient.

✔ There is much evidence that many patients have poor control of both pain and nausea and vomiting while in hospital. Many healthcare professionals have a poor understanding of the mechanisms of pain and nausea and vomiting and of how best to help patients to manage or prevent their symptoms. Some of this is due to their values and beliefs about pain and the drugs available, particularly the opioids.

✔ Extensive surgery, and accompanying insults to homeostasis, increases the risk of deep vein thrombosis and pulmonary embolism, which can be life-threatening.

✔ Emergency bowel surgery carries a very high risk of infection. Therefore, in addition to using standard precautions for preventing infection in hospitals, prophylactic measures are taken pre- and postoperatively by administering an antifungal and an antibacterial.

REFERENCES

Audit Commission (1997) *Anaesthesia Under Examination: The Efficiency and Effectiveness of Anaesthesia and Pain Relief Services in England and Wales*. London: Audit Commission.

Ballantyne J C (2007) Regulation of opioid pre-scribing. *British Medical Journal* **334**, 811-812.

Bird A and Wallis M (2002) Nursing knowledge and assessment skills in the management of patients receiving analgesia via epidural infusion. *Journal of Advanced Nursing* **40**, 522-531.

Boon N A, Colledge N R, Walker B R and Hunter J A A (2006) *Davidson's Principles and Practice of Medicine*, 20th edn. Edinburgh: Churchill Livingstone Elsevier.

Boore J (1978) *A Prescription for Recovery*. London: Royal College of Nursing.

Callesen T, Bech K and Kehlet H (1999) Prospective study of chronic pain after groin hernia repair. *British Journal of Surgery* **86**, 1528-1531.

Caplan G, Board N, Paten A, Tazaelaar-Molinia J, Crowe P, Yap S J and Brown A (1999) Decreasing lengths of stay: the cost to the community. *Australian and New Zealand Journal of Surgery* **69**, 433-437.

Carlisle J B (2006) Preventing postoperative nausea and vomiting: prevention in context. *British Medical Journal* **333**, 448.

Carper B (1978) Fundamental patterns of know-ing in nursing. *Advances in Nursing Science* **1**, 13-23.

Carr E C J, Thomas V N and Wilson-Barnet J (2005) Patient experiences of anxiety, depression and acute pain after surgery: a longitudinal per-spective. *International Journal of Nursing Studies* **42**, 521-530.

Chumbley G M, Hall G M and Salmon P (2002) Patient controlled analgesia: what information does the patient want? *Journal of Advanced Nursing* **39**, 459-471.

Clancy J, McVicar A J and Baird N (2002) *Preoperative Practice. Fundamentals of Homeostasis*. London: Routledge.

Coulling S (2005) Nurses' and doctors' knowl-edge of pain after surgery. *Nursing Standard* **19**, 41-49.

Department for Constitutional Affairs (DfCA) (2005) *Mental Capacity Act*. London: The Stationery Office.

Descartes R (1662) *De l'homme*. Translated by Hall T S (1972) *Treatise of Man*. Cambridge, MA: Harvard University Press.

Dihle A, Bjolseth G and Helseth S (2001) The gap between saying and doing in post-operative pain management. *Journal of Clinical Nursing* **15**, 469-479.

Drayer R A, Henderson J and Reidenburg M (1999) Barriers to better pain control in hospitalised patients. *Journal of Pain and Symptom Control* **17**, 434-440.

Edwards H E, Nash R E, Najman J M, *et al*. (2001) Determinants of nurses' intention to administer opi-oids for pain relief. *Nursing and Health Sciences* **3**, 149-159.

Gallagher E J, Esses D, Lee C, Lahn M and Bijur P E (2006) Randomized clinical trial of morphine in acute abdominal pain. *Annals of Emergency Medicine* **48**, 150-160.

Greenstein B and Gould D (2004) *Trounce's Clinical Pharmacology for Nurses*, 17th edn. Edinburgh: Churchill Livingstone.

Hayward J (1975) *Information: A Prescription Against Pain*. London: Royal College of Nursing.

Higgins I, Madjar I and Walton J (2004) Chronic pain in elderly nursing home residents: the need for nursing leadership. *Journal of Nursing Management* **12**, 167-173.

Hudcova J, McNicol E, Quah C and Carr D B (2006) Patient controlled opioid analgesia versus conventional opioid analgesia for postoperative pain. *Cochrane Database of Systematic Reviews* (4), CD003348.

Jackson M (2003) *Pain: The Science and Culture of Why We Hurt*. London: Bloomsbury Press.

Kapur P A (1991) The big, little problem. *Anesthesia and Analgesia* **73**, 243-245.

Kirkevold M, Gortner S R, Berg K and Saltvold S (1996) Patterns of recovery among Norwegian heart surgery patients. *Journal of Advanced Nursing* **24**, 943-951.

Lachaine J (2006) Therapeutic options for the prevention and treatment of postoperative nausea and vomiting: a pharmacoeconomic review. *Pharmacoeconomics* **24**, 955-970.

Lyon C and Clark D C (2006) Diagnosis of acute abdominal pain in older patients. *American Family Physician* **74**, 1537-1544.

Macario A, Claybon L and Pergolizzi J V (2006) Anesthesiologists' practice patterns for treatment of postoperative nausea and vomiting in the ambulatory post anesthesia care unit. *BMC Anesthesiology* **6**, 6.

MacIntyre P E, Upton R N and Ludbrook G L (2003) Acute pain management in the elderly patient. In: Rowbotham D J and MacIntyre P E (eds). *Acute Pain: Clinical Management*. London: Arnold.

Marieb E N (2005) *Essentials of Human Anatomy and Physiology*, 8th edn. San Francisco, CA: Benjamin Cumming.

McCaffrey M and Pasero C (1999) *Pain: Clinical Manual*, 2nd edn. St Louis, MO: Mosby.

McGavock H (2005) *How Drugs Work: Basic Pharmacology for Healthcare Professionals*, 2nd edn. Oxford: Radcliffe.

Melzack R and Wall P (1965) Pain mechanisms: a new theory. *Science* **150**, 971-979.

Melzack R and Wall P (1983) *The Challenge of Pain*. New York: Basic Books.

Moore S M (1999) Effects of interventions to promote recovery in coronary artery bypass surgical patients. *Journal of Cardiovascular Nursing* **12**, 59-70.

National Statistics Online (2008) *Population Estimates*. www.statistics.gov.uk/cci/nugget.asp? ID=6).

Newall C A, Anderson L A and Phillipson J D (1996) *Herbal Medicines: A Guide for Healthcare Professionals*. London: Pharmaceutical Press.

Nunes Q M and Lobo D N (2005) Acute abdomen: investigations. *Emergency Surgery* **23**, 199-204.

Pert C B (1999) *The Molecules of Emotion*. London: Pocket Books.

Pert C and Snyder S (1973) Opiate receptor: demonstration in nervous tissue. *Science* **179**, 1011-1014.

Phillips J, Murray P and Kirk P (2001) *The Biology of Disease*. Oxford: Blackwell Science.

Prowse M (2006) Postoperative pain in older people: a review of the literature. *Journal of Clinical Nursing* **16**, 84-97.

Rang H P, Dale M M, Ritter J M and Moore P K (2003) *Pharmacology*, 5th edn. Edinburgh: Churchill Livingstone.

Royal College of Anaesthetists (RCA) and Pain Society (2003) *Pain Management Services: Good Practice*. London: Royal College of Anaesthetists and Pain Society.

Royal College of Surgeons (RCS) and Royal College of Anaesthetists (RCA) (1990) *Commission on the Provision of Surgical Services: Report on the Working Party on Pain After Surgery*. London: Royal College of Surgeons and Royal College of Anaesthetists.

Schafheutle E I, Cantrill J A and Noyce P R (2001) Why is pain management sub-optimal on surgical wards? *Journal of Advanced Nursing* **33**, 728-737.

Schillinger D (2006) Misunderstanding medication labels: the genie is out of the bottle. *Annals of Internal Medicine* **145**, 926-928.

Shojania K G, Duncan B W and McDonald K M (2001) *Making Health Care Safer: A Critical Analysis of Patient Safety Practices*. Evidence report/technology assessment no. 43:2001. Rockville, MD: Agency for Healthcare Research and Quality.

Simonsen T, Aarbakke J, Kay I, Coleman I, Sinnott R and Lysaa R (2006) *Illustrated Pharmacology for Nurses*. London: Hodder Arnold.

Sweeney B (2007) Postoperative nausea: prevention, drugs, treatment. *British Medical Journal* **33**, 313-314.

Sykes N (2007) Morphine kills the pain not the patient. *Lancet* **369**, 1325-1326.

Tcherny-Lessenor S, Karwowski-Soulier F, Lamarche-Vadel A, Ginsburg C and Vidal-Trecan G (2003) Management and relief of pain in an emergency department from the adult patients' perspective. *Journal of Pain and Symptom Control Management* **25**, 539-546.

Vincent C (2006) *Patient Safety*. Edinburgh: Churchill Livingstone.

Vingoe F J (1994) Anxiety and pain: terrible twins or supportive siblings. In: Gibson H B (eds) *Psychology, Pain and Anaesthesia*. London: Chapman & Hall.

Wallenborn J, Gelbrich G, Bulst D, *et al.* (2006) Prevention of postoperative nausea and vomiting by metaclopramide combined with dexamethasone: randomised double blind multicentre trial. *British Medical Journal* **333**, 324-327.

Wille-Jørgensen P, Rasmussen M S, Andersen B R and Borly L (2004) Heparins and mechanical methods for thromboprophylaxis in colorectal surgery. *Cochrane Database of Systematic Reviews* (1), CD001217.

World Health Organization (WHO) (2006) *Mortality Country Fact Sheet 2006.* **www.who.int/ whosis/mort/profiles/mort_euro_gbr_unitedking dom.pdf.**

Wright D, Paterson C, Scott N, Hair A and O'Dwyer P J (2002) Five year follow up of patients under going laparoscopic or open groin hernia repair: a randomised control trial. *Annals of Surgery* **235**, 333-337.

Zalon M L (2004) Correlates of recovery among older adults after major abdominal surgery. *Nursing Research* **53**, 99-106.

Chapter 12

Epilepsy:
a young woman with a long-term condition: epilepsy

Hippocrates was the first person to write about epilepsy. Beliefs at this time, approximately 400 years BC, appeared to focus upon epilepsy being 'handed down' by the Gods. Treatments could include 'exorcism, bleeding, castration or drinking the blood of fallen gladiators' (Tugwell, 2003).

This chapter introduces Katie Johnson, a young woman with epilepsy, whose condition is normally well controlled by her medication. However, following a party at a friend's house, she has had a convulsion. The chapter explores the scenario, the treatment that Katie is receiving and issues related to alcohol and unprotected sex.

✔ Learning outcomes

At the end of this chapter you should be able to:

✔ Give an overview of epilepsy
✔ Discuss the potential impact of epilepsy on an individual
✔ Identify pharmacological approaches to the management of seizures
✔ Discuss the actions and effects of sodium valproate related to the specific patient scenario
✔ Identify the nursing knowledge needed in order to manage this patient and her epilepsy
✔ Identify supporting nursing interventions for this patient.

Chapter at a glance

Overview of epilepsy
Anatomy and physiology of nerve transmission
Pathophysiology of epilepsy
Pharmacological interventions used to manage epilepsy
Nursing implications
Professional guidance
Quick reminder
References

Katie Johnson

Katie Johnson is 15 years old. She lives with her parents and twin brothers, Jack and Sam, who are 10 years old, in a small three-bedroomed end-terraced house. She has had epilepsy since childhood, diagnosed at the age of 11 years. She suffered from frequent tonic–clonic seizures. However, she has been maintained successfully on sodium valproate 200 mg twice a day. She has now been free of seizures for 3 years.

Katie used to be the centre of attention in her family, particularly after her epilepsy was diagnosed; however, recently it is the twins who have been the focus of her parents' attention, as they are aware that the boys have been bullied and are anxious about changing schools in September.

For the past 7 months, there have been lots of rows between Katie and her parents. She has been staying over at a friend's house once or twice a week, 'just to have some space'. Her latest school report highlights that she is not doing as well this year as her teachers had predicted, and she has had a lot of absences.

Her parents are shocked and have tried to discuss this with Katie, but these discussions always end in rows, with Katie storming to her room, shouting that they only care about the boys. Katie's parents are even more anxious when her teacher suggests that Katie's friend Jodie may not be a good influence on Katie.

Jodie is almost 16 years old and has had a regular boyfriend for 3 months, with whom she is sexually active. Jodie's parents are very busy and are unaware of the nature of this relationship and that Jodie uses both alcohol and drugs. At a recent party, Jodie encouraged Katie to drink a mixture of vodka and rum shots. Although Katie doesn't remember much about the party, she thinks she also took some 'white tablets' that John, one of Jodie's friends, offered her. She was very ill the next day, hungover and vomiting.

She had a seizure later that week. Her parents are very concerned about this, but she has an appointment to see her nurse specialist next month. Katie is more concerned that her period is now 10 days late.

OVERVIEW OF EPILEPSY

Epilepsy is a relatively common condition, affecting approximately 450 000 people in the UK (National Society for Epilepsy, 2002). It affects more men than women. Epilepsy is a disorder of the nervous system that results in the patient experiencing seizures (also referred to as convulsions or fits). The World Health Organization (WHO), (2001) defines epilepsy as a disorder 'characterised by ... recurrent seizures' resulting from 'sudden, usually brief, excessive electrical activity in a group of brain cells (neurons)'. The word 'epilepsy' is derived from the Greek for 'to seize' or 'to attack'. Patients are diagnosed as having epilepsy if they have repeated seizures (two or more within a short timeframe) that originate within the brain.

Related knowledge Causes of seizures

- *Pyrexia*: Seizures may occur in children under 5 years old as a consequence of a high body temperature, referred to as 'febrile seizures' (previously known as 'febrile convulsions').

- *Disease processes*: Relating to respiratory, hepatic or renal failure, or resulting in hypoxia, pyrexia, hypoglycaemia or electrolyte imbalance.

- Medicines or the withdrawal of medicines
(Brooker and Waugh, 2007; Lanfear, 2002).

ANATOMY AND PHYSIOLOGY OF NERVE TRANSMISSION

In health, messages to coordinate and control all body functions, for example movement and emotions, are transmitted via nerve cells (neurons) within the brain. These neurons behave like a small electrical source and produce a purposeful and controlled nervous activity (impulse) to generate a required action such as movement. There is always more than one neuron involved in the transmission of the impulse: the nerve impulse is generated within the cell of the neuron, passes along the nerve fibre to the nerve endings and then jumps to another neuron across a synapse (Figure 12.1).

The neuron is the fundamental unit of the nervous system. The dendrites are tree-like extensions of the body of the neuron; they contain neurotransmitter receptors that receive chemical input from other nerve cells. This transmission can be helped (excitatory mechanism) or hindered (inhibitory mechanism) by the assistance of neurotransmitters (chemicals produced at nerve endings) such as gamma-aminobutyric acid (GABA). GABA is probably the most common **inhibitory** substance in the central nervous system.

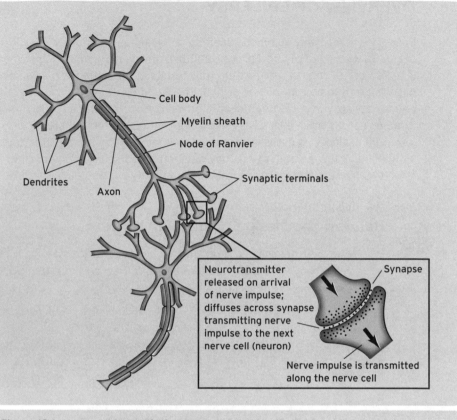

Figure 12.1 Neuronal transmission

PATHOPHYSIOLOGY OF EPILEPSY

A seizure occurs when the nerve impulses in one part of the brain are uncoordinated and many more are produced than are required. They spread to other parts of the brain, causing a burst of abnormal discharge that results in uncontrolled stimulation of the cells. This results in a disturbance of behaviour, emotion, motor activity or sensation: a seizure.

A seizure is defined as 'a sudden burst of abnormal neuronal activity within the brain' (Prosser *et al.*, 2000). Seizures are thought to be a result of a dysfunction of the inhibitory action of GABA, which is found within the central nervous system. A seizure starts with abnormal, high-frequency firing of a group of neurons. When GABA is not available to damp down this activity, other neurons become involved and the abnormal electrical activity spreads. Standard medicines used in epilepsy (**anticonvulsant** therapy) act by preventing the transmission of the nerve impulse, either by enhancing GABA action, which then suppresses the synaptic transmission, or by stopping the transmission by interfering with the spread of this excessive neuronal activity (Downie *et al.*, 2003).

The neurons affected, and the area of the brain that the impulse spreads to, determine the type of seizure that the patient experiences. Seizures are therefore classified according to their characteristics – partial or generalised. These classes can be further categorised, thus:

- *Partial (focal)*:

  - *Simple partial*: The seizure arises from a specific, localised part (limited to a small area) of the brain. This probably involves both movement (motor neurons), usually in one limb, and sensation, although it may be either motor or sensory, determined by the part of the brain affected. It is usually short-lasting and the patient does not lose consciousness. It may be preceded by a warning sign or aura, such as a smell or taste.

  - *Complex partial*: The seizure starts as a simple partial seizure but then spreads throughout the brain to become generalised, with the patient losing consciousness. It may be associated with strange and inappropriate behaviour, such as lip-smacking or chewing. The patient may experience an aura.

Both simple and complex partial seizures may develop into generalised tonic-clonic seizures.

- *Generalised*:

  - *Absence*: This seizure occurs commonly in childhood, often clearing up after puberty. It consists of brief periods of unconsciousness, or lack of awareness and motor activity. This seizure used to be referred to as 'petit mal'.

  - *Myoclonic*: This is a brief loss of consciousness accompanied by uncontrollable involuntary muscular jerking of the limbs or body.

  - *Tonic-clonic*: This is the most common type of seizure. It has identifiable stages, and used to be referred to as 'grand mal'. There may be an aura. The patient experiences loss of consciousness, rigidity (tonic phase) and jerking of the limbs (clonic phase). The patient then loses consciousness, often for as long as an hour. On regaining consciousness, confusion is common. The patient may also be incontinent of urine and/or faeces during the tonic phase (Downie *et al.*, 2003; Prosser *et al.*, 2000; Whittaker, 2004).

Personal and professional development 12.1
Further reading

Some textbooks give a much more comprehensive overview of seizures. You may wish to do some further reading. *Disorders and Interventions* by Norma Whittaker (2004) has a useful explanation of seizures on pages 183-186. Alternatively, visit the website of the WHO **www.who.org**.

Suffering seizures such as those discussed above can be very distressing for the patient and for observers. It may also interfere with aspects of the patient's life, such as driving. Seizures, once they have begun, cannot be stopped, although they are usually short-lasting. There is a potential for the patient to be injured during a seizure. Nursing interventions include observation, to keep the patient safe during the seizure, and providing care for the patient after the seizure until consciousness returns (Brooker and Waugh, 2007).

We do not understand fully why epilepsy occurs, and there is no cure. However, with treatment, some 70–80% of people with epilepsy can become seizure-free, and half are able to discontinue their medication (Chappell and Crawford, 1999). Epilepsy, depending upon the reference source consulted, is described variously as a condition, as a term covering a range of conditions or as a symptom (McIntosh and Berkovic, 2005).

If the epilepsy is a symptom of an underlying disease process, then it may be possible to treat the cause, such as an infection, trauma or a tumour. In most cases, it is not possible to identify a cause; this is referred to as 'idiopathic epilepsy' and is said to account for 60% of epilepsy (Whittaker, 2004). If a patient goes on to experience seizures for more than 5 years, it is described as 'chronic epilepsy'.

PHARMACOLOGICAL INTERVENTIONS USED TO MANAGE EPILEPSY

Indications for treatment are a confirmed diagnosis or a history of more than one seizure in 12 months. Consideration must also be given to the severity and frequency of seizures (Trost et al., 2005). Other factors, such as the patient's age, gender (it is suggested that there is a link between seizures and oestrogen levels: www.drugtopics.com) and intellectual profile, should also be considered (20% of people with learning difficulties have epilepsy), as should the patient's ability to adhere to treatment. The majority of patients can be controlled well with a single anticonvulsant medicine (monotherapy).

The aim of treatment is to control the seizures so that patients such as Katie can maintain their lifestyle. However, with any treatment regime, the prescribed dose will reflect one that controls or manages symptoms: the main aim is to reduce or eliminate seizures without impairing mental or motor function, and with minimum adverse effects.

As a principle, we tend to start with the minimum recommended prescribed dose, which is increased gradually until the seizures are controlled effectively – that is, the patient is seizure-free. It is not always possible to eliminate seizures with treatment, but it is usually possible to reduce the number and severity (Tugwell, 2003). Unfortunately, adverse reactions are 'a major issue' with anticonvulsants, and thus the choice of medication in relation to the type of seizure experienced and increasing the dose gradually are crucial (Tugwell, 2003).

The medication is monitored by talking to Katie and her parents. Blood monitoring is often used to establish circulating levels of a medicine in the bloodstream. However, this is not thought to be helpful in relation to Katie's prescribed medication, as the concentration of sodium valproate in the plasma is not a useful indication of its efficiency. Nurses need to remember that blood monitoring is an invasive technique and so should be kept to a minimum.

Pharmacological knowledge The choice of medicine to be used

The choice of medicine depends upon:

- the condition;
- the type of seizure;
- patient factors, such as age, gender, occupation, alcohol and/or caffeine intake, and their ability to comply with/adhere to their treatment. We also need to consider other aspects of the patient's condition and the way it affects the patient, such as the presence of fatigue and stress;
- the cost of the medicine.

Nursing implications Patient information

If a patient is taking anticonvulsant medication, the use of other medicines, alcohol, caffeine and recreational drugs can increase their risk of seizures. It is thought that alcohol and caffeine can trigger a seizure.

Katie has been maintained successfully on sodium valproate 200 mg twice a day.

Sodium valproate

Sodium valproate is classified as an anticonvulsant medicine, effective against all types of seizures but thought to be particularly effective against tonic–clonic seizures (and also absence and myoclonic seizures). It is therefore the medicine of choice for Katie. Despite much research, the mechanism of action of anticonvulsants is still not fully understood (Rang *et al.*, 2003).

Sodium valproate is an example of a medicine that enhances GABA action. This group of medicines act by suppressing the focus of neuronal discharge by enhancing the activity of neurotransmitters such as GABA, which act by blocking the synaptic transmission to result in the reduction or abolishment of excessive discharge. Examples of these medicines are sodium valproate and phenobarbitone.

Sodium valproate is an analogue of the inhibitory neurotransmitter GABA. It leads to an increase in the concentration of GABA at the synapse. It is thought that it produces its anticonvulsant action by reducing excessive neuronal discharge. It is effective against a variety of seizures, especially myoclonic.

According to the BNF (**www.bnf.org**), the usual dose of sodium valproate is 100–200 mg taken orally once or twice daily. In young children, the dose is weight-related.

Sodium valproate also has another action, it inhibits the secondary phase of platelet aggregation, and so consideration needs to be given to other medication (prescribed and OTC) that the patient may be taking and that has a similar effect, such as aspirin.

It is contraindicated in patients with liver disease. Liver function can be affected, and it is therefore advisable that patients at risk and taking sodium valproate have liver function tests carried out regularly.

Personal and professional development 12.2
Learning needs

Take a moment to think about how familiar you are with the information presented thus far. You might wish to:

- do some further reading about epilepsy;
- undertake some research about the normal physiology of the central nervous system;
- remind yourself of the principles of pharmacodynamics and pharmacokinetics outlined in Chapter 4.

Pharmacodynamics Sodium valproate

Anticonvulsant. Potentiates the inhibitory effect of GABA through an action on the further synthesis or metabolism of GABA.

Pharmacokinetics Sodium valproate

Absorption: Absorbed well orally.

Distribution: Strongly protein-bound. Crosses the placenta and enters breast milk.

Metabolism: Metabolised in the liver. Plasma half-life is 8–20 hours.

Elimination: Via the kidneys in the urine.

Compared with most anticonvulsants, sodium valproate is relatively free of unwanted effects. According to the BNF, the adverse effects include:

- effects on the gastrointestinal tract, such as nausea, gastric irritation, diarrhoea and weight gain;
- increased alertness, aggression, hyperactivity, behavioural disturbances and increased appetite;
- thinning and curling of the hair, **ataxia** (shaky movements and unsteady gait) and tremor;
- thrombocytopenia (a reduction in the number of platelets, which can result in bruising and bleeding);
- liver failure.

A fuller list can be found at **www.bnf.org**.

These adverse effects may result in Katie being reluctant to take her medication.

Personal and professional development 12.3
Using pharmacological information: the nurse's role

It is important that experienced nurses 'use' information. We introduced the principles of pharmacodynamics and pharmacokinetics in Chapter 4. Using this information, can you draw any conclusions from the information given above about sodium valproate?

In reality

Sodium valproate is still classified in the BNF (**www.bnf.org**) as an anti-epileptic, but some authors suggest that 'anticonvulsant' is a better term for encouraging patient adherence because the label is more acceptable.

Inhibition of sodium channel function

Another group of medicines that are commonly used to treat epilepsy inhibit sodium channel function (sodium is necessary for the generation of the nerve impulse). This group of medicines works by preventing the spread of neuronal excitation. They have a blocking action on the high frequency of nervous discharge that occurs in a seizure, but they do not interfere with the low-frequency neuron activity that is necessary for other body functions. They exert a stabilising effect on excitable cell membranes by reducing the transport of sodium ions across the neuronal cell membrane. Examples of medicines in this category are carbamazepine and phenytoin.

Current approaches

The current trend is toward monotherapy, as anticonvulsant medicines may interact with each other in two ways:

- Alteration in the metabolism of the other medicine
- A change in the ability of the medicine to bind to plasma proteins, which increases the potential for toxicity.

Although sodium valproate and carbamazepine are described as 'the two most commonly used first line treatments' (Tugwell, 2003), there are newer medications available. These include gabapentin and lamotrigine (NICE, 2004).

Gabapentin may be prescribed in combination with other medicines when epilepsy is not being controlled effectively. The mechanism of action of gabapentin is not known (Rang *et al.*, 2003), but it may inhibit calcium channels and bind to a specific site in the brain. It is relatively free of adverse effects.

Lamotrigine has similar effects to phenytoin and carbamazepine. It acts by inhibiting sodium channels. It has a broader therapeutic profile than the traditional treatments and is particularly useful in the treatment of absence seizures. Adverse effects include hypersensitivity.

NURSING IMPLICATIONS

Stigma

The concept of stigma goes back to ancient Greek culture, when the term referred to physical blemishes that marked some people as being different and therefore 'not normal'. Nowadays the term is often applied to things that we cannot see and perhaps do not understand, but to which we attach labels, such as chronic disease. The person with epilepsy may be perceived as being flawed or having defects; sadly, this perception of people with conditions such as epilepsy is found in healthcare professionals as well as the general public (Alexander *et al.*, 2006). The person may feel as if they are treated differently and unfairly as a result. This can have an effect on the way people see themselves and make them feel devalued. As a consequence, people with epilepsy may be reluctant to disclose that they have the condition, and thus avoid behaviours that draw attention to their epilepsy, such as taking tablets.

Compliance

Compliance can be defined as:

> ... the extent to which a person's behaviour (in terms of taking medications, following diets or executing other lifestyle changes) coincides with medical or health advice.
>
> (Haynes *et al.*, 1979)

Although this definition in several years old, it is used still in modern textbooks as it is clear and succinct. However, contemporary authors are critical of this approach. It is now strongly recommended that we use the term 'adherence' or 'concordance' when referring to a patient's ability to follow treatments or advice. The reason for this is that the term 'compliance' is felt to imply a paternalistic approach on the part of the health professional, that 'doctor knows best'. Adherence and concordance, on the other hand, imply a patient/healthcare professional relationship with the patient as an equal partner who has an active part in the decision-making process.

In reality

The term 'compliance' is still frequently used. This might be because we are more familiar with this term. If we wish to investigate the literature on the topic, using 'compliance' as a keyword yields more results than using 'concordance' or 'adherence'.

There is a lot of evidence to suggest that patients with epilepsy do not comply with their medication (McIntosh and Berkovic, 2005). There are many reasons for this such as:

- the patient does not feel ill;
- the adverse effects of the treatment are unpleasant;
- the patient feels stigmatised: if a patient is seen taking tablets, it inevitably attracts questions - and, as noted previously, there is still a stigma attached to epilepsy.

If there is a long gap between seizures, the patient may believe that the original diagnosis was wrong or that they have been cured. Some patients stop their treatment to test whether they still have seizures; if stopping the treatment results in the patient experiencing a seizure, this can have unfortunate consequences for their lifestyle, for example their entitlement to hold a driving licence.

Downie *et al.* (2003) suggest that 'a major cause of treatment failure is poor compliance' and that patients should therefore understand the implications of their treatment. One way of managing adherence is to consider patient factors such as lifestyle. For example, complex treatment regimes make adherence difficult, and so anything that makes the regime easier may improve adherence. In Katie's case, we could consider how often she takes her tablets and then try to limit her treatment to one medicine only.

It can take several weeks for the full pharmacological action of anticonvulsants to occur. Therefore, Katie might feel quite despondent when she first takes her medicine, especially if she is also coming to terms with her diagnosis. Katie would need a lot of support to encourage her to persevere with her treatment.

The major reason for non-compliance with a range of conditions is the unwanted, often distressing adverse effects that accompany some treatments. We have already considered the adverse effects of anticonvulsants and provided information about how the medicine works. We now need to translate this into appropriate nursing strategies.

The nurse's role

- *Careful assessment of the patient*: This helps to exclude factors in the patient's history that would mean the medicine is contraindicated, such as problems with liver function, pregnancy or breastfeeding.

- *Consideration of other medications that the patient could be taking*: This includes other anticonvulsants (e.g. phenytoin, carbemazepine) – although note that Katie is only receiving monotherapy – also medicines that Katie uses to self-medicate (e.g. aspirin) and other prescribed medicines (e.g. erythromycin (an antibiotic), antidepressants) (**www.bnf.org**).

- *Patient education*: The medicine should be taken with food or be gastro-resistant. For younger children, it can be given in syrup form. Patients should be advised to avoid the consumption of alcohol and to consult with a nurse or doctor before taking OTC medicines. Patients should understand that stopping or changing treatment can result in a return of the seizures, and so treatment should be altered only if advised by the prescriber. The patient should inform all other medical personnel (e.g. dentist, surgeon) that they are taking epilepsy medication. It is useful for the patient to carry a card or wear specialised jewellery indicating their condition and the medication taken.

- *Monitoring the effectiveness of the medication*: The nurse should note the alertness of the patient and take note of any adverse effects, such as jaundice, light-coloured stools, vomiting and diarrhoea, that would indicate liver failure.

Patient education

Alcohol

Alcohol use by adolescents may result in risk-taking (Alcohol Concern, 2002a). In the case of Katie, it appears to have resulted in unprotected sex and drug taking. The vodka and rum that Katie has been drinking contain ethyl alcohol, which is a psychoactive substance that affects the central nervous system. Although young people such as Katie and Jodie drink alcohol to 'get high', it actually exerts a depressant effect

(Rassool and Winnington, 2003). Jodie and Katie are more likely to get drunk than their male friends, as females do not metabolise alcohol as efficiently as men do (Alcohol Concern, 2002b). The type of drinking displayed by Katie, even though it was on only one occasion, is now often referred to as '**binge drinking**' – that is, occasional but heavy drinking. It may well be that Jodie, on the other hand, has an alcohol problem – dependence. Alcohol Concern (2001) defines binge drinking as 'drinking sufficient alcohol to reach a state of intoxication on one occasion, or in the course of one drinking session'. This can also be referred to as 'risky single occasion drinking' (Murgraff *et al.*, 1999).

However, alcohol is also thought to have beneficial effects on health. For example, it has been suggested that certain components of red wine may help to prevent cancer (**http://info.cancerresearchuk.org**). Therefore, it is important that advice about appropriate consumption of alcohol is given (**www.nhsdirect.nhs.uk**; **www.alcoholconcern.org.uk**). The advice for women is to drink no more than 14 units per week, and no more than 3 units per day. A unit is defined as a drink containing 8 g of absolute alcohol and refers to a 'standard' drink, such as a regular glass of wine or a half-pint of lager. The body takes about 1 hour to eliminate 1 unit of alcohol. Although we do not know exactly how much Katie drank, one bottle of spirits, such as vodka, contains about 30 units of alcohol (Alexander *et al.*, 2006). As well as the potential health effects caused by excessive drinking, alcohol can interfere with the action of many prescribed medicines and, as we saw in Katie's case, can trigger seizures.

Katie does not remember much of the party, and so we can assume that she also experienced disinhibition, relaxation and a feeling of excitement caused by the alcohol (Rassool and Winnington, 2003). Goodwin (1994) does suggest that alcohol has a 'unique' affect compared with other drugs, in that it produces a 'blackout' – that is, the person cannot recall what they did. Goodwin suggests that this effect is more likely to occur in alcoholics rather than social drinkers. In Katie's age group, up to 13% of first sexual experiences are related to alcohol (Alcohol Concern, 2002a).

Unprotected sex

Alcohol

We do not know yet whether Katie is pregnant, but we do know that continued use of alcohol during pregnancy can affect the unborn baby. When connected to drinking large amounts of alcohol, this is called fetal alcohol syndrome. The baby could have growth deficiencies, developmental problems, joint and heart problems and altered physical features such as specific facial features (Alexander *et al.*, 2006). Unfortunately, if Katie is pregnant, then her baby could also be affected by the treatment that she has been taking to manage her epilepsy.

Anticonvulsants

Sodium valproate is potentially teratogenic – that is, it can cause abnormalities in the foetus. The fertilised ovum is sensitive to medicines even in the first 2 weeks of pregnancy, although the greatest risk is between the third and eleventh weeks of pregnancy, as that is when the foetal cells start to develop into organs. If Katie is pregnant, her baby might already be at risk, and therefore her treatment would need to be reviewed. The best advice for any woman with epilepsy planning to have a family is to discuss her treatment with her doctor before she conceives. Some anticonvulsants are available that are not so problematic as sodium valproate, but any change would have to be under medical supervision so that withdrawal seizures do not occur. Medicines pass across the placenta in much the same way that medicines pass into body organs and tissues – that is, by simple diffusion from a high concentration to a low concentration. Pregnancy can affect how medicines are used by the body (medicines and pregnancy are discussed in Chapter 4).

> ## Personal and professional development 12.4
> ### The nurse's role
>
> Consider the nurse's role in relation to Katie if her pregnancy is confirmed.

Infections

Unprotected sex does not only carry the risk of unplanned pregnancy. It can also result in the contraction of a sexually transmitted disease, most commonly chlamydia. This disease is particularly problematic because it is relatively symptom-free but can result in sterility if untreated. Chlamydia is a bacterial infection and can be treated with azithromycin, an antibiotic. Azithromycin inhibits protein synthesis within the bacterial cell, thus resulting in cell death.

Katie Johnson

Katie keeps her appointment with her nurse specialist. Katie is still concerned that she might be pregnant. She discloses this to the nurse, who is reassuring and supportive; the nurse immediately carries out a pregnancy test, which proves to be negative. The nurse provides Katie with a lot of information about the implications of unprotected sex and the effects of epilepsy medication on an unborn baby. She suggests that Katie sees her GP about contraception. Katie thinks that this is quite a good idea but is concerned about what her parents will say when they find out about it.

Consent

The Children's Act of 1989 established the child's right to participate in decisions about their care and to give consent to treatment if they were deemed to be mature enough to understand the consequences. This was challenged by a Mrs Gillick in the early 1980s, when she discovered that one of her daughters had been given advice about contraception without her knowledge. Her challenge gave rise to the term 'Gillick competence', used to describe a child's ability to play a part in decisions about their own care. Following the House of Lords' judgment in the Gillick case, Lord Fraser issued some criteria considered to be the basis of good practice for health professionals and commonly referred to as the Fraser Guidelines. New guidance was issued in 2004 that does not change this legal framework but clarifies what advice the person under age 16 years should receive in relation to contraception. Further details can be obtained by accessing the revised guidance at **www.dh.gov.uk**.

Katie Johnson

Katie is relieved to find out that, at age 15 years, she can express her own wishes about contraception. She is not planning on needing a contraceptive, as she has no regular boyfriend, but she is frightened about the risk, however small, of having a 'damaged' baby. She sees her GP and he suggests that if she wishes to use contraception, it would be possible to prescibe her a contraceptive pill, such as Microgynon® 30. He suggests that she gives this some thought, as it would require a review of her anticonvulsant treatment.

Contraception
The combined oral contraceptive pill contains the hormones oestrogen and progesterone. It is a prescription-only medicine (PoM). Oral contraceptives are considered both appropriate and practical for most women. Oestrogen suppresses the development of the ovarian follicle, while progesterone is used to thicken the mucus at the cervix, making it difficult for sperm to enter.

Microgynon 30 contains the oestrogen ethinyloestradiol and levonorgesterol, a synthetic hormone similar to progesterone. It is taken daily for 21 days and then repeated after 7 pill-free days. During this 7-day period, withdrawal bleeding occurs.

Women prescribed a combined contraceptive pill should be assessed carefully in order to reduce the risks associated with their use, such as venous thromboembolism, arterial disease and migraine (**www.bnf.org**).

It is often necessary to prescribe higher doses of oral contraceptives to women who are also prescribed anticonvulsants; however, sodium valproate does not interact with hormonal contraception.

Morning-after pill
An option for Katie, if she had approached a healthcare professional earlier, would have taken to take a 'morning-after pill' such as Levonelle™. This is a synthetic hormone similar to progesterone; it can be given as part of a combined oral contraceptive, but it also used as emergency postcoital contraception. It should be taken within 72 hours after sex to be effective, although it may be used (with reduced efficacy) up to 120 hours after sex (**www.bnf.org**). Levonelle interacts with many other medicines, including anticonvulsants.

Medicine interactions

Several of the traditional anticonvulsants, such as carbemazepine and phenytoin, can reduce the effectiveness of hormonal contraception. However, the newer treatments gabapentin and lamotrigine do not cause changes in hormones, and therefore do not cause hormonal contraception failure; they may also be safer to use in pregnancy (**www.drugtopics.com**).

Katie Johnson

After discussing all the issues related to contraception with the nurse specialist, Katie decides that it is not appropriate for her to take a contraceptive pill until she is in a relationship. The nurse specialist also points out that Katie should attend the GP surgery regularly over the next few months to monitor the effects of her medication. The seizure she experienced could have been related to the alcohol that she drank, but in addition anticonvulsant medications can become less effective over time. The other reason for regular checks in the short term is that sodium valproate can cause amenorrhoea (lack of periods) and irregular periods. It may be necessary to change Katie's treatment to one of the newer therapies if this is the case.

PROFESSIONAL GUIDANCE

National Institute for Health and Clinical Excellence (NICE)

NICE has issued guidelines for the treatment of epilepsy. It acknowledges that 'drug therapy is the mainstay of management of people with epilepsy'. NICE (2004) makes the following recommendations:

- Monotherapy should be used wherever possible.
- Where monotherapy has not been successful in preventing seizures, combination therapy can be considered.
- Patient involvement is essential in treatment decisions in women of childbearing age because of the potential interactions of some treatments with oral contraceptives and the potential for harm to an unborn child.
- Regular treatment review.
- Referral to an appropriate specialist as soon as possible after a first seizure to enable timely diagnosis and treatment.

Quick reminder

✔ Epilepsy can be a symptom or a condition.

✔ The patient with epilepsy experiences seizures that can be classified as partial or generalised.

✔ There are traditional appraches to treatment using anticonvulsants such as sodium valproate and phenytoin.

✔ There are newer medicines available, such as lamotrigrine and gabapentin.

✔ Often, patients find adherence to treatment difficult.

✔ Alcohol is a recreational drug that can have adverse effects, e.g memory loss and disinhibition.

✔ It is important to review treatment regularly, particularly in young women who may be considering pregnancy.

✔ Some anticonvulsant therapies have distressing side effects and interact with other medicines.

REFERENCES

Alcohol Concern (2001) *Binge Drinking.* Factsheet 2.0. London: Alcohol Concern.

Alcohol Concern (2002a) *Young People's Drinking.* Factsheet 1. London: Alcohol Concern.

Alcohol Concern (2002b) *Women and Alcohol: A Cause for Concern?* Factsheet 2. London: Alcohol Concern.

Alexander M F, Fawcett J N and Runcimann P J (2006) *Nursing Practice: Hospital and Home – The Adult,* 3rd edn. Edinburgh: Churchill Livingstone.

Brooker C and Waugh A (2007) *Foundations of Nursing Practice: Fundamentals of Holistic Care.* Edinburgh: Mosby.

Chappell B and Crawford P (1999) *Epilepsy at Your Fingertips.* London: Class Publishing.

Downie G, Mackenzie J and Williams A (2003) *Pharmacology and Medicines Management for Nurses.* Edinburgh: Churchill Livingstone.

Goodwin D (1994) *Alcoholism the Facts,* 2nd edn. Oxford: Oxford University Press.

Haynes R B, Taylor D W and Sackett D L (1979) *Compliance in Health Care.* London: Johns Hopkins Press.

Lanfear J (2002) The individual with epilepsy. *Nursing Standards* **16**, 43-53.

McIntosh A M and Berkovic S F (2005) Treatment of new-onset epilepsy: seizures beget discussion. *The Lancet* **365**, 1985-1987.

Murgraff V, Parrott A and Bennett P (1999) Risky single-occasion drinking amongst young people: definition, correlates, policy and interventions - a broad overview of research findings. *Alcohol and Alcoholism* **34**, 3-14.

National Institute for Health and Clinical Excellence (NICE) (2004) *Epilepsy: The Diagnosis and Management of Epilepsy in Children and Adults.* London: National Institute for Health and Clinical Excellence.

National Society for Epilepsy (2002) *Seizures.* London: National Society for Epilepsy.

Prosser S, Worster B, MacGregor J, Dewar K, Runyard P and Fegan J (2000) *Applied Pharmacology: An Introduction to Pathophysiology and Drug Management for Nurses and Healthcare Professionals.* Edinburgh: Mosby.

344

Rang H P, Dale M M, Ritter J M and Moore P K (2003) *Pharmacology,* 5th edn. Edinburgh: Elsevier.

Rassool G H and Winnington J (2003) Adolescents and alcohol misuse. *Nursing Standard* **17**, 43–52.

Trost III L F, Wender R C, Suter G C, *et al.* (2005) Management of epilepsy in adults: treatment guidelines. *Postgraduate Medicine* **118**, 29–33.

Tugwell C (2003) Current and future aspects of the drug therapy of epilepsy. *Hospital Pharmacist* **10**, 296–302.

Whittaker N (2004) *Disorders and Interventions.* Basingstoke: Palgrave.

World Health Organization (WHO) (2001) *The World Health Report: Epilepsy.* Geneva: World Health Organization.

Chapter 13

Alzheimer's disease:
an older man who has Alzheimer's disease, primary hypertension and constipation

It often seems that dementia has taken the place of cancer and death in our society as a disorder to be feared and somewhat of a taboo to talk about. Many people, often jokingly, seem to associate dementia with forgetfulness. The impairment that results from dementia, however, is much more than simple forgetfulness. Dementia is extremely distressing both for the person experiencing it and for their family and friends. Most commonly, dementia is seen with increasing age. Not all dementias are the same, either in their effects or in their management; this chapter will consider only the dementia introduced in the patient scenario of Mr Harry Black, Alzheimer's disease.

Using the patient scenario of Mr Harry Black, an older man, allows the medicines management issues that are present in Alzheimer's disease to be discussed. Like many people of Mr Black's age, he also has other heath problems; therefore, the common conditions of primary hypertension and constipation are examined as well. The issues that come to light in this scenario are informed consent, covert administration and herbal medicine. This chapter also considers the nursing implications and interventions that arise in relation to the medications that can be used to treat these conditions.

Learning outcomes

At the end of this chapter you should be able to:

✔ Give an overview of Alzheimer's disease, primary hypertension and constipation

✔ Discuss the potential impact of Alzheimer's disease, primary hypertension and constipation on an individual

✔ Identify pharmacological approaches to the management of Alzheimer's disease, primary hypertension and constipation

✔ Discuss the actions and effects of the medicines identified in this patient scenario, namely rivastigmine, verapamil and laxatives

✔ Describe the nursing knowledge needed relating to medicines management for this patient and his condition

✔ Identify supporting nursing interventions for this patient

✔ Discuss the dilemmas raised by using medicines to manage challenging behaviours.

Chapter at a glance

Alzheimer's disease: setting the scene
The nature of Alzheimer's disease
Pharmacological interventions used to manage Alzheimer's disease
Nursing dilemmas
The nature of primary hypertension
Pharmacological interventions used to manage primary hypertension
The nature of constipation
Pharmacological interventions used to manage constipation
Quick reminder
References

Mr Harry Black

Mr Harry Black, a 72-year-old ex-miner, has moved into a nursing home as his wife of 50 years, Mabel, was unable to look after him any longer. He has a form of dementia known as Alzheimer's disease. His changing behaviour, over the previous 7 years or so, has become extremely distressing for Mabel and their children, Sally, Jane and Liz, as previously they knew only a very patient, placid and unassuming Harry. All of the members of Mr Black's immediate family find that one of the most distressing parts of his condition is that on most occasions he doesn't know who they are. He talks about his family members frequently, but he seems completely unaware that when he is with them they are the people that he is thinking and talking about. Until he developed Alzheimer's disease, he had had little contact with health services. He has no medical history of note, other than when he first visited his GP because of his memory problems, about 7 years ago, it was noted that his blood pressure was 175/105 mmHg. This was investigated and he was diagnosed with primary hypertension. He was initially prescribed atenolol 50 mg daily. However, he began to fall asleep frequently and to complain of cold hands and feet. His medication was then changed to verapamil 80 mg three times a day; this seems to have successfully kept his blood pressure within normal limits. Once he was diagnosed with Alzheimer's disease, he was also prescribed rivastigmine 6 mg twice daily.

ALZHEIMER'S DISEASE: SETTING THE SCENE

Alzheimer's disease is a relatively common disease of old age (Griffiths and Rooney, 2006) and results in the slow and progressive development of dementia. Dementia brings with it cognitive defects that eventually have an enormous effect on the individual's capacity to function physically, socially and emotionally. This leads ultimately to the person being unable to cope with the environment around them, leaving them vulnerable and often bewildered (confused). This confusion often results in inappropriate reactions because the person is able neither to recognise their inabilities nor to compensate for them (Williams, 2006).

> **Essential terminology**
>
> **Cognitive**
> The ability to perceive, understand and visualise ideas or sensations.

Related knowledge User viewpoint

On the Alzheimer's Society website, Rebecca explains what having dementia is like for her:

> To me, it's like knitting with a knotted ball of wool. Every now and again I come to a knot. I try to unravel it but can't, so I knit the knot in. As time goes by, there are more knots.

Extract from the Alzheimer's Society Real Lives project.

Personal and professional development 13.1

Consider whether you have ever left an appointment with your GP with a prescription and later not been able to remember some aspect of the your discussion with the GP or perhaps not been sure how to take the medication prescribed. Make a note of what it was about the consultation that may have affected your memory of the events.

THE NATURE OF ALZHEIMER'S DISEASE

Alzheimer's disease is a chronic, progressive brain disorder that affects the way that a person's brain works. The disease becomes gradually worse over a period of about 5-10 years. Although it eventually has a major impact on the person's life, the person ultimately dies from another cause, such as aspiration pneumonia (Griffiths and Rooney, 2006). The main effects of Alzheimer's disease

> ... are similar to those of normal ageing to begin with, then memory for recent events, fluency of speech and orientation in space and time declines. Mood swings can also develop. The deterioration of the nerves and neurotransmitters in the brain, which are critical for memory, causes these symptoms to appear.
> (www.alzheimers.co.uk)

Related knowledge Pathophysiology

Alzheimer's disease produces characteristic widespread plaques and tangles of what were brain cells, which have deposits of amyloid protein in them. These plaques and tangles are always accompanied by extensive loss of brain tissue, which explains the progressive symptoms resulting from deteriorating memory. Unfortunately, these plaques and tangles can be revealed only on post-mortem examination of the brain, and so a definitive diagnosis of Alzheimer's disease can be made only after death and post-mortem (Cayton *et al.*, 2002; Mera, 1997).

The nature of memory

How we remember things is an extremely complicated process that relies on the brain being able to sort, file and recollect all of the information that is showered on us continually. There are three main stages involved in memory: registering information, storing information and recalling information. There are five stages involved in information storage:

- *Short-term*: Data are retained here for a short time. We use short-term memory for actions such as doing mental arithmetic and remembering conversations that we had earlier in the day.
- *Procedural*: This enables us to remember how to carry out skills such as brushing our teeth, administering an injection or playing a sport.
- *Episodic*: This stores the memories of things that don't happen very often, such as personal events, a family holiday or falling in love.
- *Semantic*: This retains most of a person's knowledge and understanding, including all of the facts, figures and rules learnt throughout your life, for example 1066 - the date of the battle of Hastings - and the spelling rule of 'i before e except after c'.

● *Prospective*: This accumulates the data that you need to carry out future tasks, such as when and where your next lecture is, when you're next going out with friends or which day and time you next have to be on duty. It helps you to remember to do things at the right time (based on Magnussen and Helstrup, 2007).

Recovering details from memory depends on both the semantic and the episodic aspects of memory. The brain deterioration that comes about as a result of dementia seems to affect mostly these two stages of memory.

The memory loss in dementia means that the demented person has little or no ability to remember information or recognise people or places. As a result, they become disoriented in time and place, misplace or cannot find things or places and are rarely able to learn anything new. They do not appear to have any understanding of their condition. In order for the person to appreciate where they are and what is happening to them, they frequently use behaviours such as asking the same question over and over again (repetitive questioning), making up stories that seem to make the situation make sense to them (confabulation) and wandering (Hecker, 2003). In the final stages of severe dementia, memory loss can seem to fluctuate to some degree. This can make some nurses and carers believe that the person with dementia has some control over their memory and is being selective about what they can and cannot recall. Hecker (2003) suggests that this may make relatives, friends, healthcare professionals and other carers harbour feelings of resentment towards the demented person.

Initially the effects are seen in the person's prospective memory – that is, the memory that helps us to do the right thing at the right time. We have to carry out some essential actions in order to commit something to memory, and we have to be able to bring it to mind at the correct time. The person with Alzheimer's disease has increasingly little or no memory for events that have happened recently, although their long-term memory may be as good as ever, so they retain the ability to remember events from their early childhood. However, long-term memory also fades with time as the disease progresses. This then has a major impact on the person's ability to live independently.

In addition to personality changes, the person with Alzheimer's disease begins to develop difficulty with ordered speech and thought. This is accompanied by an increasing lack of ability to remain oriented to reality. As a result, the person frequently appears confused and disoriented in time and place. At the same time, the person gradually loses the ability to perform motor skills. Eventually, the person with Alzheimer's disease is unable to lead any social life or to care for themselves; the person also becomes doubly incontinent as all learned behaviour becomes forgotten and brain activity reduces. The process is almost like that of childhood development in reverse, which to many adults in the UK seems unattractive, unpleasant and unappealing – unlike the process of child development itself, which is often considered as engaging, charming and fascinating.

In the early stages of the disease, most people with Alzheimer's disease are aware that there is something wrong. Therefore, it is not surprising that many people in the early stages of Alzheimer's disease experience a range of emotions because of their insights, including anger and irritability; affected individuals frequently develop reactive depression (Cayton et al., 2002).

Reaching a diagnosis of Alzheimer's disease is fraught with much difficulty. This seems to be for two main reasons: there is not a specific diagnostic laboratory test for the disease and, as forgetfulness affects all individuals from time to time, the person's GP has to rule out all the other causes of forgetfulness and confusion. Common causes of forgetfulness and confusion include the following:

- A person with anxiety, stress or depression frequently has poor concentration. As a result, they may not take in all of the available information.
- People who are vision- or hearing-impaired are unable to take in all of the available information; consequently, their memories are not laid down clearly. Their memory is there but they may find recall difficult.
- Many drugs affect memory, causing confusion and disorientation. Examples include alcohol, narcotic analgesics (opium and its derivatives) and trycylic antidepressants (**www.bnf.org.uk**).

Because there are a number of reasons for forgetfulness and periods of confusion, Mr Black's GP will have had to rule out all of the frequent causes of impaired memory and confusion and other causes of dementia. This can be quite time-consuming and frustrating, for the patient, the GP and family members. It is only possible for an accurate diagnosis to be reached on post-mortem examination of the brain.

The nature of dementia

Dementia has been classified into four stages by the Roth et al. (1988):

- *Minimal*: At this stage the person will probably still be living without help and be able to care for themselves, but they will have some difficulty in bringing to mind events that have happened recently and will frequently be unable to find things.
- *Mild*: Here, the process has moved on to include difficulty bringing to mind all kinds of recent information. There will be some degree of disorientation in time and place. The person's ability to manage activities of daily living, solve problems and think logically will be affected.
- *Moderate*: The signs and symptoms of mild dementia become worse, so that the person is not able to manage most aspects of everyday life on their own. Their speech becomes slightly indistinct and they may have occasional episodes of incontinence.
- *Severe*: In this final stage, the person is completely unable to live independently, as they have little memory or ability to think and reason. They will be unable to speak and will be mostly doubly incontinent. They will rarely recognise members of their close family and will be totally disoriented, lethargic and almost immobile.

Although classifying dementia like this suggests that these stages are clear-cut, in practice it is often difficult to tell when one stage finishes and the other begins.

Griffiths and Rooney (2006) describe dementia as 'the loss of intellectual activity'. However, the brevity of this definition disguises the slowly advancing eradication of the person's mental ability, which eventually has a major impact on all aspects of their life. Dementia is recognised by changes in the person's mental abilities that influence both their cognitive and **perceptual** abilities. These changes affect the person's personality, so that they begin to display personality traits that are new to them; for example, they may become very angry and aggressive.

> **Essential terminology**
>
> **Perceptual**
> Having insight.

There are a number of causes of dementia, but in the Western world, Alzheimer's disease is by far the most common (Griffiths and Rooney, 2006). The following lists the various causes:

- Alzheimer's disease ⎫ most common cause

- Lewy body dementia, vascular dementia, multiple infarct dementia
- Combination of multiple strokes and Alzheimer's disease
- Parkinson's disease

⎫ reasonably common causes

- Acquired immunodeficiency syndrome (AIDS)
- Huntington's disease
- Creutzfeldt-Jakob disease
- Pick's disease
- Thyroid disease
- Chronic infection of the nervous system
- Brain tumours

⎫ less common causes

(Adapted from Cayton *et al.*, 2002; Griffiths and Rooney, 2006; and Mera, 1997).

Unfortunately, the aetiology of Alzheimer's disease is still far from being fully understood. We have various pieces of information about the disorder, but these are like the pieces of a jigsaw, and the final picture is still to be revealed. There are some genetic markers, but those found so far are not specific enough to characterise the disease as a genetic disorder; rather, it seems that people with these abnormal genes are more susceptible to Alzheimer's disease compared with the rest of the general population. There is also a very rare form of Alzheimer's disease that is inherited and is the result of a single gene disorder; this form of the disease occurs in people who are much younger than Harry Black. Despite the fact that there are families who seem to have a strong family history of Alzheimer's disease, this must be interpreted with caution. Such information demonstrates that although these family members may be more likely than the general population to develop the disorder, it has to be remembered that Alzheimer's disease is also very common in the general population (Diamond *et al.*, 2003; Griffiths and Rooney, 2006). The majority of cases of Alzheimer's disease appear to have genetic and environmental factors influencing the onset of the disease. The environmental factors that have been implicated include smoking, contact with aluminium and nutritional influences; for example, evidence is coming to light high-lighting the apparent preventive effects of drinking fruit and vegetable juices, with the protective mechanism thought to lie in the chemicals found in the skin of fruit and veg-etables known as polyphenols (Dai *et al.*, 2006; Lahiri, 2006).

There is currently little information that reliably identifies the incidence and preva-lence of Alzheimer's disease. There are two main reasons for this: such studies are extremely complex to carry out, and the criteria that doctors use to reach a diagnosis of Alzheimer's disease are not precise, which produces a diversity of findings. For example, until relatively recently, most people in the UK who had Alzheimer's disease were diagnosed with presenile dementia, but this is changing fairly quickly as the dis-order becomes more widely understood (Griffiths and Rooney, 2006). In order to find some agreement about criteria that differentiate Alzheimer's disease from other dementias, Ferri and colleagues (2005) carried out a Delphi study in Western Europe and found that 'in people aged over 60 the prevalence is around 5% whilst the approx-imate incidence is nearly 9 per 1000 population'.

Like most chronic diseases, there is no cure for Alzheimer's disease. The focus of med-ical and nursing interventions is to manage rather than improve the condition. As memory, reasoning and emotion are located primarily in the cerebral cortex, the drugs that are available to manage the disorder aim to improve the function of the cerebral cortex and consequently prevent memory from deteriorating further.

Personal and professional development 13.2

Write short notes about the way that acetylcholine works in the nervous system. Consider how comfortable you would feel about explaining this to Mr Black and his wife. Do any of the feelings that you identify from this activity suggest that you need to understand the process of neurotransmission more fully? If so, use your professional portfolio to identify three strategies that you will use to help you do this and record your learning.

Related knowledge Pathophysiology

In Alzheimer's disease, there appears to be a loss of a chemical called acetylcholine in the areas of the brain responsible for memory. This loss of acetylcholine is probably due to the widespread destruction of brain cells, which means that there are fewer cells available to make and store acetylcholine.

Acetylcholine is essential to the efficient functioning of brain cells and other aspects of the central, peripheral and autonomic nervous systems. In health, acetylcholine and a number of other chemicals, such as noradrenaline, histamine, dopamine, glutamate and gamma-aminobutyric acid (GABA), enable nerve impulses to pass around the cerebral cortex. As these chemicals allow information to be passed between nerve cells (neurons) in the brain, they are known as 'central neurotransmitters'; however, they are also found in other parts of the body, with acetylcholine being an important neurotransmitter of both the parasympathetic and sympathetic divisions of the autonomic nervous system. Acetylcholine is found at many synapses and is responsible for one of the ways that information is transmitted from one neuron to another - neurotransmission. Information is passed along the neurons using very weak electrical charges that are generated by the movement of positively and negatively charged chemicals (ions). This chemical transmission means that that information can 'jump' across the synapses that lie between the ends of each neuron.

Acetylcholine is made up of two parts, both of which are recognised in its name - acetyl (derived from acetic acid) and choline (an ammonia compound). It is stored in tiny blisters, known as vesicles, that lie in each neuronal synapse that uses this form of neurotransmission. When the electrical discharges approach the neuronal synapse, this acts as a trigger to the vesicles to release acetylcholine into the synapse. The newly released acetylcholine then assists the transmission of the electrical discharge across the synapse to the receptors of the adjoining neuron (Simonsen *et al.*, 2006).

The drugs that increase the action of acetylcholine are most commonly described as being cholinergic because of their actions. Their effects are similar to those of the cholinergic part of the sympathetic nervous system. The drugs are sometimes referred to as parasympathomimetic drugs because their actions mimic those that happen when the parasympathetic nervous system is stimulated. The cholinergic drugs are classified into two groups, based on whether they are:

- agonists, i.e. they stimulate the receptors and so imitate the action of acetylcholine; these are known as cholinergic agonists;
- antagonists, i.e. they block access to the acetylcholine receptor sites within the synapses thus preventing the destruction of acetylcholine within the synapses; these are known as acetylcholinesterase inhibitors.

PHARMACOLOGICAL INTERVENTIONS USED TO MANAGE ALZHEIMER'S DISEASE

Acetylcholinesterase inhibitors

Mr Black was prescribed rivastigmine 6 mg twice daily. In the early stages of Alzheimer's disease, the synapses that are left in the brain are thought to need more acetylcholine. The drugs that are used to do this are those that help to prevent acetylcholine being destroyed; rivastigmine, galantamine and donepezil. They do this by blocking the action of the enzyme acetylcholinesterase. This enzyme is found in some neuronal synapses where it helps to break down acetylcholine. Acetylcholinesterase also recycles some acetylcholine by returning it to the vesicles in the synapses. Inhibiting the action of acetylcholinesterase will ensure that the amount of available acetylcholine in the synapses will increase. It must be remembered that while the person keeps taking the drug, the amount of acetylcholine will continue to rise in the synapses for as long as the medication is taken (Greenstein and Gould, 2004; Rang *et al.*, 2003; Simonsen *et al.*, 2006).

> ### Personal and professional development 13.3
>
> Consider what may happen to the cholinergic receptors if the levels of acetylcholine in the central nervous system keep on rising.

This can eventually cause overstimulation of the cholinergic receptors, which results in the overstimulation of the organs that have a parasympathetic nerve supply. This adverse effect may be so great that the medication may have to be discontinued or the patient may simply stop taking it.

The parasympathetic nervous system (the craniosacral division of the autonomic nervous system) is involved with protecting, conserving and restoring the body's resources. Stimulation of the parasympathetic nervous system slows the heart; accelerates peristalsis; increases secretions of the lachrymal, salivary and digestive glands; causes the release of insulin and bile; dilates peripheral and visceral blood vessels; and constricts the pupils of the eyes, the oesophagus and the bronchioles.

In the early stages of Alzheimer's disease, there is evidence that the anticholinesterases have some effect for about half of the people with the disorder. This effect is enough to cause a 'moderate improvement' for a period of time, usually within 18 months (**www.bnf.org**). The person's cognitive deterioration is slowed down but not halted. However, the effect of these drugs does wear off, probably because more and more neurons disappear and more and more plaques and tangles appear. These medicines are therefore recommended for mild to moderate Alzheimer's disease in patients whose Mini-Mental State Examination (MMSE) score is between 10 and 20 points (NICE, 2007).

Related knowledge Pharmacology

In the UK, the medicines available on the NHS to manage Alzheimer's disease are limited to four: donepezil, galantamine, rivastigmine and memantine. The first three are acetylcholinesterase inhibitors while memantine blocks the neurotransmitter glutamate (**www.bnf.org**).

There is considerable doubt over whether it is cost-effective to use these medicines to treat the early stages of Alzheimer's disease, given the negligible improvements demonstrated: less than 50% of treated people see any improvement, and any improvement is for only a limited time. During the autumn of 2006, following a review of the evidence, NICE withdrew the guidelines recommending that acetylcholinesterase inhibitors were of benefit only to people in the early stages of Alzheimer's disease and should therefore be prescribed only for these people. This was widely interpreted as refusing treatment to people with Alzheimer's disease that may help them stave off the effects of the disease for a while (**www.bbc.co.uk**; **www.telegraph.co.uk**; **www.guardian.co.uk**; **www.timesonline.co.uk**). Understandably, this announcement was met with much controversy and public debate. The pharmaceutical company that makes one of the medicines for Alzheimer's disease and the Alzheimer's Society requested a judicial review of the NICE guidance preventing people from accessing medication that may improve their condition; following the judicial review in August 2007, NICE's decision was upheld.

Pharmacodynamics Rivastigmine

The acetylcholinesterase inhibitors work by slowing down the breakdown of acetylcholine at the synapse of the neurons in the brain that are still functioning normally. The levels of acetylcholine available in the neurons are increased as a result of taking rivastigmine and other acetylcholinesterase inhibitors (Greenstein and Gould, 2004; Rang *et al.*, 2003; **www.emc.medicines.org.uk**).

Pharmacokinetics Rivastigmine

Absorption: Rivastigmine is absorbed rapidly and completely. Peak plasma concentrations are reached within about 1 hour. Giving the drug with food delays absorption by about 1.5 hours if capsules are taken and a little more than an hour when the liquid form is taken (**www.emc.medicines.org.uk**).

Distribution: 40% bound to plasma proteins. Crosses the blood–brain barrier quickly.

▶

> ▶ *(continued)*
>
> ***Metabolism:*** Quick and extensive metabolism in the liver in laboratory experiments.
>
> ***Elimination:*** Rivastigmine metabolites are excreted by the kidneys (www.bnf.org.uk; www.emc.medicines.org.uk).

The undesirable effects of acetylcholinesterase inhibitors are a direct result of the increase in acetylcholine in the neurons. These effects include dizziness, nausea, vomiting, anorexia, weight loss, agitation, confusion, depression and diarrhoea (www.bnf.org.uk; www.emc.medicines.org.uk).

Mr Harry Black

Before Mr Black moved into the nursing home, his wife Mabel was supervising Harry taking ginkgo biloba, which she bought from the local health food store.

Ginkgo biloba

A number of herbs have long been reputed to improve memory, such as sage, lemon balm, ginseng and gingko biloba (Ernst, 2000; Kennedy and Scholey, 2003; Kennedy *et al.*, 2002). The evidence for the effectiveness of ginkgo biloba is extremely sparse, 'inconclusive and characterised by methodological deficiencies' (Diamond *et al.*, 2003). These methodological problems of the research studies that are available hinder the prescribing of ginkgo biloba by NHS doctors to help manage Alzheimer's disease. Similar reasons also influence the use of most herbal medicines, other than St John's wort – reasons that Diamond *et al.* (2003) attribute to 'small sample sizes and inadequate controls'. This is not to say that ginkgo biloba is not effective but rather that we do not have any reliable or valid evidence to demonstrate either its effectiveness or non-effectiveness. However, a large amount of anecdotal evidence claims that ginkgo biloba does aid memory (Ernst, 2000).

Mr Harry Black

Since moving into the nursing home, Mr Black has become increasingly disorientated and aggressive. It is the end of his second week in the nursing home and his primary nurse is administering his medicines. It looks as though he is about to swallow the medicines when he suddenly spits two of his three tablets at the nurse. Despite much encouragement, he is adamant that he doesn't want them.

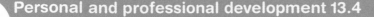

Personal and professional development 13.4

1. Reflect on how you would feel if you were the nurse in this situation.

2. Identify three possible reasons for Mr Black's behaviour.

3. List three possible nursing actions that could be taken as a result of this situation.

NURSING DILEMMAS

There are several reasons for Mr Black spitting out his tablets, such as having difficulty swallowing and refusing consent to treatment. Many healthcare professionals assume that people with dementia have no ability to make decisions or find it very difficult to make decisions. This stereotype is often so strong that many healthcare professionals discuss the patient's healthcare with the patient's family rather than with the patient. Typically, when a person with Alzheimer's disease makes a decision about their own healthcare, such as refusing to take further medication, many healthcare professionals think that such a decision is unreasonable and therefore the patient must be incapable of making a decision (Seedhouse and Gallagher, 2002).

Situations such as that described above are fraught with difficulties for the nurse. This incident, although it does not require an understanding of pharmacology, highlights a frequent medicines management issue faced by many nurses and carers everyday. Being spat at by someone can provoke a range of feelings, such as fear, anger, embarrassment, hurt and surprise. It is therefore important that nurses have the ability not only to recognise such feelings but also to be able to deal with these emotions.

Personal and professional development 13.5

1. Think about how you deal with emotions such as anger, disgust, embarrassment, horror and fear.

2. Is this an appropriate way of dealing with your emotions?

3. If you use inappropriate means of dealing with your emotions, spend some time exploring how you could change your responses and use your professional portfolio to record your learning.

Understanding why Mr Black is behaving in this way is crucial in ensuring that nurses make the correct decisions about managing such events. It is difficult to identify accurately why people in Mr Black's situation behave in such a way, but there are some very

obvious reasons that can lead to such behaviour, including pain, distress, lack of understanding, and an inability to satisfy basic human needs such as eating, drinking and
safety (cited in Maslow, 1968). This behaviour may be part of the deterioration process
of the disorder, which means that Mr Black now understands neither what medicines
are nor the condition for which his medicines have been prescribed.

People with Alzheimer's disease frequently become intimidating and aggressive. Such
behaviour is rarely deliberate and seems to be mostly because of the individual's lack
of ability to communicate effectively. Their behaviour reflects their feelings of frustration. Unfortunately, this often results in unacceptable and antisocial behaviour. The
people caring for an aggressive patient sometimes focus on the behaviour rather than
the cause of the behaviour. Pulsford and Duxbury (2006), in a literature review of
aggressive behaviour by people with dementia in residential care settings, identify a
number of studies that suggest that many nurses and carers have such views because
they have a limited understanding of dementia or how to use what Kitwood (1997) calls
a 'person-centred approach' to care.

Nursing knowledge Nursing implications

The feelings produced in situations such as that described arise frequently in
nursing. Nurses have to learn how to deal with their own emotions so that they
can not only help their patients and their families more effectively but also
protect themselves from psychological stress and burnout. Having the skills that
help you to successfully manage these feelings and be sensitive to the needs of
others is known as 'emotional intelligence' (McQueen, 2004). The psychological
work that you have to do in order to best manage these feelings is called
'emotional labour' (Hochschild, 1985; Smith, 1992).

Personal and professional development 13.6

What do you understand by the term 'person-centred approach' (Kitwood,
1997)? Consider whether you need to know more about it. If you do need to
learn more about it, then identify in your professional portfolio how you will
achieve this and what you learn as a result.

This could be because of insufficient education or resources to help nurses and carers
prevent or manage behaviour such as this, or other challenging behaviours such as
wandering, shouting or of agitation. As a result, the patient may be labelled as violent
and aggressive. They may then be seen to need some kind of control in order to prevent their antisocial behaviour. This can result in physical restraint, but more often

drugs are used to manage and prevent the behaviour, thus making the patient more amenable and malleable for the staff; this practice is known as 'chemical restraint' (Kow and Hogan, 2000; Middleton *et al.*, 1999; Thurmond, 1999).

Chemical restraint: patient benefit or chemical control

Considerable concern has been expressed over the years regarding the misuse of sedatives by healthcare professionals, especially in the care of older people and patients who are confused and disoriented (Burstow and Stokoe, 2001; Kow and Hogan, 2000; Pulsford and Duxbury, 2006). There are a number of reasons for this misuse:

- Ageist and sexist attitudes
- Lack of understanding of dementia and the ageing process
- Lack of suitable staff and resources
- Sedated people are easier to manage and control
- Sedated people need fewer and less well trained staff to care for them
- Emergency care valued over supportive care
- Caring for old people commonly perceived to need few skills.

In a number of studies, both professionals and carers say that it is much easier to manage a sedated patient than to deliver the complex and holistic care that patients with dementia need (Burstow and Stokoe, 2001; Kow and Hogan, 2000; Kwasny *et al.*, 2006; Thurmond, 1999).

To some healthcare professionals, working with older people or people with mental health problems is seen as 'unglamorous'. Such beliefs seem to reflect some of the negative stereotypical images of older people common today. Sadly, in modern society, older people, especially those with mental health problems, are often perceived to be unattractive (Bachrach-Lindstrum *et al.*, 2007; Campbell 2005a, b; McKinlay and Cowan, 2003, 2006; Nelson, 2005; Schofield *et al.*, 2005; Slevin, 1991). Moreover, Kwasny and colleagues (2006), McKinlay and Cowan (2006) and Slevin (1991), among others, go so far as to suggest that the negative views of older people seen in society pervade medicine, nursing and the allied professions. This, they suggest, results in many healthcare professionals having ageist attitudes.

Related knowledge User viewpoint

The relative's comments that follow are not unusual. Carers find it difficult to understand why medicines are used to sedate people when simple measures are frequently all that are needed to calm patients. The following account is an all too frequent story of families' experiences.

▶

▶ *(continued)*

Throughout my father's five year decline into advanced dementia I have seen him in every possible mood and I have witnessed the manner and approach of many different healthcare professionals. The common view, to varying degrees, has been that my father has been difficult and that drug therapy is the solution.

My torment and frustration have been immense. To me it has been obvious that what he has needed, as have so many like him, is kindness, sympathetic handling and an understanding of his condition. Unfortunately, staff in homes and hospitals seem to find it easier to cope if all their patients are docile and bed- or chair-bound. Those who wander or display unusual behaviour are reported to doctors as agitated and in need of medication.

All patients should be treated as individuals but my experience of the last five years has shown me that elderly people, and especially those with dementia, are lumped together as a constipated group in need of something to confine them to their chairs. (**www.alzheimers.co.uk**)

Consent to treatment

Mr Black may have spit out his tablets because he no longer wants to take some or all of his prescribed medication. He is well within his rights, both ethically and legally, to withdraw his consent to treatment at any time if he no longer wishes to continue taking medication, for whatever reason. Adult patients who are mentally competent have the right to refuse treatment, even when the suggested treatment would improve their health or refusal could lead to their death (DfCA, 2005). The only exception to this rule is where the treatment is for a mental disorder and the person is detained under the Mental Health Act 1983 (DfCA, 2005). As Mr Black is not detained under the Mental Health Act 1983, the nurses administering his medication must consider him to be competent to consent unless they can demonstrate otherwise.

Assessing Mr Black's capacity to consent can be fraught with difficulty and is not something that should be devolved to any one healthcare professional. The assessment requires an overview of Mr Black's behaviour over time and includes tools such as the Mini-Mental State Examination (MMSE) (Folstein *et al.*, 1975). The responsibility for deciding whether a person has the capacity to consent (i.e. is mentally able to consent) lies with the multidisciplinary team. Such decisions should be taken only after every healthcare professional involved has had the opportunity to present their perspective. The decision of the team must be discussed and agreed on by Mr Black's next of kin. Evidence of the decision-making process and the resulting actions must be documented in Mr Black's notes (DfCA, 2005; NMC, 2007a).

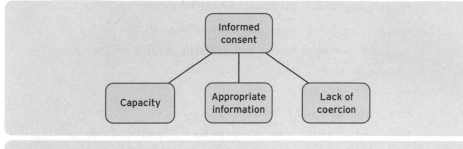

Figure 13.1 Constituents of informed consent

Legally, in order to make a decision and give informed consent to treatment, a number of factors must be followed by the healthcare professionals (Figure 13.1) (DfCA, 2005, 2007; NMC, 2007a).

In October 2007 the Department for Constitutional Affairs (DfCA) was absorbed into the newly established Ministry of Justice. This led to the setting up of the Office of the Public Guardian with the Public Guardian there 'to help protect people who lack capacity from abuse' (**www.publicguardian.gov.uk**).

Dysphagia

Another reason that Mr Black may have spat out his tablets is that he may have dysphagia (difficulty in swallowing). Older people are more at risk of dysphagia compared with younger people.

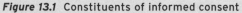

Personal and professional development 13.7

List five signs that you may observe that would suggest to you that Mr Black might have dysphagia.

There may be a number of reasons for Mr Black's dysphagia, including the following:

- The physiological processes involved in swallowing frequently become less efficient with advancing age; for example, the salivary glands commonly produce less saliva (Morris, 2005).

- Following stroke or other neurological disease, the swallowing mechanisms may be disabled. Many people, particularly those in nursing homes, have dysphagia as a result of stroke or neurological disease (Morris, 2005).

- Drinking insufficient fluid leads to dehydration, which results in a dry mouth, making it very difficult to swallow.

Essential terminology

Neurological
Concerned with the nervous system.

Signs that may indicate dysphagia in a patient include the following:

- Keeping food in the mouth and doing nothing with it
- Difficulty chewing or moving food to the back of the mouth
- Spitting out lumps of food
- Refusing food or drink
- Coughing/choking on solids or liquids
- Complaints of food being stuck in the back of the throat
- A 'wet' or 'gurgly' voice after swallowing
- Dribbling
- Recurring chest infections or chronic chestiness
- Regurgitation after swallowing (Morris, 2005).

Sticky/glutinous capsules

A dry mouth makes it very difficult for the patient to swallow capsules. The soft (usually gelatinous) covering of the capsule may stick to the mucous membranes of the mouth and the tongue, rather like glue.

As Mr Black is unable to communicate verbally to the staff that he is experiencing discomfort with swallowing, he will communicate in the only way he can - by spitting out the capsules. Although nurses must observe carefully all of the people that they care for, in situations such as this it is important to be particularly vigilant as Mr Black's ability to respond to verbal questioning is limited. In different circumstances, the nurse may be able to question the patient in order to elaborate on their observations and widen their assessment.

Hiding medicines

There is evidence that after being administered medicines, some people in nursing homes hide their tablets or capsules in their mouth, usually under the tongue or in the cheek pocket (Barnes *et al.*, 2006; Burstow and Stokoe, 2001; Cowan *et al.*, 2002). When the patient thinks they are not being observed, they remove the medicines from their mouth. Patient may do this consciously or subconsciously. If this is a conscious decision, then they are within their legal rights to do so; however, it would be appropriate to discuss with the patient their hoarding of medicines and then discontinue the prescription if that is their wish. If the patient is acting subconsciously, then their capacity to consent to treatment must be brought into question, investigated properly and documented carefully.

Inability to swallow tablets

Many people who are not dysphagic find tablets and capsules difficult to swallow. Mr Black may be one of these people, although we are not provided with this information.

His wife or family may be able to give this information. When such information is not volunteered by the family or carer of a patient who cannot communicate verbally but who is able to swallow, the nurse should ask about it during the admission assessment.

Nursing knowledge Nursing actions

If a person finds it difficult to swallow tablets or capsules, they are best advised to take their medicine in as upright position as possible. If the patient is unable to position him- or herself, the nursing staff should ensure that the patient is in this optimum position before administering the medication. The nurse should ensure that the patient has moistened their mouth by taking a sip of fluid. If the patient is able, ask them to put the tablet or capsule as far back on their tongue as they can, without making themselves gag, and then to take as large a drink of water as they can. This should wash the tablet or capsule into the pharynx, making it easier for the patient to swallow with the next drink. The patient should continue taking drinks of water until they have swallowed at least half a glass of water. This process should be repeated with each tablet or capsule. If the patient is unable to do this, the nurse should place the tablet or capsule on to the back of the patient's tongue, taking care not to make the patient gag. The nurse should then give the patient drinks of water until the tablet or capsule is swallowed.

Altering the form of tablets and capsules

Crushing tablets or emptying the contents of capsules seems to be a relatively common practice. Wright (2002), in an observational study undertaken in independent nursing homes in the UK, found that over 60% of nurses crushed tablets or opened capsules before administration of medicines. His study revealed that this practice happens in 80% of nursing homes at least once a week. Altering the form of tablets or opening capsules is to be discouraged, for two reasons:

- It may change the rate of action of the drug by it being absorbed in a different part of the gastrointestinal system from what it was designed to do. This is especially so with gastro-resistant (sustained-release or enteric-coated) medicines.

- Changing the form of the medicine breaks the medicine's product licence and therefore the pharmaceutical company will no longer be liable for any difficulties that the patient may have with the medicine. The legal recourse passes to the person who altered the presentation of the medicine (Dimond, 2004).

Palatability of medicines

It could be that Mr Black does not like the taste of tablets, or a particular tablet. Most adults swallow tablets, even when they taste unpleasant, as they have conscious control over their actions. However, Mr Black's deteriorating condition could mean that he knows only that he has something that tastes unpleasant in his mouth. Therefore, in order to get rid of the unpleasant taste as quickly as possible, he may react by immediately spitting out the medicine. If he has difficulty swallowing tablets or capsules, they will be in his mouth for a longer time than usual and may become quite unpalatable in both taste and texture.

Nursing knowledge Nursing actions

When Mr Black spat his medicines out, a number of actions could have been taken by the nurse. The nurse would have to consider all of these in the decision-making process in order to judge which would be the most appropriate for the situation. The possible actions include the following:

- Try to ascertain the reasons for the patient's behaviour.

- Try to minimise other distractions in the environment. Mr Black has limited concentration and so will find other activities, such as television, radio and people chatting, a major distraction. He may not understand why the medicines are being offered if he is focusing on something that the nurse considers to be in the background and has ignored.

- See whether Mr Black will take some of the tablets. He could be objecting to one tablet rather than them all.

- In order to help Mr Black swallow more easily, ensure that he is in as upright a position as possible. Encourage him to put the tablets as far back on his tongue as he can without invoking the gag reflex (if he cannot do this, the nurse will have to do this for him), and then ask him to drink the full glass of water that has been given to him to help him swallow the tablets.

- Ask Mr Black to put one tablet in his mouth at a time and swallow each one with at least half a glass of water. Half a glass of water is the minimum amount of fluid that should be used to swallow tablets. When not being used for swallowing, the oesophagus collapses in on itself, and so a reasonably large amount of fluid is needed to open up the oesophagus and help to wash down the tablets or capsules. Without a reasonable amount of water, it is difficult for the oesophagus to push small items through the system by **peristalsis**.

- Ask the doctor to change the prescription to a form that Mr Black might find more acceptable. Many medicines are available in an alternative form, most commonly liquid, which many people find easier to swallow than tablets.

Although not every medicine is available in liquid form, Wright (2002) states that 'there is at least one drug in each drug family that is available in liquid form'. Other forms of medication that could also be considered are patches, inhalers and suppositories. However, changes in the skin as a result of the ageing process may mean that patches are unreliable for older people.

- Arrange a medication review. This will ensure that Mr Black is prescribed only those medicines that are really needed. Many people continue taking medicines that they no longer need as they continue to obtain a supply of medicines by using the repeat prescription service offered by their GP. The taking of many medicines – polypharmacy – can lead to difficulties for some people.

- Assess Mr Black's understanding of his medication and give any appropriate information.

- Record on the medicine sheet that Mr Black refused his medication.

- Document Mr Black's behaviour in his patient records.

- Arrange a multidisciplinary team meeting to discuss Mr Black's possible deterioration.

Essential terminology

Peristalsis
Waves of involuntary contractions of the muscular wall that move along the gastrointestinal tract, pushing the contents through the gastrointestinal tract to the rectum.

Covert administration

The practice of disguising medication (covert administration) in food and/or drink by nurses caring for adults is thought to be a common practice, both in the UK and in other countries (Kirkevold and Knut, 2005; Scott and Williams, 1997; Treloar *et al.*, 2000, 2001; Wong *et al.*, 2005). There is very little medical or nursing literature about covert administration. However, our experience seems to reflect that of others: when discussing this practice with both student nurses and qualified nurses, working in NHS and private acute and long-term care facilities (adult, learning disability and mental health), we heard much anecdotal evidence to suggest that covert administration is relatively common, despite nursing's professional body prohibiting it except in very defined situations (NMC, 2007a, b).

There are a number of ethical and legal issues underlying covert administration. Many nurses and doctors seem to think that covert administration of medicines is an acceptable practice, as it utilises the ethical perspective of beneficence. However, if the patient is not consulted regarding their medication, how can the healthcare professional know that it is in the best interests of the patient to take the prescribed medication?

THE NATURE OF HYPERTENSION

Hypertension (*hyper* = above normal, *tension* = pressure), or high blood pressure, describes blood-pressure readings that are higher than those considered normal for the person's age. Hypertension is a very common disorder in the Western world today. In the UK it is estimated that 20% of people have elevated blood pressure of more than 140/90 mmHg, which warrants treatment or monitoring (BHS and NICE, 2006). Constantly high blood pressure readings are of concern because this is a major risk factor in the development of atherosclerosis, a condition in which fatty deposits, known as plaques, are laid down in the lining of the arteries. These plaques lead initially to a narrowing of the internal diameter of the affected arteries and eventually to total occlusion (blockage). Three important organs feel most of the effects of atherosclerosis: the heart, the brain and the kidney. Atherosclerosis is responsible for the development of coronary heart disease, transient ischaemic attacks and renal failure. Coronary heart disease and stroke are the two leading causes of morbidity and mortality in the Western world today (DH, 2000). Hypertension is thought to contribute to 66 000 deaths as a result of coronary heart disease and stroke in people aged under 75 years (BHS and NICE, 2006).

Related knowledge Pathophysiology

Blood pressure is maintained by two factors:

- The amount of blood pumped out of the heart into the arterial circulation (cardiac output)
- The force caused by the narrowing of the arterioles (peripheral resistance).

Blood pressure can be raised when the circulating volume of blood increases or as a result of increasing resistance in the arterioles. There are two systems that normally work in tandem to ensure that blood pressure is kept within normal limits. These systems are the hormonal (i.e. the renin-angiotensin-aldosterone mechanism) and the autonomic nervous system controls.

When hypertension is persistent, the continued high pressure has an effect on the layer that lines the inside of the arteries/arterioles (endothelium). This results in the arterial/arteriole walls becoming thicker. One of the major effects on the arteries/arterioles of this thickening from hypertension is the loss of elasticity. This loss of elasticity means that the affected vessels find it increasingly difficult to dilate or constrict in order to accommodate the ever-changing volumes of blood circulating around the body. The less elastic the vessels become, the more they resist blood flow. Eventually, if this goes untreated, in an effort to overcome this resistance to blood flow, the left ventricle of the heart makes more and more effort to pump blood around the body. This increased workload will eventually lead to thickening (hypertrophy) of the muscle wall (myocardium) of the left ventricle. This maintains homeostasis for a time, but eventually the hypertrophied myocardium weakens and becomes unable to eject enough blood through the aorta into the arterial circulation to meet the demands of the body. Heart failure then results (Boon *et al.*, 2006).

Essential terminology

Dilation

Broadening of the diameter of an artery. This wider diameter permits a larger volume of blood to flow through the artery. The consequence of this is lower pressure inside the blood vessel.

Constriction

Narrowing of the diameter of an artery. This results in a smaller volume of blood flowing in the artery, resulting in higher pressure inside the vessel.

Hypertension is classified into three types:

- *Primary hypertension*: Idiopathic (has no obvious cause). This was previously called essential hypertension.

- *Secondary hypertension*: The result of a particular factor or disease.

- *Malignant hypertension*: Occurs, rapidly, with blood pressure levels that have the potential to cause life-threatening events such as cerebral oedema (swelling of the brain due to too much fluid in the brain cells). When such a hypertensive crises happen, they are most commonly due to pre-eclampsia or secondary to some medicines, such as monoamine oxidase inhibitors (a type of antidepressant). This form of hypertension is rare.

Most affected people do not know that they have primary hypertension, as it often has no obvious symptoms (asymptomatic), especially in the early stages of its development. The commonly used description of primary hypertension as the 'silent epidemic' demonstrates both its consequences and its hidden nature, given that it is a major factor in the development of coronary heart disease and stroke in the Western world.

Causes of secondary hypertension include the following:

- Use of certain medicines, e.g. non-steroidal anti-inflammatory drugs, oral contraceptives, steroids, liquorice, sympathomimetics, some cold cures
- Renal disease
- Renovascular disease (affecting the blood vessels of the kidney)
- Phaeochromocytoma (a normally benign tumour of the adrenal gland)
- Conn's syndrome (a disorder of excessive production of the hormone aldosterone in the adrenal gland)

● Coarctation of the aorta (narrowing of the aorta distal to the exit of the left subclavian artery)

● Cushing's syndrome (a cluster of symptoms that occur when the level of steroid hormones in the body is consistently too high; this can happen as a result of disease in the adrenal glands or if the patient is taking corticosteroids to treat a medical condition). (Adapted from Williams *et al.*, 2004.)

Mr Black's hypertension has been controlled well for a number of years with lifestyle changes and medication. However, if he were newly diagnosed with primary hypertension today, his management plan would probably be very different. Current NICE (2006) clinical guidelines suggest that for 'persistent raised blood pressure above 140/90 mmHg (millimetres of mercury)' the following advice should be followed:

● Lifestyle interventions should be offered initially and then periodically to patients undergoing assessment or treatment for hypertension.

● Establish cardiovascular risk and eliminate secondary causes of hypertension such as kidney disease.

● Offer drug therapy to: patients with persistent high blood pressure of 160/100 mmHg or more, and patients at increased cardiovascular risk with persistent blood pressure of more than 140/90 mmHg.

● In hypertensive patients aged 55 years or older or black patients of any age the first choice for initial therapy should be either a calcium channel blocker or a thiazide type diuretic. For this recommendation, black patients are considered to be those of African or Caribbean descent, not mixed race, Asian or Chinese.

● In hypertensive patients younger than 55, the first choice for initial therapy should be an angiotensin-converting enzyme (ACE) inhibitor (or an angiotensin-II receptor antagonist if an ACE inhibitor is not tolerated).

In reality

Many people may have been prescribed medication to control their blood pressure before the publication of the NICE (2006) guidelines. If they feel well, they may be continuing with this medication. Some of these people will have been asked to return to their GP for a medication review but may not yet have done so. As a result, nurses may be involved in caring for a number of people whose treatment does not conform to the latest NICE guidelines.

Having to lower a patient's blood pressure as an emergency is rare. When this does need to be done, it is carried out by a doctor and so is not within the scope of this chapter. More usually, lowering a patient's blood pressure is carried out over a period of time, and both medication and advice about non-pharmacological methods to lower blood pressure are offered. Some people are able to lower their blood pressure to within normal limits without resorting to the use of medication.

> ## Personal and professional development 13.8
>
> Which of the following pieces of information would you give to a patient to help them reduce their blood pressure by non-pharmacological means?
>
> - Eat a diet that is low in saturated fat.
> - Stop smoking.
> - Take up running.
> - Reduce salt intake.
> - Eat at least five portions of fruit and vegetables a day.
> - Drink only moderate amounts of alcohol.
> - Drink a litre and a half of water a day.
> - Walk for a minimum of 30 minutes at least three times a week.

Mr Black was initially prescribed atenolol 50 mg daily when his hypertension was diagnosed 7 years ago. Atenolol was discontinued when he complained of falling asleep and having cold hands and feet. These are well-recognised adverse effects of atenolol (**www.bnf.org**). Pharmacological knowledge and understanding of medicine changes constantly as science develops. As a result of such knowledge, this group of medicines is no longer used for primary hypertension as it can increase the person's chance of developing type 2 diabetes. Atenolol is one of a number of medicines known as beta-blockers.

PHARMACOLOGICAL INTERVENTIONS USED TO MANAGE HYPERTENSION

Beta-blockers

This group of medicines capitalise on the way that the neurotransmitters adrenaline and noradrenaline function at the synapses of the autonomic nervous system. These neurotransmitters use two main types of **adrenergic** receptor: alpha (α) and beta (β). Both of these receptors are found in glands (e.g. salivary glands, lachrymal glands), cardiac muscle and smooth muscle.

Essential terminology

Adrenergic
Producing the hormone adrenaline or a chemical that has similar properties to adrenaline.

In uncomplicated primary hypertension, the role of beta-blockers has become increasingly controversial in recent years. The BNF has changed its advice in an effort to 'clarify the role of beta-blockers for hypertension'. Studies re-evaluating the benefits of beta-blockers (e.g. Carlberg *et al.*, 2004) have led to changes in the advice regarding atenolol. The BNF now advises that **antihypertensive** drugs other than beta-blockers are usually more effective for reducing the incidence of stroke, myocardial infarction and cardiovascular mortality. This is consistent with NICE (2006) guidance, which states that beta-blockers are no longer preferred as routine initial therapy for hypertension. Furthermore, beta-blockers (especially if combined with a thiazide diuretic) are best avoided if there is concern about diabetes. However, the BNF states that there is a role for beta-blockers in angina, in the management of patients who have had a myocardial infarction, and in heart failure.

Most people newly diagnosed with hypertension nowadays are not prescribed beta-blockers. Those who are already taking beta-blockers for hypertension may be reluctant to change their medication if it works well and suits them. Other patients on beta-blockers may avoid attending medication reviews and so continue with their treatment. Consequently, many nurses will come across people taking beta-blockers for hypertension for many years to come.

Related knowledge Pharmacology

There is a wide variety of drugs available to lower blood pressure. The antihypertensives recommended for use by the British Hypertensive Society and NICE (2006) are:

- angiotensin-converting enzyme (ACE) inhibitors;
- calcium channel blockers;
- thiazide-type diuretics.

There is also another group of blood-pressure-lowering medicines: the angiotensin-II receptor antagonists.

Verapamil

Verapamil is a **calcium channel blocker**, a group of medicines used to treat primary hypertension.

Pharmacodynamics Verapamil

Calcium channel blockers work by preventing the flow of calcium ions across the cell membrane of the smooth muscle cells of the coronary and systemic arteries. This reduces the flow of calcium into the muscle cells and as a result the muscle cells relax. In primary hypertension, this is particularly useful as it prevents the constriction of the arteries that raises blood pressure.

Verapamil has a number of adverse effects, including constipation, headache, nausea, vomiting, dizziness and occasional flushing (**www.emc.medicines.org.uk**; Greenstein and Gould, 2004; Rang *et al.*, 2003).

Pharmacokinetics Verapamil

Absorption: Absorbed rapidly. Reaches its greatest plasma concentration within 2 hours after administration. Food intake does not appear to influence absorption.

Distribution: 90% of verapamil is bound to plasma proteins.

Metabolism: Metabolised primarily in the liver.

Elimination: 70% of the dose is excreted by the kidneys and 16% is excreted in the faeces (**www.emc.medicines.org.uk**).

Grapefruit flesh and juice have been reported to increase verapamil levels in the blood, which may lead to hypotensive episodes. Not only should patients taking verapamil be advised to avoid both the flesh and the juice of grapefruit, but this advice should be given to everyone taking calcium channel blockers. Grapefruit, both flesh and juice, interacts with a variety of drugs, including warfarin (a commonly prescribed anticoagulant). For a full list of the drugs that interact with grapefruit, refer to the BNF, Appendix 1.

Verapamil also interacts with digoxin, beta-blockers, alcohol, inhaled anaesthetics, carbamazepine, rimfampicin and cimetidine (Greenstein and Gould, 2004; Rang *et al.*, 2003; **www.emc.medicines.org.uk**).

Mr Harry Black

Over the next few days, Mr Black gradually becomes more and more agitated and is frequently found wandering about, aimlessly pacing the floor. He has become more verbally aggressive. The nursing staff have noticed that Harry's bowel habits seem to have changed since his admission to the nursing home.

Mr Black could be in pain or distress as a result of constipation. Constipation often occurs when a person's environment changes, for example on holiday. This may be due to the individual eating different food, which has a profound effect on the gastrointestinal system for some people, causing either constipation or loose stools (diarrhoea). For Mr Black, finding himself in a new and unfamiliar environment will probably be disorienting as he tries to make sense of where he is and what is happening to him with fewer and fewer cerebral abilities to help him do this. He will probably not have the same visual prompts that he had at home that reminded him about where he was, when to eat and drink, where the toilet is located, and what time and day it is. In addition, the nature of Alzheimer's disease means that Mr Black will eventually forget to fulfil all of what Roper *et al.* (2000) call his 'activities of living'. Constipation is also an adverse effect of taking verapamil.

THE NATURE OF CONSTIPATION

Related knowledge Pathophysiology

Most people understand the term 'constipation' to mean that the affected person is having difficulty with defecation (the emptying of faeces from the rectum). However, the term is rather imprecise and can mean anything from incomplete emptying of the rectum to infrequent action of the bowel. Norton (2006) suggests that when a patient states that they are constipated, the nurse must clarify what the person actually means. The updated Rome diagnostic criteria is often used as a definition: 'persistently difficult, infrequent or seemingly incomplete defecation, on the basis of criteria such as the incidence of straining, hard stools or incomplete evacuation' (Thompson *et al.*, 1999). Constipation can result in abdominal, pelvic and anal pain as well as discomfort and bloating. It can also cause headache, nausea, vomiting and fatigue. Norton (2006) points out that constipation can also cause worry and apprehension: bowel habits are very private affairs in the UK, and so it can be very difficult for a person to talk to a doctor or nurse about constipation. There seems to be a misunderstanding that people always become constipated as a result of growing older, but Harari (2002) clearly identifies that healthy older people are no more likely to be constipated than healthy young people. However, certain disorders that cause constipation are more common in old age, leading to constipation being more widespread in the older population.

Constipation is a symptom rather than a disease. Consequently, any signs that suggest that any patient is constipated should always be investigated fully. Many disorders and diseases affect the way the bowel works, while a diet lacking in roughage and water can also lead to constipation. Social and environmental factors, such as immobility, lack of privacy and ignoring the need to defecate because the person finds it difficult to get to the toilet, can also result in constipation in the older person (Firth and Prather, 2002). It is necessary to rule out bowel disease, such as diverticular disease, in the constipated patient. Diverticular disease reduces colonic transit time, the amount of time it takes faecal matter to travel through the colon (large bowel). It is also necessary to identify whether constipation is an adverse effect of medicines that the person is taking, as many medicines have a constipating effect, e.g. antacids, iron, opiates and sedatives.

Factors that may lead to constipation include the following:

- Medication, including prescribed, OTC and herbal medicines
- Dehydration

- Physical inactivity
- Diet low in roughage
- Changes in bowel physiology as a result of increasing age
- Difficulties accessing the toilet (social, environmental, physical)
- Result of disease (e.g. hypothyroidism)
- Regularly delaying the urge to defecate.

PHARMACOLOGICAL INTERVENTIONS USED TO MANAGE CONSTIPATION

Once it has been confirmed that Mr Black's constipation is not a result of a bowel disorder, there are a number of ways that it can be managed. He may need a pharmacological intervention in the short term, but he will also need to have non-pharmacological measures for long-term prevention of constipation.

Nursing knowledge Interventions

There are a number of non-pharmacological interventions that the nurse can include in Mr Black's care plan. These interventions are aimed at improving Mr Black's ability to pass soft stools; they include the following:

- Increase fluid intake to about 2 litres a day.
- Increase the amount of exercise taken.
- Increase the fibre intake by eating wholegrain cereals, wholemeal bread and more fruit and vegetables (**www.food.gov.uk**; Wisten and Messner, 2005).
- Ensure that he has as much privacy as possible and that the toilet environment is as warm and comfortable as possible, with sufficient toilet paper, handwashing facilities and ventilation.
- Review his medication, looking for medicines that have the unwanted effects of constipation, such as iron, aluminium and diuretics, and seek possible alternatives if needed.

Laxatives

The management of constipation is best considered as acute or chronic. The BNF outlines four groups of medicines that can be used to manage constipation: three groups of laxatives (bulk-forming, stimulant, osmotic) and faecal softeners. There are also preparations used for bowel cleansing before investigations and surgery.

- *Bulk-forming laxative*: These increase the volume of faeces, so stimulating peristalsis in the gut. However, an adequate intake of fluid (2 litres per day) must be maintained. Achieving the maximum effect can take a number of days. The increase in faecal mass can have the unwanted effects of abdominal distension (bloating), flatulence and gastrointestinal obstruction. These drugs are useful when it is difficult for the patient to increase fibre in their diet (**www.bnf.org**; Rang *et al.*, 2003).

- *Stimulant laxatives*: These medicines work by decreasing gastrointestinal transit time by speeding up intestinal motility. Examples include bisacodyl and senna. This type of laxative is usually the first choice of medication for the treatment of acute constipation. They usually have an effect within 12 hours and so are best given at night before sleep. Because of their mode of action, they can cause abdominal pain due to gastrointestinal spasm (**www.bnf.org**; Rang *et al.*, 2003). Stimulant laxatives actively increase the contractions of the bowel wall, so moving the faecal content of the bowel towards the rectum. As a result, people using this type of laxative often experience colic (pain/discomfort from the spasmodic stimulation of the colon) as the colon tries to move faecal content along the bowel.

- *Osmotic laxatives*: Using the principle of osmosis, these medicines change the way that, in normal circumstances, water is absorbed back into the gut wall from faecal matter. This results in a more hydrated and softer stool, which then stimulates peristalsis. The hydration (additional water) of the faecal bowel content has two actions: softening and increasing the bulk of the faeces. These medicines can cause abdominal distension and discomfort. A commonly used example is lactulose (**www.bnf.org**; Rang *et al.*, 2003). Osmotic laxatives are considered to be fairly safe because their action depends purely on their ability to attract water into the bowel content from the cells of the gut.

Bowers (2006) points out that there have been few randomised controlled trials for the treatment or prevention of constipation. The few studies that have been published are trials funded by pharmaceutical companies, and Bowers (2006) points out that they may be methodologically unsound. Bowers also draws attention to the fact that the individuals in the study samples used were all relatively young and healthy. Given that many of the people who need to use medication for constipation are older people, some of whom are frail and many of whom frequently have complex diseases, it is not possible to generalise the results from trials such as these.

Personal and professional development 13.9

Suggest three non-pharmacological measures that could improve a patient's constipation.

Pharmacological knowledge

Many drugs have the undesirable effect of causing constipation. Prescribed medicines that have this effect include antidepressants, iron supplements, opioids and antiparkinsonian drugs (**www.bnf.org**; Greenstein and Gould, 2004; Rang *et al.*, 2003).

Using the patient scenario of Mr Harry Black has enabled a discussion about medicines management issues for some common disorders. Working in clinical practice addressing some of the dilemmas faced by many nurses on a day-to-day basis can be fraught with difficulty. Exploring useful strategies that realistically keep the patient as the focus of care has highlighted the depth of knowledge and understanding needed by nurses.

Quick reminder

✔ Alzheimer's disease, a common form of dementia, brings about memory loss, as a result of the decline in brain function.

✔ It is difficult to be precise about how common Alzheimer's disease is in the UK. Its incidence increases with age.

✔ Diagnosing Alzheimer's disease in its early stages is difficult.

✔ NICE guidelines for the management of dementia recommend that people with a suspected diagnosis of dementia be referred to a memory assessment service.

✔ Following a judicial review, the NICE guidelines for the prescribing of acetylcholinesterase inhibitors remain unchanged: acetylcholinesterase inhibitors such as rivastigmine are recommended only for people with a moderate degree of Alzheimer's disease.

✔ Although these drugs aim to improve cognitive function and prevent further memory loss, they become less and less effective over time.

✔ Some herbal therapies, such as ginkgo biloba, are claimed to improve memory, but there is no robust evidence for this.

✔ As the disease progresses, increasing memory loss affects the person's ability to function on an everyday level and affects their reasoning abilities and emotions. It can also result in profound personality changes. This may result in challenging behaviours, which may be managed by administering drugs, raising ethical and legal issues such as chemical restraint, informed consent, capacity to consent, crushing tablets and covert administration.

▷

✔ 20% of people in the UK are thought to have hypertension.

✔ Lifestyle interventions can lower raised blood pressure.

✔ NICE guidelines for managing hypertension include calcium channel blockers such as verapamil.

✔ Constipation may be acute or chronic. Treatment includes dietary advice, increasing fluid intake and pharmacological interventions. The latter include faecal softeners and laxatives, which may be bulk-forming, stimulant or osmotic.

REFERENCES

Audit Commission (2000) *Forget Me Not: Mental Health Services for Older People*. London: Audit Commission.

Bachrach-Lindstrum M, Jensen S, Lundin R and Christensson L (2007) Attitudes of nursing staff working with older people towards nutritional nursing care. *Journal of Clinical Nursing* **16**, 2007-2014.

Barnes L, Cheek J, Nation R L, Gilbert A G, Paradiso L and Ballantyne A (2006) Making sure the residents get their tablets: medication administration in care homes for older people. *Journal of Advanced Nursing* **56**, 190-199.

Boon N A, Colledge N R, Walker B R and Hunter J A A (2006) *Davidson's Principles and Practice of Medicine*, 20th edn. Edinburgh: Churchill Livingstone Elsevier.

Bowers B (2006) Evaluating the evidence for administering phosphate enemas. *British Journal of Nursing* **15**, 378-381.

British Hypertension Society (BHS) and National Institute for Health and Clinical Excellence (NICE) (2006) *Hypertension: Management of Hypertension in Adults in Primary Care*. London: National Institute for Health and Clinical Excellence.

Burstow P and Stokoe R (2001) *Keep Taking the Medicine: Antipsychotics and the Over Medication of Older People – Its Causes and Consequences*. Report commissioned by Paul Burstow, Liberal Democrat MP, Liberal Democrat Party, London.

Campbell S L (2005a) Conceptual model of attractiveness as a factor influencing quality of care and outcomes of residents in nursing home settings. *Advances in Nursing Science* **28**, 107-115.

Campbell S L (2005b) Resident attractiveness as an influential factor in the provision of quality care in nursing homes. *Journal of Gerontological Nursing* **31**, 18-25.

Carlberg B, Samuelsson O and Lindholm L H (2004) Atenolol in hypertension: is it a wise choice? *Lancet* **364**, 1684-1689.

Cayton H, Graham N and Warner J (2002) *Dementia: Alzheimer's and Other Dementias*. London: Class Publishing.

Cowan D, While A, Roberts J and Fitzpatrick J (2002) Medicines management in care homes for older people: the nurse's role. *British Journal of Community Nursing* **7**, 634-638.

Dai Q, Borenstein A R, Wu Y, Jackson J C and Larson E B (2006) Fruit and vegetable juices and Alzheimer's disease: the Kame project. *American Journal of Medicine* **119**, 751-759.

Department for Constitutional Affairs (DfCA) (2005) *Mental Capacity Act*. London: The Stationery Office.

Department for Constutional Affairs (DfCA) (2007) *Mental Capacity Act (2005) Code of Practice*. London: The Stationery Office.

Department of Health (DH) (2000) *National Service Framework for Coronary Heart Disease*. London: Department of Health.

Diamond B J, Johnson S K, Torsney K, Morodan J, Prokop B J, Davidek D and Kramer P (2003) Complementary and alternative medicines in the treatment of dementia: an evidence based review. *Drugs and Aging* **20**, 981-998.

Dimond, B (2004) *Legal Aspects of Nursing*, 4th edn. London: Pearson Education.

Ernst E (2000) *Herbal Medicine: A Concise Overview for Professionals*. Boston, MA: Butterworth-Heinemann.

Ferri C P, Prince M, Brayne C, *et al*., (2005) Global prevalence of dementia: a Delphi consensus study. *Lancet* **366**, 2112-2117.

Firth M and Prather C M (2002) Gastrointestinal motility problems in the elderly patient. *Gastroenterology* **122**, 1688-1700.

Folstein M F, Folstein S E and Mc Hugh P R (1975) Mini-Mental State: a practical method for grading the cognitive state of patients for the clinician. *Journal of Psychiatric Research* **12**, 169-198.

Greenstein B and Gould D (2004) *Trounce's Clinical Pharmacology for Nurses*, 17th edn. Edinburgh: Churchill Livingstone.

Griffiths C and Rooney C (2006) Trends in mortality from Alzheimer's disease, Parkinson's disease and dementia, England and Wales, 1979-2004. *Health Statistics Quarterly* **30**, 6-14.

Harari D (2002) Epidemiology and risk factors for bowel problems in frail older people. In: Potter J, Norton C and Cottenden A (eds) *Bowel Care in Older People*. London: Royal College of Physicians.

Hecker J (2003) Memory loss. In Hudson R (ed.) *Dementia Nursing: A Guide to Practice*. Abingdon: Radcliffe Medical Press.

Hochschild A R (1985) *The Managed Heart: Commercialization of Human Feeling*. London: University of California Press.

Kennedy D O and Scholey A B (2003) Ginseng potential in the enhancement of cognitive performance and mood. *Pharmacology, Biochemistry and Behavior* **75**, 687-700.

Kennedy D O, Scholey A B and Wesnes K A (2002) Modulation of cognition and mood following administration of single doses of ginkgo biloba, ginseng and a ginko/ginseng combination to healthy young adults. *Physiology and Behavior* **72**, 739-751.

Kirkevold Ø and Knut E (2005) Concealment of drugs in food and beverages in nursing homes; cross sectional study. *British Medical Journal* **330**, 20-24.

Kitwood T (1997) *Dementia Reconsidered*. Buckingham: Open University Press.

Kow J V and Hogan D B (2000) Use of physical and chemical restraints in medical teaching units. *Canadian Medical Association Journal* **162**, 3939-3940.

Kwasny P, Hagen B and Armstrong-Esther C (2006) Use of major and minor tranquilisers with older patients in an acute care hospital: an exploratory study. *Journal of Advanced Nursing* **55**, 135-141.

Lahiri D K (2006) Where the action of environment (nutrition), gene and protein meet: beneficial role of fruit and vegetable juices in potentially delaying the onset of Alzheimer's disease. *Journal of Alzheimer's Disease* **10**, 359-361.

Magnussen S and Helstrup T (2007) *Everyday Memory*. Hove: Psychology Press.

Maslow A H (1968) *Towards a Psychology of Being*. London: New York: Van Nostrand.

McKinlay A and Cowan S (2003) Student nurses' attitude towards working with older patients. *Journal of Advanced Nursing* **43**, 298-307.

McKinlay A and Cowan S (2006) If you're frail you've had it: a theory of planned behaviour study of student nurses' attitudes towards working with older patients. *Journal of Applied Social Psychology* **36**, 900-917.

McQueen A C (2004) Emotional intelligence in nursing work. *Journal of Advanced Nursing* **47**, 101-108.

Mera S L (1997) *Understanding Disease: Pathology and Prevention*. Cheltenham: Stanley Thornes.

Middleton H, Keene R G, Johnson C, Elkins A D and Lee A E (1999) Physical and pharmacological restraints in long term care facilities. *Journal of Gerontological Nursing* **25**, 26-33.

Morris H (2005) Dysphagia, medicines and older people: the need for education. *British Journal of Nursing* **10**, 419-420.

National Institute for Health and Clinical Excellence (NICE) (2006) *Hypertension: Management of Hypertension in Adults in Primary Care*. NICE guideline 34. London: National Institute for Health and Clinical Excellence.

National Institute for Health and Clinical Excellence (NICE) (2007) *Donepezil, Galantamine, Rivastigmine and Memantine for the Treatment of Alzheimer's Disease*. Technology appraisal III (amended). London: National Institute for Health and Clinical Excellence.

Nelson T D (2005) Ageism: prejudice against our feared future self. *Journal of Social Issues* **61**, 207-221.

Norton C (2006) Constipation in older patients: effects on quality of life. *British Journal of Nursing* **15**, 188-192.

Nursing and Midwifery Council (NMC) (2007a) *Standards for Medicines Management*. London: Nursing and Midwifery Council.

Nursing and Midwifery Council (NMC) (2007b) Covert administration of medicines: disguising medicines in food and drink. In: Nursing and Midwifery Council. *A-Z of Advice*. London: Nursing and Midwifery Council.

Pulsford D and Duxbury J (2006) Aggressive behaviour by people with dementia in residential care settings: a review. *Journal of Psychiatric and Mental Health Nursing* **13**, 611-618.

Rang H P, Dale M M, Ritter J M and Moore P K (2003) *Pharmacology,* 5th edn. Edinburgh: Elseivier.

Roper N, Logan W W and Tierney A J (2000) *Roper-Logan-Tierney Model of Nursing: Based on Activities of Living*. Edinburgh: Churchill Livingstone.

Roth M, Huppert F A, Tym E, Mountjoy C Q, Diffident-Brown A and Shoesmith D S (1988) *The Cambridge Examination for Mental Disorders of the Elderly: CAMDEX*, 1st edn. Cambridge: Cambridge University Press.

Schofield I, Tolson D, Arthur D, Davies S and Nolan M (2005) An exploration of the caring attributes and perceptions of work place change among gerontological nursing staff in England, Scotland and China (Hong Kong). *International Journal of Nursing Studies* **42**, 197-209.

Scott J and Williams E R L (1997) Concealed administration of drug treatment may represent thin edge of the wedge. *British Medical Journal* **314**, 299-300.

Seedhouse D and Gallagher A (2002) Undignifying institutions. *Journal of Medical Ethics* **28**, 368-372.

Simonsen T, Aarbakke J, Kay I, Coleman I, Sinnott R and Lysaa R (2006) *Illustrated Pharmacology for Nurses*. London: Hodder Arnold.

Slevin O (1991) Ageist attitudes among young adults: implications for a caring profession. *Journal of Advanced Nursing* **16**, 1197-1205.

Smith P (1992) *The Emotional Labour of Nursing*. London: Palgrave Macmillan.

Thompson W G, Longstreth G F, Drossman D A, *et al*. (1999) Functional bowel disorders and functional abdominal pain. *Gut* **45** (suppl. 2), 1143-1147.

Thurmond J A (1999) Nurses' perceptions of chemical restraint in use in long term care. *Applied Nursing Research* **12**, 159-162.

Treloar A, Beats B and Philpot M (2000) A pill in the sandwich: covert medication in food and drink. *Journal of the Royal Society of Medicine* **93**, 408-411.

Treloar A, Philpot M and Beats B (2001) Concealing medication in patients' food. *Lancet* **357**, 62-64.

Welsh S and Deal M (2001) Covert medication: ever ethically justifiable? *Psychiatric Bulletin* **26**, 123-126.

Williams B, Poulter N R, Brown M J, *et al*. (2004) British Hypertension Society guidelines for hypertension management 2004 (BHS-IV): summary. *British Medical Journal* **328**, 634-640.

Williams M (2006) *Dementia*. In: R L Gregory (ed.) *The Oxford Companion to the Mind*. Oxford: Oxford University Press.

Wisten A and Messner T (2005) Fruit and fibre (Pajala porridge) in the prevention of constipation. *Scandinavian Journal of Caring Science* **19**, 71-76.

Wong J G W S, Poon Y and Hui E C (2005) I can put the medicine in his soup, Doctor. *Journal of Medical Ethics* **31**, 262-265.

Wright D (2002) Medication administration in nursing homes. *Nursing Standard* **16**, 33-38.

Chapter 14

Diabetes mellitus:
an adult with type 2 diabetes, depression and hypothyroidism

Diabetes mellitus affects more than 2 million people in the UK (National Institute for Health and Clinical Excellence (NICE), (2007), and the figure is increasing on a yearly basis. It is possible that a similar number of people may have undiagnosed diabetes. Wickens (2005) estimates that up to 90% of people with diabetes have type 2 diabetes. This chapter introduces a patient with type 2 diabetes mellitus.

Learning outcomes

At the end of this chapter you should be able to:

✔ Give an overview of diabetes mellitus
✔ Discuss the potential impact of diabetes mellitus on an individual
✔ Identify pharmacological approaches used to manage diabetes mellitus
✔ Discuss the actions and effects of insulin related to the specific patient scenario
✔ Identify nursing knowledge needed to manage this patient and his diabetes
✔ Identify other therapies, related to the patient scenario, used to treat risk factors that increase the risk of cardiovascular disease
✔ Describe the features of depression
✔ Outline some treatment approaches for depression
✔ Recognise the potential implications of depression on the patient's ability to manage his diabetes successfully
✔ Define hypothyroidism
✔ Discuss the impact of hypothyroidism on this patient's condition
✔ Identify supporting nursing interventions for this patient.

Chapter at a glance

The nature of diabetes mellitus
Pharmacological interventions used to manage diabetes mellitus
The nature of depression
Pharmacological interventions used to manage depression
The nature of hypothyroidism
Pharmacological interventions used to manage hypothyroidism
Quick reminder
References

Mr Ronnie Middleton

Mr Middleton was diagnosed as having type 2 diabetes mellitus at 46 years old. He is now 62 years old. His diabetes was discovered at a routine medical examination, when he applied for a new job. He had gradually put on weight, which he couldn't seem to lose, even though he watched his diet and tried to take a bit more exercise. He had also started to get up during the night to pass urine, but he assumed that this was because he was getting older.

He managed his diabetes quite successfully on metformin 500 mg three times per day, gliclazide 80 mg once a day before breakfast, acarbose 50 mg three times daily and a 'healthy' diet. However, since his wife died 4 years ago, he has struggled to 'see the point of all this fuss', doesn't always take his medication as directed and has put on weight.

This is a somewhat classic picture of the development of type 2 diabetes mellitus. The onset is gradual and the patient often finds other explanations for the symptoms. NICE (2007) defines diabetes mellitus as a 'chronic metabolic disorder characterised by elevated blood glucose levels resulting from a lack of the hormone insulin or resistance to its action'. Insulin is responsible for the control of glucose, fat and amino acid metabolism. Thus, patients with diabetes mellitus have difficulty with blood sugar control: without insulin, glucose cannot enter the cells and stays in the bloodstream. The elevated blood sugar (hyperglycaemia) results in biochemical abnormalities.

THE NATURE OF DIABETES MELLITUS

Diabetes mellitus is a disorder characterised by hyperglycaemia (a high blood sugar level) as a consequence of some degree of insulin lack. The aetiological factors (causes) and presentation of the disorder vary.

Anatomy and physiology

Carbohydrates (starches and sugars) are taken into the body in the diet. They are used by body cells to produce energy. In order to do this, carbohydrates need to be broken down by digestion into glucose and then to cross the cell membrane, facilitated by the hormone insulin (Hand, 2000).

The pancreas contains endocrine tissue – the islets of Langerhans – which secrete substances directly into the bloodstream. These islets produce two hormones: insulin (produced by beta cells) and glucagon (produced, in much smaller quantities, by alpha cells). Insulin and glucagon are produced as required in response to eating or fasting.

Insulin is a complex hormone with a key role in the regulation of carbohydrate, fat and protein metabolism. It maintains normal blood glucose levels by:

- promoting glucose uptake by the cells, involving the transport of glucose through the cell membrane;
- converting glucose to glycogen for storage in the liver and muscles (glycogenesis);
- promoting protein synthesis;
- converting glucose to triglycerides for storage as body fat.

Glucagon increases blood sugar. In response to low blood sugar, it:

- promotes the conversion of stored glycogen to glucose (glycogenolysis) and its release from the liver;
- promotes fat breakdown (lipolysis) and protein breakdown (gluconeogenesis) to provide an alternative source of glucose;
- in the absence of insulin generates the production of ketones bodies (weak acids produced as a consequence of fat breakdown) in the absence of insulin (Alexander *et al.*, 2006).

Insulin and glucagon work in harmony to maintain blood sugar levels. When blood sugar levels fall when fasting, such as between meals, glucagon is produced; when blood sugar levels rise after eating, insulin is produced. The body needs to be able to maintain its systems in a state of equilibrium, despite fluctuations such as falling blood glucose levels between meals. This constant interplay between the two hormones maintains **homeostasis** (the constancy of the body's internal environment).

The liver plays a key role in maintaining blood glucose levels. In the presence of hyper-glycaemia, glucose is converted to glycogen (glycogenesis) and stored as either glycogen or fat (stimulated by insulin), thus reducing blood glucose levels (this also occurs in muscle cells). In the presence of **hypoglycaemia**, glycogenolysis occurs (glycogen is broken down into glucose, controlled by adrenaline/epinephrine and glucagon), increasing blood glucose levels.

Pathophysiology

In the absence of insulin, glucose cannot move from the bloodstream into the cells. As a result, the level of glucose in the bloodstream rises. Eventually the glucose is transported to the kidneys. When the glucose levels in the kidney tubules exceed the renal threshold (9.9-11.1 mmol/litre), glucose is excreted by the kidneys (glycosuria). Some glucose remains in the kidney tubule and begins to exert an osmotic effect, drawing water into the tubule. This in turn increases urinary output, so the patient produces large volumes of urine (polyuria) and experiences urinary frequency, which may involve getting up during the night to pass urine (nocturia). Ultimately this may result in dehydration, and the patient experiences thirst as a consequence.

Because the cells are not able to use glucose for energy, energy has to be produced from non-carbohydrate sources such as proteins and fats. In patients with type 1 diabetes, this results in increased appetite and weight loss.

> ### Essential terminology
>
> **Diabetes**
> From the Greek for 'siphon' or 'to pass through'.
>
> **Mellitus**
> From the Latin for 'honey sweet' (Wickens, 2005).

The patient with diabetes experiences tiredness as a result of lack of energy (inability to utilise glucose) and increased appetite. The body tries to eliminate the elevated blood sugar, which results in excessive thirst (polydipsia). These features are subtle in patients with type 2 diabetes but can be much more obvious in patients with type 1 diabetes.

Related knowledge Pathophysiology

There is another form of diabetes – diabetes insipidus. This condition occurs as a consequence of the pituitary gland failing to produce the hormone vasopressin (antidiuretic hormone), which is responsible for the reabsorption of water by the kidneys. Desmopressin (a synthetic, more specific derivative of vasopressin) is used as replacement therapy and administered orally.

Diabetes refers to any condition in which the patient produces large quantities of urine and experiences excessive thirst.

The World Health Organization (WHO) has reclassified the methods and criteria for diagnosing diabetes mellitus (**www.diabetes.org.uk**). The diagnosis should be based on the patient's history (presence of polyuria, polydipsia, unexplained weight loss) and blood glucose measurement, a fasting blood glucose of 7.0 mmol/litre (normal fasting blood glucose for an adult is 4-6 mmol/litre) or oral glucose tolerance test. If the blood glucose level 2 hours after taking oral glucose is greater than 11.1 mmol/litre, then diabetes mellitus is confirmed.

Type 1 diabetes

Type 1 diabetes mellitus is thought to be an autoimmune disease resulting in the destruction of the beta pancreatic cells, which are responsible for the production of insulin (Dixon, 2002). Patients with type 1 diabetes need replacement insulin for their lifetime.

Successful blood glucose management is assessed using measurements of glycosylated haemoglobin (HbA_{1c}), the percentage of haemoglobin bound to glucose (NICE guidelines suggest that this should be 2.3-6.5%). Glucose binds irreversibly to haemoglobin for the life of the red blood cell (approximately 90 days). Monitoring the haemoglobin gives an indication of the average blood glucose concentration for the previous 2-3 months; this helps the healthcare professional assess control over a period of time. Other measurements, such as urine testing and blood monitoring (testing a drop of capillary blood by placing it on a reagent strip), reflect the blood glucose level only a few hours before the urine test or at the immediate time of blood monitoring.

Blood monitoring by the patient at home using a blood-monitoring kit is a more accurate way of identifying patterns or trends, such as highs and lows rather than an average (Dixon, 2002). Patients are advised to maintain a blood glucose level of 4-9 mmol/litre (**www.bnf.org**).

Type 1 diabetes mellitus is usually characterised by:

- onset before age 30 years;
- autoimmune response;
- weight loss;
- immediate effects;
- absolute lack of insulin;
- ketosis;
- requirement for insulin replacement (adapted from Phillipe and Whittaker, 2004).

Type 2 diabetes

Unlike in type 1 diabetes, which is associated with absolute insulin deficiency, people with type 2 diabetes have *some* insulin deficiency (Bhattacharyya, 2001). This deficiency is thought to be due to a combination of factors, such as insulin resistance and a loss of secretory function by the pancreatic cells. Type 2 diabetes has an insidious (subtle) onset,

---

and the presenting symptoms such as thirst are often explained away by other reasons. As a consequence, patients with this type of diabetes may have already developed long-term complications before presenting; in fact, the presence of such complications may be what initiates the patient to visit the doctor. As the disease progresses, less insulin is produced, which can result in the requirement for increased doses of oral antidiabetic drugs (OADs)/hypoglycaemic medicines, additional medicines and insulin in order to maintain glycaemic control (Lowey, 2005).

Type 2 diabetes mellitus is usually characterised by:

- onset after age 40 years;
- reduction in insulin production;
- insulin resistance;
- no autoantibodies detected;
- slow onset;
- familial pattern;
- obesity;
- treatment aimed at improving insulin production (adapted from Phillipe and Whittaker, 2004).

Related knowledge Pathophysiology

There are some other, less common forms of diabetes mellitus:

- *Gestational diabetes* occurs in some women during pregnancy but usually disappears after birth; treatment may include insulin and modification of diet.
- *Diabetes secondary to other diseases and treatments*, e.g. pancreatic disease, stress, treatment with corticosteroids.

Short-term complications of diabetes mellitus

Hypoglycaemia (low blood sugar)

The blood glucose is lower than the normal fasting range, but symptoms do not usually appear until the blood glucose falls below 3 mmol/litre. In this situation, the patient may experience a range of symptoms, such as sweating, dizziness, palpitations, hunger and deteriorating conscious level. However, there is a direct correlation between symptoms and treatment; onset with insulin results in a full-blown symptomology and fast deterioration within 5–15 minutes depending upon the type of insulin used. Mr Middleton is at risk from hypoglycaemic attacks related to his gliclazide. This is the most common adverse effect of this medicine. The hypoglycaemic attack can be both severe and prolonged (Rang *et al.*, 2003). Although hypoglycaemia is usually a response to treatment, particularly insulin (but also oral diabetic agents), in people with type 1 diabetes it can be a consequence of unexpected exercise.

Hypoglycaemia requires a prompt response. Treatment consists of administration of glucose, Hypostop® or glucagon:

- *Glucose* is administered orally by giving a drink containing sugar, by eating something sugary such as a chocolate bar or fudge, by taking dextrose tablets if the patient is conscious, or by giving an intravenous injection of glucose 50% (this latter intervention involves a healthcare professional).

- Hypostop® is a gel containing 40% glucose monohydrate. It is applied to the buccal mucosa and then the cheek is massaged. This treatment offers a rapid response.

- Glucagon may be given by intramuscular or subcutaneous injection. This is a useful strategy for diabetic patients who have recurrent hypoglycaemic attacks. Family members can give this treatment following appropriate training (Downie *et al.*, 2005).

Hyperglycaemia (high blood sugar)

This presents with symptoms of fatigue, thirst, passing large quantities of urine and hunger. It may be seen in undiagnosed diabetic people. In type 2 diabetes, these symptoms may occur over a long period of time and be explained away by other factors, such as 'getting old' and so missed. In type 1 diabetes, the symptoms appear before diagnosis. After the commencement of insulin, hyperglycaemia can lead, if untreated, to ketoacidosis, a serious medical emergency.

Ketoacidosis

When glucose is not utilised fully, fat metabolism is increased in order to compensate. Oxidation of fatty acids in the liver leads to the formation of energy-rich compounds but also produces compounds called ketones (Hand, 2000). If this production of ketones continues, ketoacidosis develops. Ketones accumulating in the bloodstream overwhelm the body's bicarbonate buffering system, which is responsible for maintaining the pH level of the blood between 7.35 and 7.45 (Hand, 2000). Diabetic ketoacidosis is a life-threatening complication of diabetes, consisting of hyperglycaemia, hyperketonaemia and metabolic acidosis. Untreated, it can result in coma and death (Palmer, 2004).

Treatment with an intravenous infusion of short-acting insulin reduces the hyperglycaemia and inhibits the production of ketones, thus correcting the acidosis. However, ketoacidosis can cause electrolyte disturbance (raised potassium levels initially, followed by reduced potassium levels as the patient is rehydrated) and dehydration, and this needs to be treated with a fast infusion of intravenous fluids, initially sodium chloride and potassium replacement, related to the patient's blood electrolyte levels.

Long-term complications of diabetes mellitus

Although the exact mechanism underlying the following changes is not fully understood, the damage to the blood vessels is thought to result from poor glycaemic control:

- *Macrovascular*: Damage to larger blood vessels – thickening and hardening of the arterial wall. Leads to atherosclerosis, stroke, heart attack (myocardial infarction) and the potential for amputation.

- *Microvascular*: Damage to small blood vessels. Thought to result from a combination of atherosclerotic changes in large vessels and microcirculation defects (Whittaker, 2004). Leads to damage to the retina (retinopathy), kidney damage (nephropathy) and nerve damage (neuropathy).

- *Diabetic foot* is a syndrome (collection of symptoms) that occurs as a consequence of vascular changes and neuropathic changes, complicated by other consequences of diabetes such as poor healing.

Unfortunately, patients with type 2 diabetes, because of the subtlety of the symptoms, may develop long-term vascular damage as a consequence of the untreated hyperglycaemia or present with the long-term complications of diabetes before the diagnosis of diabetes is made (Downie *et al.*, 2003).

Mr Middleton has type 2 diabetes mellitus.

Aims of treatment

The aims of treatment for type 2 diabetes are:

- correction of symptoms;
- prevention of complications;
- maintenance of health, including normal weight and body mass index (BMI), blood pressure and lipid levels.

Diet and nutrition

Diet is considered to be vital in the management of diabetes (Mason, 2002). When a patient is newly diagnosed, consideration of diet (including the need for weight loss) and activity related to the patient's lifestyle is the priority. Treatments, whether oral hypoglycaemic agents or insulin, are seen as 'extras'.

In patients with type 2 diabetes, the emphasis is on weight reduction followed by the adoption of a healthy diet – high in fibre, and low in sugar, fat and salt (Downie *et al.*, 2003). As such a diet is recommended for the general population, it is suggested that this helps patients adhere with the diet, as it does not have to be different from that of family and friends. However, it is important that the patient with diabetes eats regular meals throughout the day.

Specific advice is given in relation to daily intake of saturated fat, which should comprise less than 10% of the total energy intake in order to reduce the risk of hyperlipidaemia (high levels of lipoproteins in the bloodstream; see Chapter 10) associated with diabetes (Vaughan, 2005). Other recommendations are to increase dietary fibre intake, reduce salt consumption and manage carbohydrates by using the glycaemic load (GL), an indication of the glycaemic index of the carbohydrate, which determines how quickly the carbohydrate enters the bloodstream in relation to quantity.

Patients with type 1 diabetes have more flexibility regarding their diet if they use blood glucose monitoring to assess their insulin needs (Vaughan, 2005), but the same dietary principles apply.

Most newly diagnosed patients are monitored for a period, usually 3 months, of dietary restriction and increased activity before starting any pharmacological treatments (Bhattacharyya, 2001; Dixon, 2002; Mason, 2002). Successful dietary modification enhances the efficiency of the prescribed medications.

It is recommended that the patient diagnosed with diabetes is referred to a dietician, so that the patient's lifestyle and individual wishes can be considered and an achievable, realistic dietary plan implemented. European and UK guidelines are available in relation to diet for people with diabetes.

Most people who present with type 2 diabetes are overweight (thought to be related to insulin resistance). Mr Middleton has stared to gain weight since the death of his wife. His diet needs to be reassessed based upon his weight and body mass index (BMI). The aims of dietary control in patients with diabetes are based upon:

- maintaining BMI within the recommended range (20-25 kg/m^2);
- maintaining normal blood glucose levels (4-8 mmol/l);
- preventing complications;
- maintaining good health;
- preventing hyperlipidaemia (Mason, 2002).

PHARMACOLOGICAL INTERVENTIONS USED TO MANAGE DIABETES MELLITUS

Oral hypoglycaemics (oral antidiabetic agents)

The main groups of hypoglycaemic agents used in the UK are:

- *Sulphonylureas*: Indicated for patients who have some pancreatic function and normal weight, e.g. gliclazide.
- *Biguanides*: Usually indicated when the patient is overweight and has little pancreatic function, e.g. metformin.

- *Thiazolidinediones (glitazones)*: Stimulate a receptor (peroxisome proliferator-activated receptor gamma, PPARγ, resulting in lowered insulin resistance.
- Alpha-glucosidase inhibitors: Reduce the rise in postprandial (occurring after meals) blood glucose, e.g acarbose (Gadsby, 2006; Lowey, 2005).

Dixon (2002) suggests that athough treatment initially may involve only one antidiabetic agent, many patients suffer a 'secondary failure of treatment'. Most patients therefore require a combination of antidiabetic medicines or insulin.

Sulphonylureas

This group of medicines acts by stimulating the beta cells of the pancreas to produce more insulin (Dixon, 2002). There are several sulphonylureas available, which have different durations of action. There is a suggestion that long-term administration may result in improved insulin activity. Sulphonylureas may be prescribed on their own or with metformin (a biguanide) or insulin and help to reduce hyperglycaemia within a few days. Gliclazide is the most commonly prescribed sulphonylurea because it rarely causes side effects and has a long duration of action. One consequence of giving patients prescribed hypoglycaemic therapy is that the patient may experience treatment-induced hypoglycaemia (see earlier). Sulphonylureas may also cause gastrointestinal upset and weight gain (Gadsby, 2006; Whittaker, 2004).

Gliclazide

Gliclazide is a sulphonylurea. Its duration of action is up to 24 hours, although it has a shorter length of action than some other sulphonylureas, e.g. glibenclamide (**www.bnf.org**). Gliclazide is a popular choice of medicine because, although it has the potential to cause hypoglycaemic attacks, they are unlikely. Gliclazide takes 4–5 hours to achieve a peak response and is taken before breakfast in order to give good cover for both lunch and the evening meal (Dixon, 2002). It is advocated for use in older patients.

Pharmacodynamics Gliclazide

Gliclazide is a hypoglycaemic sulphonylurea. It enhances the first phase and, to some degree, the second phase of insulin secretion.

It reduces platelet adhesiveness and aggregation and increases fibrinolytic

Pharmacokinetics Gliclazide

Absorption: Well absorbed. Food intake does not affect the rate or degree of absorption.

Distribution: Peak plasma levels are reached within 1 hour; plasma protein binding is approximately 95%.

Metabolism: Metabolised primarily in the liver and so should be used with caution in patients with hepatic dysfunction. Metabolised to inactive products.

Elimination: Excreted mainly by the kidneys. If the patient has renal impairment, the medicine stays in the body longer (**www.emc.medicines.org.uk**).

Biguanides

The only biguanide available in the UK is metformin (Gadsby, 2006). It acts by inhibiting gluconeogenesis and increasing peripheral utilisation of glucose (Bhattacharyya, 2001); it possibly reduces appetite. Metformin is effective only if some insulin is produced. It is the medicine of choice for obese patients (NICE, 2002) as it reduces adverse macrovascular outcomes (Gadsby, 2006). Metformin should always be introduced slowly and the dose increased over a period of weeks. It can cause gastrointestinal side effects, but the most serious, albeit rare, side effect is **lactic acidosis** (build-up of lactic acid in the blood, which can cause muscle cramp), usually in the presence of renal impairment. The patient's serum creatinine levels should be checked to test renal function (see Chapter 4), and metformin should be discontinued if the serum creatinine level rises above 150 mmol/litre (Gadsby, 2006). Side effects can be reduced by starting on a low dose such as 500 mg daily and then increasing the dose over several weeks. Metformin is often given in conjunction with sulphonylureas and insulin.

Pharmacodynamics Metformin

Metformin is a biguanide with antihyperglycaemic effects. It lowers basal and postprandial glucose. It is thought to act by:

- reducing hepatic glucose production;
- slightly increasing insulin sensitivity in muscle, improving peripheral glucose uptake and utilisation;
- delaying intestinal glucose absorption.

Pharmacokinetics Metformin

Absorption: The presence of food slightly delays absorption.

Distribution: Metformin has a half-life of 3 hours. Plasma protein binding is negligible.

Metabolism: Not metabolised.

Elimination: Excreted unchanged in the urine (Rang *et al.*, 2003).

Alpha-glucosidase inhibitors

Acarbose is the only alpha-glucosidase inhibitor available in the UK. It was previously considered useful for diabetics who could not manage their blood sugar by diet alone, or where other hypoglycaemic agents were not effective, and in obese patients, but its use is limited because of its side effects. It is an oral hypoglycaemic agent that reduces the high blood glucose that occurs after meals (postprandial hyperglycaemia); it is thought that this results in a reduced insulin demand. Acarbose is a complex carbohydrate molecule and competes with disaccharides and polysaccharides so that they cannot be broken down into monosaccharides and absorbed in the intestine. The medicine achieves this effect by inhibiting the enzyme alpha-glucosidase in the intestine, which is responsible for breaking down carbohydrates into monosaccharides. Since carbohydrates are absorbed as monosaccharides, the absorption of glucose is therefore reduced. The carbohydrates pass further down into the large bowel, thus inhibiting the absorption of starch and sucrose. This may result in flatulence and diarrhoea. To avoid this side effect, the medicine is started in a low dose.

Pharmacodynamics Acarbose

The action of acarbose is based on the competitive inhibition of intestinal enzymes. Glucose derived from these carbohydrates is released and taken up into the blood more slowly. Acarbose reduces the postprandial rise in blood glucose, thus reducing blood glucose fluctuations.

Pharmacokinetics Acarbose

Absorption: Absorbed systemically.

Metabolism: Degraded to inactive metabolites by the intestinal or bacterial enzymes of the gastrointestinal tract.

Elimination: Metabolites are excreted in the faeces.

Mr Ronnie Middleton

Mr Middleton is being seen every 3 months by the diabetes nurse specialist, as she is concerned about how he is managing his diabetes. At the clinic, he has his HbA_{1c} checked; the results indicate a lack of adequate glycaemic control. He has not lost any weight. On checking his weight and comparing it with his height on a BMI chart, the nurse identifies that he has a BMI of 31 kg/m^2, indicating that he is obese (obesity is defined by a BMI of 30 kg/m^2 or more) (NICE, 2006). Mr Middleton admits to having difficulty managing his blood sugars and his medication. He confesses that he discontinued the acarbose some time ago because of an 'upset stomach' and bloating. It is decided to start him on a small dose of insulin. NICE (2002) guidelines recommend that insulin should be commenced when the patient experiences inadequate control with other medications.

Insulin

Insulin binds to the cell membrane, increasing the permeability of the cell to glucose and thus permitting the uptake of glucose by the cell (Hand, 2000). According to Dixon (2002), approximately 50% of patients with diabetes require insulin as the beta cells of the pancreas become 'exhausted'. Patients with type 2 diabetes mellitus may need larger doses of insulin than patients with type 1 (Lowey, 2005). However, the dose of insulin can be reduced if combined with metformin.

> **Essential terminology**
>
> **Recombinant DNA technology**
> This uses DNA that is produced as a consequence of deliberately combining genetic material (DNA) from different sources – that is, genetic engineering. In the case of insulin, this usually involves adding a human insulin gene to the genetic material of a non-disease-producing laboratory strain of the bacterium *Escherichia coli* (Galbraith *et al.*, 2007).

Wherever possible, insulin treatment should copy the insulin production from a normal pancreas - that is, maintain a basal or background level of insulin in the bloodstream and supply insulin as required at mealtimes, in order to prevent hyperglycaemia or hypoglycaemia (Gummerson, 2006).

There are many insulin products available. Most are human insulins, specifically developed by recombinant DNA technology using bacteria (**www.bnf.org**). Insulin is inactivated by gastrointestinal enzymes, and so replacement insulin is given by injection (NICE, 2007).

Insulin can be short-acting, intermediate-acting or long-acting. Modern treatment regimes are based upon a combination of regular injections of short-acting insulin at mealtimes and longer-acting insulin given one or twice per day (e.g. early morning and evening).

Short-acting insulins

Also referred to as soluble insulin and non-analogue insulin, short-acting insulins are used to cover mealtimes, when an extra bolus of insulin is required to cope with the rise in blood glucose. Insulin is administered by subcutaneous injection. It is recommended that short-acting insulin is administered 30 minutes before eating (Gummerson, 2006). There are also some rapidly acting insulin analogues that are absorbed faster (within 15 minutes) and so can be given just before or even after a meal. The dose can be adapted to the carbohydrate content of the meal, giving the patient a greater level of control, particularly if they have irregular mealtimes. Rapidly-acting insulin analogues have fewer side effects such as hypoglycaemia and weight gain compared with non-analogue standard insulins.

An insulin analogue is an insulin molecule that has been altered so that it retains its biological effect but has some advantage over standard human insulin (Gummerson, 2006).

Longer-acting standard insulins

A substance such as zinc is added to insulin (Lowey, 2005) to slow the absorption of insulin. Slow-release insulins are used to maintain 24-hour basal control. They include both intermediate-acting and long-acting insulins. Slow-release insulins cause peaks of action (5-7 hours after dosing for the intermediate-acting insulin) and patients' reactions vary (Gummerson, 2006).

Long-acting insulin analogues

These provide a more sustained and therefore predictable basal insulin supply (Gummerson, 2006).

Biphasic insulin analogues

These are premixed formulations of a fast-acting, and therefore shorter-duration, insulin and a longer-acting insulin analogue. They manage the need for insulin at mealtimes and also maintain a basal insulin level (Gummerson, 2006).

Nursing knowledge Nursing interventions

Because of the need for repeated injections of insulin, there is a risk of local problems such as fat hypertrophy (increase in size of tissue), loss of sensitivity, and impaired or erratic absorption. In order to avoid these problems, patients should be advised to rotate sites for injection. Insulin is given by subcutaneous injection. When the patient self-administers, the injection sites need to be easily accessible; the usual sites are the upper arm, outer thigh and abdomen. However, insulin is absorbed more readily from certain sites, such as the abdomen and arm. Alexander *et al.*, (2006) suggest that the same sites should be used in relation to particular times of the day, e.g. the arm/abdomen for morning injections and the thigh for evening injections.

Personal and professional development 14.1
Patient education

Insulin is given by subcutaneous injection. What advice could you give the patient about the following?

- Suitable sites for injection
- Rotating sites for injection
- Care of the skin
- Care and storage of insulin, syringes and needles

- Obtaining further supplies of insulin and equipment.

You may wish to access a website such as **www.diabetes.org.uk**, which is designed for people with diabetes mellitus, to see what advice they offer.

Insulin delivery

Pen devices are helpful to patients who have a needle-phobia (Dixon, 2002). Insulin pens are popular and easy to use. They use a cartridge containing 3 ml of insulin. Pen types require specific cartridges as there is no compatibility between manufacturers (Wiffen *et al.*, 2007).

Insulin can also be given by insulin pump, which enables a continuous basal infusion and mealtime top-ups activated by the patient. This is known as a continuous subcutaneous insulin infusion (CSII). The device contains a reservoir of insulin, which connects to the patient via a catheter and a cannula inserted under the skin. The cost-effectiveness of CSII is being investigated by NICE (2007), which has recommended it for specific groups of patients with type 1 diabetes – those in whom current treatment has failed and those who have the 'commitment and competence to use it'.

Pharmacological knowledge Associated treatments

Because of the well-documented risks associated with diabetes, such as heart disease, the National Service Framework (DH, 2001) recommends a range of associated treatments to minimise these risks, particularly in relation to type 2 diabetes.

- *Antihypertensives*: Up to 70% of patients with type 2 diabetes also have hypertension (DH, 2001), which is often difficult to control. Medicines used include ACE inhibitors, beta-blockers (see Chapters 10 and 13) and calcium channel blockers. Treatment of hypertension reduces mortality and protects sharpness of vision (visual acuity). N.B. ACE inhibitors can increase the risk of hypoglycaemia during the first weeks of treatment. If the patient has renal impairment, beta-blockers can blunt the signs of hypoglycaemia (**www.bnf.org**).

- *Statins*: More than 70% of patients with type 2 diabetes have raised cholesterol levels (DH, 2001).

- *Aspirin*: This is given for primary and secondary prevention of myocardial infarction.

- *Obesity treatments*: Patients who are obese may be prescribed orlistat or sibutramine (see Chapter 16) (**www.bnf.org**).

New developments

Dixon (2002) suggests that there are three potential strategies for the future for people with diabetes: better delivery systems for insulin, new treatments and the possibility of a cure.

Better delivery systems for insulin

An inhaled rapid-acting insulin has been produced. However, NICE (2006) has recommended that this should not be a routine treatment and should be used only where patients (with type 1 or 2 diabetes) are having difficulty controlling their blood sugar by usual methods and are unable to start or increase insulin (related to needle-phobia or problems with injection sites).

New treatments

Transplantation of pancreatic cells may be considered (primarily for people with type 1 diabetes, as there is a limited supply of pancreatic cells). Islet cells are infused into the liver via the hepatic portal vein (Wickens, 2005). A successful adult transplant requires about 1 million islet cells, and there is the possibility of rejection. Alternatively, transplantation of the pancreas (rather than pancreatic cells) was first carried out in 1966 with some considerable success, and an 82% survival rate (Bhattacharyya, 2001). Donor organs are in short supply and transplantation is not usually undertaken in type 2 diabetes, mainly due to the patient's age and the existence of other problems.

Research is being undertaken into the development of oral insulin, an insulin 'pill', although this is in its early stages. It is thought that a large insulin dose will be required (Diabetes UK, 2007).

A cure?

Although we have already explained that human insulin is in fact produced by genetic engineering, there are some newer developments that are gene therapies. This means that the genome (which contains the genes for a cell - around 30 000 genes) has been altered to treat a medical condition. An example of this is the research undertaken by Dr Ann Simpson and her team in 2001 in Australia, who successfully inserted the human insulin gene into the genome of liver cells (in the laboratory, using cell cultures), resulting in the production and storage of insulin. It is hoped that if this is successful in humans, it could allow the body to self-regulate just as in the person who does not have diabetes mellitus (**www.diabetes.org.uk**).

Patient education

Because of the complex nature of diabetes, it is important that the patient plays an active part in the management of their own condition. Management of diabetes must be seen as a multidisciplinary responsibility and there needs to be a designated leader to effectively identify and coordinate the input of the different professionals.

Diet and nutrition

The approach to nutrition and diet in diabetes is based upon a healthy diet that the whole family can adhere to and that falls within contemporary nutritional advice to maintain health. The patient's diet is not different from that of the rest of the family and can be followed relatively easily if eating out. Guidelines for patients with diabetes include the following:

- Eat regular meals.
- Reduce fat intake.
- Increase fibre intake.
- Eat at least five portions of fruit and vegetables every day.
- Reduce salt intake.
- Reduce sugar intake; use sweeteners instead if necessary.
- Drink alcohol only in moderation.
- 'Diabetic' foods are expensive and unnecessary (Mason, 2002; NICE, 2000).

Alcohol

For patients treated with insulin or sulphonylureas and who choose to drink alcohol, alcohol should always be taken with food, as these treatments have the potential to cause hypoglycaemia. Advice about alcohol consumption for diabetic patients is the same as that for the general public (Vaughan, 2005): drink no more than 14 units per week for women, or 21 units for men, and have one or two days each week with no consumption of alcohol.

Monitoring responses to therapy

Urinalysis is a simple, inexpensive and non-invasive way of testing for the presence of glucose and ketones in the urine. It requires some manual dexterity and an ability to interpret colour when using the urine reagent strips. It also requires a willingness to undertake the test (some patients are unhappy about handling their own urine) and an ability to act upon the results. Blood glucose monitoring has largely replaced this method of monitoring glycaemic control, but it is still useful for some patients.

The availability of portable blood monitoring kits for patients to use at home has made this method much more acceptable and accessible and provides a more accurate measurement. Patients can become much more active in their management, adjusting the dose of insulin in response to the blood results and so having more flexibility. Available kits include a finger-pricking device (lancet), a reagent strip and a meter to interpret the results. The patient needs to be motivated to use this test. It is an invasive procedure, which some patients might find uncomfortable or painful. It also requires dexterity and the ability to interpret and act upon results. The patient needs to be advised about the safe disposal of lancets.

Managing long-term complications

In order to manage the complications of diabetes effectively, the patient should be advised to:

- maintain regular contact with their diabetes nurse specialist;
- attend regular check-ups as required with their diabetic physician;
- have regular blood pressure checks;
- see their optometrist and GP regularly in order to test for the presence of eye disease;
- have an annual test for the presence of protein in the urine; if necessary, this should be followed up by a serum creatinine test. If this is positive, the patient requires an ACE inhibitor, even if their blood pressure is within normal parameters (**www.bnf.org**);
- attend their podiatrist regularly to have foot care managed effectively.

Patient empowerment

Diabetes is a lifelong disease, and so it is important to empower the patient to manage their diabetes effectively (Meetoo, 2004). Managing diabetes can be a challenge for the patient, and the success of management is often determined by the patient's health beliefs. Becker's (1974) health belief model is still used by healthcare professionals to help them understand and facilitate adherence/concordance in patients with chronic conditions. This model suggests that patients may see the cost of treatment as too high – for example, the impact on their lifestyle or the experience of unpleasant side effects – and that they weigh up the costs and benefits of the treatment. The trigger for patients 'conforming' to treatments and advice is the perceived 'threat' – that is, the effect of, and the risks posed by, the condition.

Patients with diabetes mellitus may have to cope with the stigma associated with having a chronic illness, the difficulties inherent in maintaining good glycaemic control and having to come to terms with having a condition for which there is currently no cure (Whittaker, 2004). Treatments such as insulin injections can be uncomfortable or painful, and the act of injecting might be misinterpreted by others. Diabetes may have an impact on the person's ability to undertake some jobs and may interfere with sexual function in men (impotence). Urine and blood glucose monitoring require the patient to have contact with body fluids in a way that they may not have experienced before. The patient therefore has to come to terms with their diagnosis as well as embarking on major changes to their lifestyle.

The role of the nurse is critical (Meetoo, 2004) in enabling the patient to make decisions. The patient needs information, skills and self-awareness, and needs to know how to access healthcare appropriately.

In the case scenario, Mr Middleton had support from his wife regarding his lifestyle modifications. The added loss and grief that he has experienced may have made these modifications even more difficult for him.

Professional guidance

The National Service Framework for Diabetes (DH, 2001) sets out series of standards relating to the recognition of diabetes and working with people with diabetes, which all healthcare professionals should follow:

- Standards 1 and 2 relate to preventing and identifying diabetes.
- Standard 3 relates to empowering people with diabetes and their carers as decision-makers in order to enable them to have more personal control on a day-to-day basis. This standard recommends patient-held records and patient education.
- Standard 4 refers to the clinical care that people with diabetes should receive in order to optimise quality of life and reduce the risk of long-term complications. A team approach is recommended.
- Standards 5 and 6 relate to the care of children and young people with diabetes.
- Standard 7 relates to the care of acute diabetic emergencies, ensuring prompt recognition and treatment by appropriately trained healthcare professionals.
- Standard 8 relates to caring for people with diabetes in hospital, ensuring consistent and high-quality care.
- Standard 9 relates to diabetes and pregnancy.
- Standards 10, 11 and 12 refer to the detection, minimisation and management of diabetic complications through early detection and effective management. This involves integrated service provision, clear referral systems and specialised secondary care services.

Mr Ronnie Middleton

At Mr Middleton's appointment with the diabetes nurse specialist, the nurse specialist becomes more concerned about his raised HbA_{1c}. She notices that he is still gaining weight but appears generally disinterested in his condition. He admits to feeling depressed most of the time, that he isn't sleeping very well and that he feels tired all the time, but he also says he is hungry and so is eating more. She refers him to his GP, who prescribes fluoxetine, a selective serotonin reuptake inhibitor (SSRI), 20 mg daily in the morning.

THE NATURE OF DEPRESSION

It is thought that at least 20% of the population develop a depressive illness at some point (Shah, 2002). Downie et al. (2003) suggest that the figure is much higher (60-70% of adults), with 1.5% requiring treatment. Depression is a difficult term to define and is complicated by a public lack of understanding. It may convey a range of situations from 'feeling down' or sadness to an underlying pathological condition (Shah, 2002). This may explain why it is also poorly treated. Depression 'involves severe emotional disturbance' (Anon, 2000), for which there may or may not be a contributory factor. Traditionally depression has been described as either endogenous (alternating bouts of mood-lowering and excitation) or reactive (a response to an adverse life event). However, there was a need to acknowledge a range of other types of mood disorder that were not classified easily, and we now describe depression as unipolar (mood swings always in the same direction) or bipolar (alternating depression and mania) (Rang *et al.*, 2003). Since the introduction of the *Diagnostic and Statistical Manual of Mental Disorders* (DSM-IV) criteria (Alexander *et al.*, 2006), diagnosis has been based upon the presence of certain symptoms for a minimum of 2 weeks. Depression may be classified as mild, moderate or severe, depending upon the symptoms.

There are several theories that to try to explain depression related to the following factors:

- *Genetic influences*: There is some evidence that depression 'runs in families', but this is difficult to verify.
- *Early childhood experiences*: Lack of acceptable parental care may be a factor.
- *Age of onset*: Possibly linked to vascular changes in adults over 65 years of age.
- *Social stress and life events*: May results in potential neuroendocrine changes related to the hypothalamic-pituitary-adrenal (HPA) axis.
- *Neurochemical changes*: The 'monoamine deficiency hypothesis' (Shah, 2002).

Pathophysiology

Normally the cells of the brain produce large enough quantities of neurotransmitters to maintain cell-to-cell transmission. The neurotransmitters are constantly reabsorbed by the enzyme monoamine oxidase. According to Prosser *et al.* (2000), depression involves 'disruption of a range of central nervous system monoamine receptors' and modulation of the stress response.

Social stress and life events

Depression can be the outcome of feelings of stress and can also lead to stress. There is a suggestion that psychosocial stress is associated with the HPA axis. The HPA becomes active as a response to chronic stress and may be abnormal in patients with depression. The HPA is under the control of a variety of neurotransmitters, including serotonin, noradrenaline (norepinephrine), acetylcholine and endogeneous opioids. Depletion of noradrenaline and serotonin at the nerve endings in the brain is associated with depression. Monoamine oxidase is an enzyme that enhances the breakdown of noradrenaline and serotonin (Prosser *et al.*, 2000).

Neurochemical changes (the monoamine deficiency hypothesis)

The monoamine theory suggests that depression occurs as a consequence of deficient monoaminergic transmission in the brain – either synaptic underactivity or underactivity of monoamines in the brain (mainly noradrenaline and/or serotonin). Monoamines are thought to be responsible for maintaining mood (discovered as a result of observing the actions of drugs such as tricyclic antidepressants and monoamine oxidase inhibitors on the brain).

PHARMACOLOGICAL INTERVENTIONS USED TO MANAGE DEPRESSION

'Depression is a broad and heterogeneous (having different elements) psychiatric disorder' (Shah, 2002) and 'the treatment and management of depression is a challenge for all healthcare professionals' (Moore and McLaughlin, 2003).

Contemporary approaches to treatment include cognitive behaviour therapy (CBT), a form of conversation therapy that helps to weaken the links between stressful situations and their usual responses to them; behavioural activation, which encourages patients to make changes; counselling; and medicines such as tricyclic antidepressants (e.g. amitriptyline) and selective serotonin reuptake inhibitors (SSRIs, e.g. fluoxetine). Medicines are still an important part of treatment for depression, but there is much debate about their use (Moore and McLaughlin, 2003). Anon (2000) suggests there is an overreliance on drugs, whether prescribed medicines or alcohol.

Fluoxetine

Fluoxetine is an example of an SSRI. This group of antidepressants inhibits the neuronal reuptake of serotonin (5-hydroxytryptamine, 5-HT) by blocking the action of the uptake pump, thus enabling the 5-HT to remain longer in the synaptic cleft, enhancing its action. SSRIs have a more selective action than tricyclic antidepressants, and so have fewer anticholinergic effects (effects upon smooth muscle, secretion of saliva, sweat and digestive juices, and pupil dilation) and cardiotoxic effects. Patients may experience hypersensitivity (e.g. rash) gastrointestinal problems such as nausea and vomiting, headaches, sleep abnormalities, dizziness, fatigue, hallucinations, agitation, urinary problems and sexual dysfunction.

Pharmacodynamics Fluoxetine

Fluoxetine is a selective inhibitor of serotonin reuptake, which probably accounts for its mechanism of action and effects.

Pharmacokinetics Fluoxetine

Absorption: Absorbed rapidly. The bioavailability is not affected by the presence of food.

Distribution: Extensively bound to plasma proteins. Steady-state concentrations are achieved after dosing for several weeks.

Metabolism: Metabolised slowly by the liver; some active metabolites.

Elimination: Excreted mainly (60%) by the kidneys. Elimination is slow – 5-6 weeks after the treatment is discontinued. Also secreted in breast milk.

Dosage should be reviewed after 3-4 weeks and adjusted as necessary. The dose can be increased gradually to 60 mg, but there is a proportional increase in the potential for adverse effects. Treatment should be continued for 6 months in order to ensure that the patient is free from symptoms. The treatment needs to be discontinued gradually, over a period of 1-2 weeks.

Pharmacological knowledge Other medicines

Tricyclic antidepressants are thought to block the reuptake of the neurotransmitters noradrenaline (norepinephrine), 5-HT (serotonin) and dopamine into the presynaptic neuron. This results in an increased amount of the neurotransmitters in the synaptic cleft (where nerve impulses are transmitted from one neuron to another, from presynaptic neuron to postsynaptic neuron).

Monoamine oxidases are a group of enzymes involved in the metabolism of serotonin, noradrenaline, dopamine and adrenaline. They exert their effects at adrenergic and dopaminergic nerve endings. Monoamine oxide inhibitors (MAOIs) used as medicines interfere with the breakdown of the neurotransmitters concerned with mood and so produce an antidepressant effect. MAOIs are used only when other treatments have failed (Wickens, 2005).

Figure 14.1 shows the action of tricyclic antidepressants and MAOIs.

Alcohol

Alcohol is frequently used as support by people trying to cope with stressful and distressing events in their life. Unfortunately, the perceived beneficial effects are temporary and may make the depression worse (Moore and McLaughlin, 2003). Alcohol depresses the central nervous system. It also interacts with many prescribed and OTC medicines. If alcohol is used with medicines that act upon the central nervous system, the effects may be enhanced. There is no evidence that fluoxetine does

Normally brain cells release sufficient quantities of excitatory chemicals (neurotransmitters) to stimulate neighbouring cells. The neurotransmitters are constantly reabsorbed into the brain cells, where they are broken down by an enzyme called monoamine oxidase. In depression fewer neurotransmitters are released. Antidepressant drugs act to raise the levels of neurotransmitters in the brain.

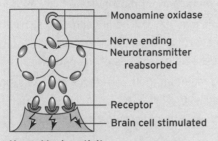

Monoamine oxidase

Nerve ending
Neurotransmitter reabsorbed

Receptor
Brain cell stimulated

Normal brain activity
In a normal brain neurotransmitters are constantly being released, reabsorbed and broken down.

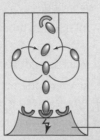

Brain cell poorly stimulated

Brain activity in depression
Fewer neurotransmitters than normal are released, leading to reduced stimulation.

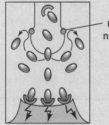

Drug blocks reabsorption of neurotransmitter

Action of tricyclics
Tricyclic drugs increase the levels of neurotransmitters by blocking their reabsorption.

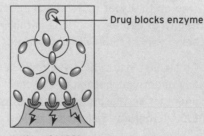

Drug blocks enzyme

Action of MAOIs
MAOIs increase the levels of neurotransmitters by blocking the action of the enzyme (monoamine oxidase) that breaks them down.

Figure 14.1 Action of antidepressants (after BMA, 1992)

interact with alcohol, but the use of alcohol while the patient is taking fluoxetine is not advised (**www.bnf.org**).

Nursing implications

Nursing the patient with depression can be difficult. The symptoms of depression may be subtle. Depression can make the patient feel hopeless and unsupported, and they may have other problems, such as eating disorders.

It is inevitable that the adults nurses come into contact with have more than one health problem. Empowering the patient to take control of their condition is important. This may involve many lifestyle changes, such as diet modification, attending clinics for monitoring, handling their own body fluids such as blood and urine, and complex treatment regimes. This difficult situation can become even more challenging if the patient has a mental health problem such as depression. Nurses are likely to meet patients with both physical and mental health problems wherever they deliver care. It is important, therefore, for nurses to acknowledge the following:

- Some 'difficult' behaviour by the diabetic patient may indicate hypoglycaemia.
- Patients with mental health problems may have difficulty adhering to treatment regimes.
- Nursing assessments should reflect the holistic needs of the patient.
- Nurses must make every attempt to maintain their knowledge and skills, and acknowledge when they need to seek specialist advice.
- Management of chronic diseae requires a multidisciplinary approach.

Mr Ronnie Middleton

At his next apppintment with the diabetes nurse specialist, Mr Middleton appears brighter. It is too soon to assume that this is a result of his treatment, because it can take up to a year to establish effectiveness of his medication, due to the subjective nature of depression. He is not losing any weight, although he is adamant that he is being very careful with his diet.

On his last vist to his GP, Mr Middleton had a range of blood tests taken to eliminate any underlying pathology. On checking these results, it is discovered that he has an underactive thyroid gland (hypothyroidism). He is initially prescibed levothyroxine 100 micrograms daily, to be reviewed in 3 months.

THE NATURE OF HYPOTHYROIDISM

An undersecretion of thyroid hormones (T_3 and T_4) from the thyroid gland leads to a deficiency of these hormones circulating in the body; this condition is known as hypothyroidism. Hypothyroidism is usually a result of a disorder of the thyroid gland itself (primary hypothyroidism), but less commonly it may be a consequence of a disorder of either the pituitary gland or the hypothalamus (secondary hypothyroidism). Primary hypothyroidism primarily affects females. The disorder can affect people at any age, but it is more common in older people. The commonest disorder causing primary hypothyroidism is Hashimoto's thyroiditis, an autoimmune thyroid disease (Boon et al., 2006). The resulting lack of circulating T_3 and T_4 has an impact on most of the metabolic processes in the body. As a result, hypothyrodism presents with a variety of often non-specific signs and symptoms. Frequently, the affected person is not fully aware of how they have changed, as this undersecretion of thyroid hormones tends to happen gradually, with the effects appearing subtly and slowly. The person's changing appearance, thought patterns and mood are often more obvious to their family and friends than to themselves.

Related knowledge Pathophysiology

The thyroid gland has two lobes separated by an isthmus. The gland lies in front of the trachea at the front of the lower part of the neck. It produces thyroid hormones (T_3 and T_4), which control the body's metabolism and consequently its production of energy. These thyroid hormones, which are secreted directly into the bloodstream, are produced when the thyroid gland is stimulated by thyroid-stimulating hormone (TSH). TSH is produced by the anterior pituitary gland when the serum levels of thyroid hormones fall below normal. TSH production is stimulated by thyrotropin-releasing hormone (TRH), which is produced by the hypothalamus.

In primary hypothyroidism autoantibodies are present in the bloodstream, and these cause the thyroid gland to become inflamed (thyroiditis). This inflammation prevents the thyroid gland from secreting thyroxine. This lack of thyroxine eventually causes the body's metabolic rate to slow down, leading to increasing tiredness, lethargy, low body temperature, scaly skin and hair loss. The ability to think and make decisions also declines as thyroxine levels fall. This leads to the classic clinical features of hypothyroidism, which include:

- increasing sluggishness and apathy;
- dry skin;
- thickening of the subcutaneous tissues as a result of oedema;
- puffy eyelids;
- enlarged tongue and lips;
- increasing weakness;
- increasing fatigue and exhaustion;
- always feeling cold;
- weight gain despite poor appetite;
- abnormally low temperature, pulse rate, respiratory rate and blood pressure;
- frequently sleeping in the day and yet always feeling tired;
- slow and dull thinking processes;
- altered menstruation, e.g. menorrhagia or amenorrhoea;
- low or no libido;
- hoarse, monotonous, slow speech;
- constipation;
- increased serum cholesterol levels;
- untreated, the individual eventually becomes comatose.

PHARMACOLOGICAL INTERVENTIONS USED TO MANAGE HYPOTHYROIDISM

Levothyroxine

Levothyroxine is a synthetic form of the thyroid hormone thyroxine, which is normally produced by the thyroid gland. It is most commonly prescribed for patients with hypothyroidism (insufficient thyroid hormone).

Pharmacodynamics Levothyroxine

Levothyroxine mimics the action of thyroxine, which increases the basal metabolic rate as a consequence of increased oxygen consumption and heat production. This has observable effects upon the heart (increase in heart rate) and kidneys (increased output of urine). Other effects include enhanced protein and carbohydrate metabolism, faster protein synthesis and improved gluconeogenesis.

Pharmacokinetics Levothyroxine

Absorption: Variable.

Distribution: Via the plasma, where thyroxine is bound to the plasma proteins (Rang *et al.*, 2003).

Personal and professional development 14.2
Using information

It is important that experienced nurses use information. We introduced the principles of pharmacodynamics and pharmacokinetics in Chapter 4. Using this information, can you draw any conclusions from the information given above?

Nursing implications

Levothyroxine (thyroxine) is prescribed as replacement therapy and controls the symptoms of hypothyroidism to ensure that all of the body's metabolic function is adequate. It is important that Mr Middleton understands two things: he must take his prescribed levothyroxine medication every day, and he must take it for the rest of his life. He should also understand that his condition should be monitored regularly (yearly) by his GP to ensure that he is receiving the correct dosage. This should be part of his health action plan. Regular medication review becomes more important with increasing age, as older people tend to metabolise and excrete drugs less efficiently than younger people and also have a greater likelihood of having diseases of the liver and kidneys, which make metabolism and excretion less effective. This leads to drug levels building up in the plasma, causing toxicity.

It is important that the nurse or doctor undertakes a medication review for Mr Middleton, as he is now on quite a lot of medicines. One particular issue to take note of is the potential interaction between levothyroxine and his antidiabetic medication, specifically insulin, as the dosages may need to be increased (**www.bnf.org**).

Quick reminder

✔ Type 2 diabetes mellitus is a complex disorder that is challenging to manage.

✔ Treatments must be tailored to the individual patient with regard to choice of medicine and delivery system.

✔ Diet and activity changes are the first step in treating the patient with type 2 diabetes.

✔ Type 2 diabetes is treated with oral antidiabetic agents initially.

✔ Insulin may become part of the treatment regime for type 2 diabetes. There are a variety of types of, and delivery systems for, insulin.

✔ The potential for both short- and long-term complications needs to be managed carefully.

✔ Diabetes requires lifestyle changes as well as medications. The patient requires a great deal of support and information.

✔ Depression is a common but poorly understood condition.

✔ There is a range of treatments available for depression, which include medication and nursing interventions.

✔ Hypothyroidism is a condition with a gradual onset, and so it is easily missed by the patient. Relatives may be the first to notice changes.

✔ Working with a patient who has a physical condition and is suffering from mental ill-health is challenging for healthcare professionals

REFERENCES

Alexander M F, Fawcett J N and Runcimann P J (2006) *Nursing Practice: Hospital and Home – The Adult*, 3rd edn. Edinburgh: Churchill Livingstone.

Anon (2000) Understanding depression. **www.pjonline.com/editorial/20000108/comment/depression.html.**

Becker M M (1974) *The Health Belief Model and Personal Health Behavior*. Thorofare, NJ. C B Slack.

Bhattacharyya A (2001) Treatment of type 2 diabetes mellitus. *Hospital Pharmacist* **8**, 10–16.

Boon N A, Colledge N R, Walker B R and Hunter J A A (2006) *Davidson's Principles and Practice of Medicine*, 20th edn. Edinburgh: Churchill Livingstone Elsevier.

Department of Health (2001) *National Service Frameworks for Diabetes: Standards*. London: The Stationery Office.

Diabetes UK (2007) Insulin pill to replace injections? **www.diabetes.org.uk/About_us/News_Landing_Page/Insulin-pill/.**

Dixon N (2002) Antidiabetic agents. *Pharmaceutical Journal* **268**, 538–539.

Downie G, Mackenzie J and Williams A (2003) *Pharmacology and Medicines Management for Nurses*. Edinburgh: Churchill Livingstone.

Gadsby R (2006) Oral hypoglycaemic agents in type 2 diabetes. *Practice Nurse* **32**, 16–18.

Galbraith A, Bullock S, Manias E, Hunt B and Richards A (2007) *Fundamentals of Pharmaology. An Applied Approach for Nursing and Health*, 2nd edn. Harlow: Pearson Education.

Gummerson I (2006) An update on insulin analogues. *Pharmaceutical Journal* **277**, 169–172.

Hand H (2000) The development of diabetic ketoacidosis. *Nursing Standard* **15**, 47–52.

Lowey A (2005) Drug treatment of type 2 diabetes in adults. *Nursing Standard* **20**, 55–64.

Mason P (2002) Diet and diabetes. *Pharmaceutical Journal* **268**, 499–500.

Meetoo D (2004) Clinical skills: empowering people with diabetes to minimise complications. *British Journal of Nursing* **13**, 644–651.

Moore K and McLaughlin D (2003) Depression: the challenge for all health professionals. *Nursing Standard* **17**, 45–52.

National Institute for Health and Clinical Excellence (NICE) (2000) *Clinical Guideline: Obesity – The Prevention, Identification, Assessment and Management of Overweight and Obesity in Adults and Children*. London: National Institute for Health and Clinical Excellence.

National Institute for Health and Clinical Excellence (NICE) (2002) *Full Guidance: Type 2 Diabetes – Management of Blood Glucose*. London: National Institute for Health and Clinical Excellence.

National Institute for Health and Clinical Excellence (NICE) (2006) *Clinical Guideline 43: Obesity – The Prevention, Identification, Assessment and Management of Overweight and Obesity in Adults and Children*. London: National Institute for Health and Clinical Excellence.

National Institute for Health and Clinical Excellence (NICE) (2007) *Final Scope for the Appraisal of Subcutaneous Insulin Infusion for the Treatment of Diabetes (Review)*. London: National Institute for Health and Clinical Excellence.

Palmer R (2004) An overview of diabetic ketoacidosis. *Nursing Standard* **19**, 42–5.

Phillipe M and Whittaker N (2004) in Whittaker N (2004) *Disorder and Intervention*. Basingstoke: Palgrave.

Prosser S, Worster B, MacGregor J, Dewar K, Runyard P and Fegan J (2000) *Applied Pharmacology: An Introduction to Pathophysiology and Drug Management for Nurses and Healthcare Professionals*. London: Mosby.

Rang H P, Dale M M, Ritter J M and Moore P K (2003) *Pharmacology*, 5th edn. Edinburgh: Elsevier.

Shah P J (2002) Aetiology and pathology of clinical depression. *Hospital Pharmacist* **9**, 219–222.

Simonsen T, Aarbakke I K, Coleman I and Sinnott R L (2006) *Illustrated Pharmacology for Nurses*. London: Hodder Arnold.

Vaughan L (2005) Dietary guidelines for the management of diabetes. *Nursing Standard* **19**, 56–64.

Whittaker N (2004) *Disorders and Interventions*. Basingstoke: Palgrave.

Wickens A (2005) *Foundations of Biopsychology*, 2nd edn. Harlow: Pearson Education.

Wiffen P, Mitchell M, Snelling M and Stoner N (2007) *Oxford Handbook of Clinical Pharmacy*. Oxford: Oxford University Press.

Chapter 15

Asthma:
a young man with asthma, eczema and Down's syndrome, who develops pneumonia

This chapter uses the patient scenario of Mr Steven Twedell, a 34-year-old man with asthma who developed community-acquired pneumonia. He also has atopic eczema and Down's syndrome. Asthma is a relatively common chronic disorder that can seriously impair breathing and can have a major impact on the person's lifestyle. Explored in this chapter are some of the medicines that would be used to treat these disorders and the medicines management issues that nurses will have to consider when helping Mr Twedell to manage asthma, eczema and community-acquired pneumonia. These issues include accurate assessment, consent, patient education, non-discriminatory practice and the prevention and management of infection.

✔ Learning outcomes

At the end of this chapter you should be able to:

- ✔ Give an overview of asthma, atopic eczema, community-acquired pneumonia and Down's syndrome
- ✔ Discuss the potential impact of asthma on an individual
- ✔ Identify the pharmacological approaches used to manage asthma, atopic eczema and community-acquired pneumonia
- ✔ Describe how anatomical and physiological differences can have an impact on respiration and inhalation techniques
- ✔ Identify the nursing knowledge needed to help this patient manage his disorders
- ✔ Identify supporting nursing interventions for this patient
- ✔ Discuss some of the legal issues related to people with Down's syndrome who become acutely ill.

Chapter at a glance

Asthma: setting the scene
The nature of Down's syndrome
The nature of asthma
Pharmacological interventions used to manage asthma
The nature of atopic asthma
Pharmacological interventions used to manage atopic eczema
The nature of pneumonia
Pharmacological interventions used to manage community-acquired pneumonia
Consent to treatment
Pharmacological interventions used to manage painful injections
Oxygen therapy
Being acutely ill and having a learning disability
Having a learning disability and accessing healthcare
Quick reminder
References

Mr Steven Twedell

Mr Steven Twedell, a 34-year-old man, has learning disability as a result of Down's syndrome. He was also diagnosed with atopic eczema when he was a young child. By the time Mr Twedell was in his late twenties, his older siblings had left home to start new lives of their own, his father had died following a stroke and his mother had remarried and moved to Portugal with her new husband. Mr Twedell's mother and stepfather had wanted him to move with them, but he didn't want to leave his wider family and friends. As he was unable to care fully for himself, he moved into a flat, where he now lives independently with minimal support. About 2 years ago, Mr Twedell was diagnosed with asthma after having episodes of acute dyspnoea (breathlessness), which became more and more frequent. These episodes seemed to be the result of Mr Twedell becoming attached to a large, very friendly Persian cat that had moved in next door with the new neighbours. The practice nurses, with the help of the community learning disability nurse, contacted by Mr Twedell's GP practice, enabled Mr Twedell to administer his prescribed medication of salmeterol and fluticasone himself using an Accuhaler device. As a result, for the past few months or so, his asthma has been reasonably well controlled using his prescribed asthma medication. Mr Twedell also uses prescribed aqueous cream for topical use daily to manage his atopic eczema.

ASTHMA: SETTING THE SCENE

Many nurses see people with asthma only when patients are hospitalised because of a severe asthma attack. As a result, many nurses believe that asthma is an acute condition. However, this is far from the truth: the majority of people with asthma live in the community, where they manage their asthma. It is only when something goes seriously wrong that some people have their asthma treated as an emergency in hospital. Nurses need to recognise that asthma is actually a chronic condition and that they have an important role to play in helping people with asthma to understand their disorder and how to get the best out of their prescribed medicines so that they can live their lives to the full. This means giving control back to the patient, so helping them to manage their disease rather than it managing them. Only when healthcare professionals fully understand asthma, the medicines used to treat it and the effects of both the disease and the medicines can they help people to self-manage their asthma (Gamble *et al.*, 2007; McDonald and Gibson, 2006; Reddel and Barnes, 2006). Exploring the knowledge and skills related to the medicines used in the scenario in this chapter will help you to do this. This will enable you to meet the healthcare needs of people with asthma and the other disorders featured in this chapter, and will also develop your ability to transfer your knowledge and understanding of the issues raised in this chapter to other situations.

Personal and professional development 15.1 Insight

Write down the first three things that you think of when you think of people with Down's syndrome. Consider what you base these ideas on. Are any of these thoughts judgemental in any way? If they are, use your professional portfolio to plan how you can change your attitudes.

Personal and professional development 15.2 Insight

Write down at least three feelings that you think you might have if you suddenly could not breathe very easily.

THE NATURE OF DOWN'S SYNDROME

Down's syndrome is a genetic disorder that results from an abnormality of one of the chromosomes. Normally, people have 46 chromosomes, however, individuals with Down's syndrome have an additional chromosome. They have three rather than two copies of chromosome 21; this is known as trisomy (derived from *tri* - three – and *soma*

- the body's cells and tissues) 21. The aetiology is unknown, but the risk of having a baby with Down's syndrome is more common in older rather than younger pregnant women. Down's syndrome is by far the most common cause of intellectual disability. Around 60 000 people in the UK are thought to have Down's syndrome (St George's London University and Down's Syndrome Association, 2002). However, it must be remembered that as there are no requirements to keep details of people with Down's syndrome, these figures are, at best, only 'guesstimates'.

People with Down's syndrome have some degree of learning disability, which can vary from very mild to extremely severe. Children and adults with Down's syndrome can often be recognised by some typical distinguishing physical features. Some of these physical features can have a significant effect on breathing, including a flattened nasal bridge, a small oropharynx and nasopharynx, and a large tongue that is inclined to protrude; this limits the amount of airflow into the main bronchus. People with Down's syndrome tend to be mouth-breathers and to produce more mucus than normal. They can also have a number of general health problems, particularly relating to their physical and social environment. Problems may be due to a lack of available and suitable exercise opportunities and the continual grouping together with other people with learning disabilities, which means they frequently 'share' infections. Lack of accessible exercise opportunities will have seriously affected Mr Twedell's cardio-vascular system and respiratory tract efficiency.

People with Down's syndrome also seem to be more prone than the rest of the population to a number of disorders, including:

- thyroid problems;
- poor immune system;
- respiratory problems, chest infections, coughs and colds;
- Alzheimer's type dementia (Martin, 2007; St George's London University and Down's Syndrome Association, 2002).

THE NATURE OF ASTHMA

Asthma is a chronic disorder of a section of the respiratory system. It affects the bronchioles (small, narrow air passages) that funnel air into and out of the alveoli (air sacs) of the lungs. Consequently, it can have a major effect on breathing. In the UK, asthma is a common disease and is becoming increasingly so, in both children and adults. Asthma is not only a problem in the Western world. World Health Organization (WHO) statistics show that, in 2005, 300 million people worldwide had asthma and 225 000 people died as a result of their asthma; the WHO suggests that over the next decade, asthma deaths will increase by 20% (WHO, 2006). Asthma is a much more complicated disorder than was once assumed, as both an element of hypersensitivity (allergy) and a genetic component may be involved. The recognition of this has given rise to a debate in the medical literature (Editorial, 2006; Wenzel, 2006) concerning the various underlying complexities and calls for asthma to be reclassified as a collection of different diseases rather than one distinctive disease.

The effects of asthma vary from person to person. The condition affects some people more severely than others, in the frequency or the intensity of the disorder or both. The main symptoms of asthma are produced by the bronchioles (small airways) being narrowed in some way (bronchoconstriction). This bronchoconstriction is due to constriction of the circular smooth muscle that lines the bronchioles, so making the lumen of the smaller bronchi and bronchioles narrower than usual. The smaller bronchi have irregularly spaced pieces of cartilage, but these do not keep the smaller bronchi as patent as do the C-shaped rings of cartilage in the larger bronchi. The bronchioles do not have any cartilage to keep them patent and so bronchoconstriction can restrict the lumen of the bronchioles considerably. Narrowing of the lumen restricts the space available for air inhalation and exhalation; thus, the usual volume of air cannot be taken into the alveoli for gaseous exchange. Consequently, the body tissues do not get the oxygen that they need in order to maintain bodily functions. As air cannot flow freely in and out of the bronchial tree, there is some degree of airflow obstruction, which can be heard by the nurse and the patient. This sound is known as wheezing. Airflow obstruction results in dyspnoea (difficulty in breathing) and a feeling of tightness in the chest.

Thus, bronchoconstriction produced by the inflammation in the bronchioles results in the classic set of symptoms that make up the disorder known as asthma: dyspnoea, wheezing and chest tightness (Boon *et al.*, 2006; Currie and Douglas, 2007).

The experience of a limited amount of air reaching the lungs, and the increased effort that must be made to try and get more air into and out of the lungs, can cause a number of feelings in the patient, such as concern, fear, alarm, worry, anxiety and panic. These feelings can then cause the person to hyperventilate (overbreathe). This can make the situation worse: breathing is used by the body as a fairly rapidly acting means of removing or retaining acids, and so the more deeply or more quickly the individual breathes, the larger the amount of CO_2 excreted in exhaled air. Losing increasing amounts of CO_2 means that carbonic acid is lost from the body and the blood pH rises (moves towards the alkaline end of the pH scale). Under normal circumstances, the body regulates this changing pH by reducing the amount of CO_2 being excreted. In the short term, the person achieves this by breathing more slowly and more shallowly. If hyperventilation continues, this loss of carbonic acid leads to muscle spasms and fainting. Over longer periods of time, the kidneys, via urine, maintain normal acid-base balance by excreting or reabsorbing acids and bases.

Personal and professional development 15.3
Patient education

Label the unlabelled diagram of the respiratory system below. Write short notes that would help you to explain to Mr Twedell the form and function of the respiratory system and the pathophysiological effects of asthma. Using your understanding of the nature of Down's syndrome, consider the methods and resources that you would use to facilitate Mr Twedell's learning, and list these.

Answers can be found at the back of the book.

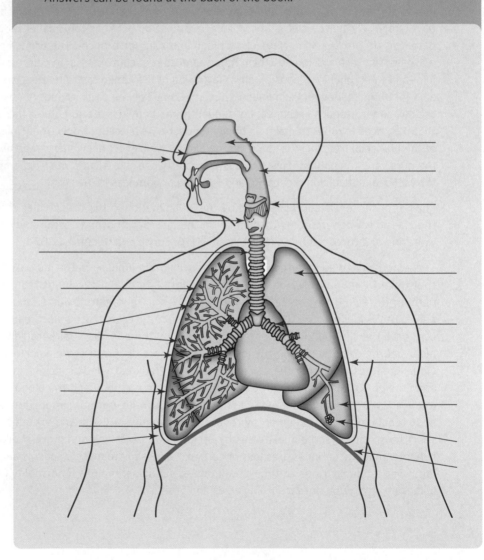

Related knowledge Pathophysiology

The altered physiology that produces the patient's signs and symptoms in asthma are a result of an inflammatory response in the small airways of the respiratory system, particularly in the bronchioles. For many people, this seems to be a response to an allergen. In asthma, the inflammatory response is localised to the smaller bronchi and bronchioles. Here, **antigens** stimulate the production of a number of immunoglobulins (antibodies) as part of the body's defence mechanism.

An asthma attack is caused when an allergen stimulates a **hypersensitivity** (allergic) reaction. The allergen stimulates the B-lymphocytes (plasma cells) to produce immunoglobulin E (IgE), one of the five immunoglobulins produced by the immune system. At the same time, the T-lymphocytes secrete lymphokines and cytokines. This leads to a cascade of reactions from the immune system, including the release of eosinophils, mast cells and macrophages. The IgE antibodies bond to mast cells, thus stimulating the release of histamine. Histamine, eosinophils and macrophages encourage rapid bronchoconstriction (narrowing of the lumen of the small bronchi and bronchioles), causing some degree of airway obstruction. They also stimulate the production of other chemical mediators, namely leukotrienes, thromboxanes and prostaglandins, which all contribute to local cellular changes. These changes in the airway cells also cause the increased production of thick mucus, which causes coughing in order to expel this excess mucus. These changes also cause vasodilation (increased diameter of blood vessels), which leads to oedema (tissue swelling caused by fluid) of the walls of the smaller bronchi and bronchioles. As a result of this oedema, further bronchoconstriction is caused and consequently there is increasing obstruction of the smaller airways (British Thoracic Society and Scottish Intercollegiate Guidelines Network, 2005; Mera, 1997; Phillips *et al.*, 2001; Tortora and Derrickson, 2006).

Figures 15.1 and 15.2 show a normal bronchiole and a bronchiole in asthma, respectively.

Essential terminology

Allergy

The response by the immune system to a substance that is unfamiliar to the body. This initial reactive response by the immune system is known as sensitivity, but in some individuals each time they are exposed to that particular substance they become more and more sensitive until the response becomes disproportionate to the stimulus. They may not realise that their immune system is responding in this way until they are hypersensitive (overly sensitive).

Antigen

Substance that produces an immune response. Antigens that produce an exaggerated (hypersensitivity) response are usually referred to as allergens.

SEE CHAPTER 9

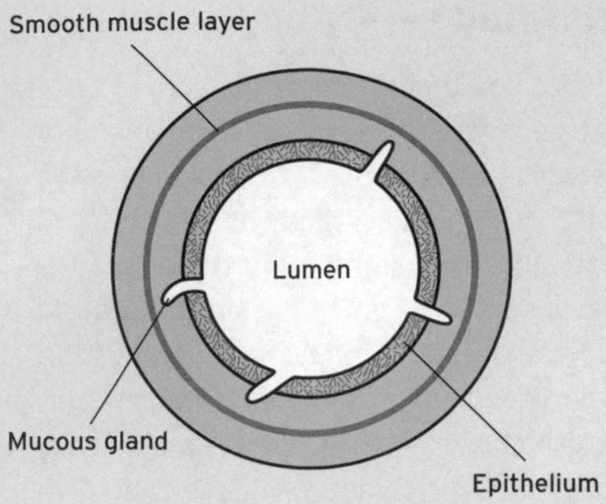

Figure 15.1 Diagram of normal bronchiole

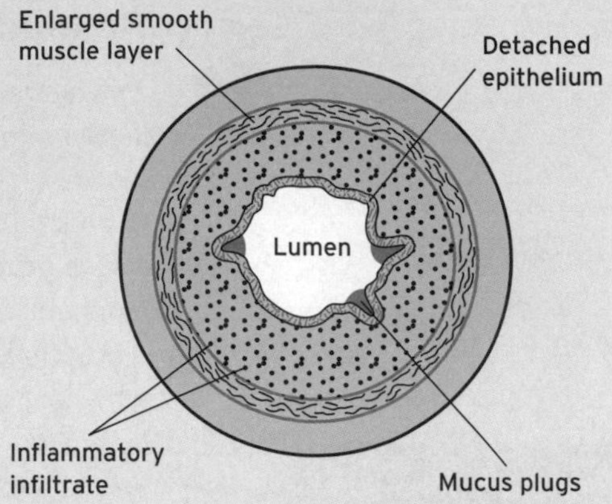

Figure 15.2 Diagram of bronchiole in asthma

The British Thoracic Society (BTS) (2006) has estimated that approximately 15% of adults in the UK have been diagnosed with asthma. Asthma is not always easy to diagnose, because its symptoms are similar to those seen in many other disorders (BTS and SIGN, 2005; Gillissen, 2004). However, cough, wheeze, chest tightness and shortness of breath that is 'variable, intermittent, worse at night, and provoked by triggers including exercise' (BTS and SIGN, 2005) are likely to be the symptoms of asthma. One of the key features of asthma is its variability (Gillissen, 2004), with the symptoms fluctuating within and between individuals. However, the one sign that is always present is of inflammation of the bronchi and bronchioles, and it is this that leads to the increased reactivity to particular triggers and that produces the symptoms of dyspnoea, wheezing and chest tightness. The reason for this inflammation is still not known, and it is not fully understood why the inflammatory response is triggered in some people and not others or why, even when it is triggered, some people develop asthma and some do not.

A number of factors can lead to an asthma attack. Much of the evidence regarding asthma is anecdotal, but more and more studies are being designed to explore these factors in relation to asthma. Asthma triggers can vary between individuals. Some people react to one trigger, while others react to a combination of a number of triggers. These triggers include:

- allergens, such as house dust mites, pet hairs, some foods (e.g. eggs, dairy produce, food colourings) and pollens (there is little reliable and valid evidence to support this yet);
- tobacco smoke (some studies suggest a possible link between smoking in mothers and wheezing in infants);
- air pollution;

- some medicines (e.g. aspirin);
- exercise;
- stress (BTS and SIGN, 2005).

Diagnosing and monitoring asthma

It is difficult to assess whether a patient's asthma is unstable or deteriorating. One useful method for both patients and staff is peak expiratory flow (PEF) rate measurement and recording. The PEF rate is also frequently referred to as peak flow. Measuring and recording of the PEF rate is helpful to the patient and the professionals involved in their care and management, as the PEF rate readings are an objective measurement of the speed that the patient is able to exhale and thus how their lungs are performing. It is also possible to monitor the effect of a particular medication strategy by measuring the PEF rate following medication. To measure the PEF, the patient inhales (breathes in); after putting their mouth around the tube attached to the respirometer, they exhale (breathe out) for as long as they possibly can. The machines that measure PEF rate are usually small enough to be used at home, although Mr Twedell has not yet been taught to monitor his symptoms in this way.

Another means of measuring the capacity of the lungs is by measuring the forced expiratory volume (FEV). The patient is asked to inhale as deeply as possible and then to forcibly exhale (breathe out as hard as they can) into a machine that measures the speed and force of the exhaled breath (expiration). The needle on the gauge indicates the volume of air exhaled, expressed in litres per minute (l/min). This reading is then recorded on a chart; following subsequent recordings, the results are shown as a graph. In health, the PEF and FEV rate vary with gender and age. Men often have larger lungs and are stronger than women and so can exhale with greater force and speed than many women; therefore, PEF rate measurements in men are generally higher than in women. Young adults have greater PEF rates than children, but with increasing age the PEF rate measurements generally decline again. The PEF rate is also affected by certain behaviours, such as smoking, as well as in asthma and obstructive airways disease (COPD).

Living with asthma

A report from Asthma UK (2007) draws attention to the fact that, for many people in England, their asthma is not well managed. This is distressing both for the individual and their family. This report estimates that inefficient management of asthma costs the NHS in England £43.7 million a year. The report also notes that some geographical areas of England have much more effective treatment and management of asthma compared with other areas of the country; for example, people with asthma in the north of England are much more likely to be admitted to hospital than those living in the south.

The NHS Improvement Plan (DH, 2004) and the chronic disease management programme (DH, 2001, 2004) recognise that increasing numbers of people are living with chronic diseases. In publishing these guidelines, the DH aims to improve the care that people with long-term conditions, such as asthma, receive from the NHS. The key suggestion is that healthcare professionals need to change their philosophy and implement patient-focused care that is proactive and, for the most part, takes place in primary care (community-based) settings rather than relying on the traditional approach, which is rooted in secondary care (hospital-based) settings and as a result is reactive. To encourage this philosophy, general practitioners are now paid to manage such patients more effectively and to institute a regular system to review their registered patients who have asthma. Many nurses working in primary care as practice nurses specialise in asthma care. The aim of this is two-pronged: first, so that they can help individuals diagnosed with asthma to understand and effectively manage their asthma; and second, to ensure that GPs meet the targets in the Quality Outcomes Framework (QOF) standard by which they all are paid.

People who have asthma exacerbations (episodes of deterioration) may die, needlessly, as a result. In order to help healthcare professionals recognise the degrees of seriousness of a particular asthma exacerbation, such episodes have been classified according to their level of significance (BTS and SIGN, 2008). This classification recognises five levels of seriousness Table 15.1.

Table 15.1 The five levels of severity of acute asthma exacerbations

Near-fatal Asthma	**Raised $PaCO_2$ and/or requiring mechanical ventilation with raised inflation pressures**
Life threatening asthma	Any one of the following in a patient with severe asthma: - PEF <33% best or predicted - bradycardia - SpO_2 <92% - arrhythmia - PaO_2 <8 kPa - hypotension - normal $PaCO_2$ (4.6 - 6.0 kPa) - exhaustion - silent chest - confusion - cyanosis - coma - feeble respiratory effort
Acute severe asthma	Any one of: - PEF 33-50% best or predicted - respiratory rate ≥ 25/min - heart rate ≥ 110/min - inability to complete sentences in one breath
Moderate asthma exacerbation	- increasing symptoms - PEF > 50-75% best or predicted - no features of acute severe asthma
Brittle asthma	- Type 1: wide PEF variability (>40% diurnal variation for >50% of the time over a period >150 days) despite intense therapy - Type 2: sudden severe attacks on a background of apparently well controlled asthma
(BTS and SIGN, 2008)	

PHARMACOLOGICAL INTERVENTIONS USED TO MANAGE ASTHMA

The medicines that are commonly used to manage asthma are often divided into two groups: those that prevent an asthma attack from starting (preventers) and those that relieve an attack if an attack begins (relievers) (**www.bnf.org**; BTS and SIGN, 2007; Medicines and Healthcare Products Regulatory Agency, 2007; National Institute for Health and Clinical Excellence, 2007). Much information available to both the public and healthcare professionals is categorised in this manner, including that from NHS Direct, Asthma UK and **www.bbc.co.uk**. Using such a classification system is useful to patients and healthcare professionals in helping them to understand when and how medicines can be used to keep asthma under control. Mr Twedell has been using an Accuhaler 50/100 μg device to help manage his asthma symptoms. This device provides 50 μg of salmeterol combined with 100 μg of fluticasone propionate in each dose provided by the inhaler device so is in essence a preventer. Mr Twedell found the education from the healthcare professionals and the short video demonstration of how to use an Accuhaler to be very useful (**http://medguides.medicines.org.uk/ai/ai.aspx?id=AI1007&name=Seretide&use=Asthma**).

Inhalation

Using the body's innate ability to inhale air is a very useful means of delivering medication. It takes advantage of the body's natural way of taking in air to deliver a particular drug in an aerosol form deep into the respiratory tract. Once in the small airways, the inhaled drug diffuses out of the air almost directly into the capillaries surrounding the alveoli without having to be absorbed first by the gastrointestinal tract. Inhaled bronchodilators act on the smooth muscle in the bronchioles and the smaller bronchi to reduce constriction of this smooth muscle. Inhaled corticosteroids reduce the inflammatory process in these small airways, so reducing oedema and the quantity and viscosity of mucus production (Greenstein and Gould, 2004; Rang *et al.*, 2003; Simonsen *et al.*, 2006). This route of administration has a great advantage over medicines taken orally, as the drug is absorbed extremely quickly and thus its effects are exerted quickly. As the difficulty in breathing is caused by bronchoconstriction, the drugs of choice for asthma are those that cause the bronchioles to dilate; these are known as bronchodilators. When a bronchodilator is inhaled, the smooth muscle lining the bronchi and bronchioles and the bronchial mucosa feel the effects very quickly. Using an inhaler means that there are a fairly small number of systemic adverse effects, as generally only very small amounts of the drug are swallowed and absorbed.

There are some disadvantages to this mode of delivery, although they may appear to be fairly minor compared with the almost immediate benefits that can result in medicines being administered in the inhaled form. These disadvantages include the following:

- In order to obtain maximum benefit, the correct technique must be used. It is suggested that 30% of adults have some difficulty using aerosol inhalers (Downie *et al.*, 2003).

- Even if the patient has an extremely efficient technique, only a small percentage of the drug actually goes into the lungs. (Inhaled medicines are designed with this in mind, however, and so although the dose delivered to the bronchioles is small compared with the dose of the same medicine administered orally, it is sufficient to produce the desired effects.) Most of the dose (almost 70%) is lost to the atmosphere and into the inhaler, while a fifth of the dose is lost in the air that is exhaled. A small percentage of the dose lands in the mouth, particularly in the nasopharynx (back of the throat) and on the tongue (Downie *et al.*, 2003; Rang *et al.*, 2003; Simonsen *et al.*, 2006).

Types of inhalation devices

There are a number of ways that inhaled medicines can be delivered to the lungs. Many people are familiar with the handheld inhaler, as this type of device is used most commonly today. This device is a metered dose aerosol inhaler (MDI).

Metered dose inhaler (MDI)

The metered dose inhaler consists of two parts: a small, usually plastic mechanism, and a small pressurised cylinder of medicine that is inserted into the inhaler mechanism. This pressurised canister contains the bronchodilator, which is mixed with an inert propellant gas under pressure so that the contents of the container can be sprayed into the mouth and nasopharynx. Usually, the patient presses a button to activate the device after inserting the MDI into the mouth and making a firm seal around the mouthpiece with the lips. The device is activated and the person inhales normally, which draws aerosols (droplets) into the respiratory system. Coordination between activating the inhaler device and normal inhalation is vital in order to ensure successful delivery of the drug into the smaller airways. Learning to use an MDI has some common principles:

1. The patient may use one or both hands, depending on what they find most comfortable.

2. Remove the protective cap and shake the device well.

3. Breathe out normally and then place the mouthpiece into the mouth and seal the lips around it.

4. At the same time as breathing in through the mouth, press the activating button to release the spray of medication. (The seal around the mouthpiece is inadequate if aerosols are seen escaping from the mouth at this point.)

5. Hold the breath while removing the inhaler from the mouth and for as long as is comfortable afterwards.

6. Breathe out slowly.

7. If further puffs of the inhaler are prescribed, keep the inhaler upright and repeat the process any time after 30 seconds or 1 minute.

▲

Personal and professional development 15.4

Consider the different anatomical features that people with Down's syndrome have. List the problems that these features may cause for Mr Twedell when he learns to use an inhaler device.

Spacer devices

The British Thoracic Society and Scottish Intercollegiate Guidelines Network (BTS and SIGN, 2007) recommend using a spacer device (e.g. Nebuhaler® or Volumatic®) in the treatment of acute asthma. However, Currie and Douglas (2007) qualify this by pointing out that it is important that a spacer device is used correctly. When a spacer is used correctly, then it is as effective as any other device for administering inhaled drugs. A spacer device is particularly useful for people who have difficulty in using an MDI effectively to manage their symptoms. These difficulties are usually a result of poor inhalation technique, as the synchronisation of inhaling and triggering the MDI is crucial in delivering the drug into the lungs. A spacer device works by providing a space between the mouth and the MDI and reduces the speed and the force of the aerosol as it hits the back of the nasopharynx. A spacer allows the propellant used in the MDI more time to evaporate.

Designs differ slightly, but a spacer device is basically a large empty reservoir, usually made of plastic or metal. Many spacers have a one-way valve. Each device has a mouthpiece at one end and an aperture at the other end into which the MDI is inserted, after removing the cap from the mouthpiece of the MDI. With the MDI attached to the spacer device, the patient puts the device into their mouth, seals their lips around the device's mouthpiece and then activates the MDI. The mist of vaporised drug is then released into the reservoir of the spacer device and the patient breathes normally, inhaling the contents of the reservoir. The delay between the patient activating the MDI and inhaling the contents of the spacer device should be kept to a minimum; Rees and Kannabar (2007) suggest that this should be no more than 30 seconds.

As well as helping people who have difficulty in coordinating inhalation and triggering the MDI, spacers help other people manage their medication more effectively. It is recommended that spacers are also used by children and other patients who:

- require higher doses of medication;
- have nocturnal asthma (drowsiness can inhibit the usual technique);
- have repeated episodes of candidiasis due to inhaled corticosteroids (**www.bnf.org**; Greenstein and Gould, 2004; Rang *et al.*, 2003).

Like any other piece of medical equipment, spacers should be kept clean. Patients should be advised to wash their spacer device once a week in warm soapy water, and then to rinse and dry it well.

Spacer devices are extremely effective for many people, but not all patients are able to use them successfully. Although coordinating breathing with activating the spray is not quite so crucial in spacer devices as in MDIs, there is only a short delay between the two actions - no more than 30 seconds (Rees and Kannabar, 2007). Other reasons for patients being unable to use a spacer include limb or hand paresis or paralysis and altered anatomical features.

The differences in Mr Twedell's airway anatomy, due to Down's syndrome, mean that he may be unable to use an inhaler effectively. He does not have as much free space in his nasopharynx compared with people without Down's symdrome, and as a consequence he is likely to breathe through his mouth rather than his nose. Also, his tongue protrudes further into his oral cavity and he produces much more saliva than is usual. Together these features make it difficult for Mr Twedell to inhale the aerosol spray from an MDI or an MDI and a spacer device effectively (**www.dsmig.org.uk/library/articles/transcript-doull.pdf**). Mr Twedell's intellectual disability may mean that it would take him longer than average to learn to use an MDI, with or without a spacer device.

Dry powder inhalers

Mr Twedell may have had to try several different types of inhaler before one was found that suited his abilities and needs. His altered anatomical features increase the likelihood of limited success when using an inhaler. The type of inhaler that has proved to be most effective for Mr Twedell is a dry powder, or breath-actuated, inhaler.

The Accuhaler® is available for use with a variety of different drugs for inhalation. This dry powder inhaler (DPI) is a handheld inhaler that contains the medicine in capsule (fine powder form). The mouthpiece is inserted into the user's mouth and actuated by the person when they inhale. The advantage of this type of inhaler, as Mr Twedell has found, is that the mouthpiece is smaller and no coordination between activating the device and normal inhalation is required. The user primes the device, breathes out as deeply as possible, puts the mouthpiece into their mouth and then breathes in quickly and deeply, using only the mouth, through the device. A click is usually heard when the device actuates, so that the patient knows that the device has been activated.

This type of inhaler device is not useful if the patient's breathing is deteriorating. At times such as these, a nebuliser may be used with an MDI.

Nebulisers

Nebulisation works on the principle that liquid can be broken down into lots of smaller parts. You can see this in action by running water through a tap and putting your finger partially over the outlet; the flow of water changes from a stream to a spray, often with many different sizes of droplets of water. You can manipulate these droplet sizes by how much or how little your finger occludes the tap outlet. When drugs are dissolved in a solution to be nebulised, the nebuliser aims to break down the fluid into smaller liquid particle sizes for inhalation. These particles are usually so small that they cannot be seen by the naked eye.

In this situation, a nebuliser is a medical device that enables a liquid form of a particular drug to be used as an inhalation. Higher doses of drugs are generated by a nebuliser than can be achieved by an MDI. Nebulisers are usually used only as last-resort treatment and in emergency situations when higher doses are required. They use either a small powered compressor or compressed gas (usually air or oxygen) or ultrasound to break down the medicinal fluid into very small particles or aerosols that can be inhaled. The compressed gas used to drive the nebuliser has to be prescribed along with the drug to be nebulised. As in any situation requiring the use of oxygen, it is imperative that patients who rely on a hypoxic drive to stimulate breathing are never given nebulised drugs using oxygen, as this will compromise their breathing by reducing their stimulus to breathe. Only a small percentage (about 10%) of the nebulised spray produced is actually inhaled (O'Callaghan and Barry, 1997); another 10% is swallowed, and the rest of the spray is vented to the outside air through the sides of the facemask. The particle size of nebulised drugs is extremely small and the spray produced is invisible to the naked eye. If a fine mist can be seen in the facemask or venting out of the sides, then the nebuliser is not working correctly. The length of time it takes for the nebulised solution to be administered depends on the type of nebuliser used, but the Asthma Society recommends up to 15 minutes.

Related knowledge Legal issue

Although the principles underpinning the design of all nebulisers are similar, different nebulisers are made by a number of manufacturers and do not operate in an identical way. As with all medical devices, the operator must know how to use the equipment and how to clean and maintain it. Nurses are bound by legal and ethical codes and must read and understand the operating, cleaning and maintenance instructions and undergo any required training before using a nebuliser. The nurse's responsibilities in relation to medicines management also mean that when a patient is to be discharged home with a piece of equipment that assists in delivering their medicine regime, such as a nebuliser, then the patient or carer must be able to use, clean and maintain it safely and effectively.

Nursing knowledge Nursing implications

In order to maximise inhalation of the nebulised particles, the patient should be assisted to sit upright, either in a chair or in bed, to maximise their lung capacity and to reduce the effort of breathing. Individuals with deteriorating severe asthma have to make great efforts to breathe, which uses up large

▶

▶ *(continued)*

amounts of energy. Being dyspnoeic means that the patient cannot replace that energy, and so they quickly become exhausted. As a result, the patient must be assisted in order to make their breathing as effortless as possible; good positioning is fundamental in this. It is important to remember, however, that if the individual finds an upright position distressing or uncomfortable, then they should be helped into their preferred position, as this will cause less distress and so require less effort to breathe.

O'Callaghan and Barry (1997) and the BTS and SIGN (2005) guidelines state that individuals with asthma should rarely need to use a nebuliser at home, as an MDI and spacer, if used correctly, is equally effective. If the patient is to be discharged from hospital with a nebuliser to use at home, then they must be helped to understand how to use it before they leave the ward.

Related knowledge Patient education

In order to use a metered dose inhaler correctly, the patient needs to follow the instructions carefully and develop an efficient technique. Placebo inhalers and manufacturers' guidelines are available to facilitate this process. As with many skills, it takes practice to perfect the inhalation technique; having a realistic timescale helps many people. It must be remembered that if the patient is using the inhaler to relieve an episode of acute breathlessness, then the patient is likely to have some degree of anxiety, which may affect their ability to use the inhaler. This is particularly likely in the early days after diagnosis, when the patient is still developing their technique. When teaching the patient to use an inhaler, observation and then supervised practice are required. This gives the patient an opportunity to see how to carry out the skill and then have someone guide them through the process.

Written instructions are useful so that the patient can refer to these at a later stage. Thought must be given to providing information in a format that is suitable for the individual. Some people cannot read very well or at all, some people have visual impairment and some people cannot understand certain written information either because they have intellectual impairment or do not understand the particular language being used. Likewise, people who are hearing-impaired may not hear what the nurse says or be able to lip-read. The nurse may need to consider presenting information in a different language, using simpler terminology, using a reader-friendly font and background, using photographs or video clips, using a T-loop, lip speaker or sign language, and sending email or text messages to the patient.

It is useful to check at regular future dates that the patient is still using the correct technique. Some patients find that a written management action plan helps them maintain an effective technique and assists them to learn to live with their asthma in the long term (BTS and SIGN, 2005; Gibson *et al.*, 2003; Haughey *et al.*, 2004).

Step approach

The pharmacological management and the resulting BTS and SIGN (2005) guidelines that are produced use a step approach (see Figure 15.3). This means that either the strength or the dosage of the patient's medications may be increased when needed and decreased when the patient improves. How and when the patient moves up and down the steps depends on how well their asthma is controlled and how severe their new symptoms are. Medication is increased until the patient's symptoms subside, and then the medication is reduced slowly. This reduction in the patient's medication must be sufficient to ensure that control of the patient's symptoms is maintained.

Step 3: Add-on therapy
1. Add inhaled long-acting β_2 agonist (LABA)
2. Assess control of asthma:
    - Good response to LABA – continue LABA
    - Benefit from LABA but control still inadequate – continue LABA and increase inhaled steroid dose to 800 μg/day* (if not already on this dose)

Step 2: Regular preventer therapy
Add inhaled steroid 200–800 μg/day*
400 μg is an appropriate starting dose for many patients
Start at dose of inhaled steroid appropriate to severity of disease

Step 1: Mild intermittent asthma
Inhaled short-acting β_2 agonist as required

* BDP, beclomethasone dipropionate.

Figure 15.3 Step management plan for asthma (after BTS and SIGN, 2005)

Salmeterol

Salmeterol is one of a group of medicines known as the selective bronchodilators, which open up the lumen of the smaller airways. Bronchodilation is widening of the lumen of the airways. These medicines open up the airways that are narrowed as a result of obstruction, so letting more air into the lungs on inspiration and more air out of the lungs on expiration. Depending on whether the selective bronchodilator in question is long-acting or short-acting, they can act as relievers or preventers. Salmeterol is prescribed for Mr Twedell because it is a beta-2 (β_2) agonist, one of the long-acting forms of the selective bronchodilators.

Pharmacodynamics β_2 agonists

The nervous system uses neurotransmitters to aid the transmission of nerve impulses between neurons (nerve cells) and between neurons and non-neural cells such as muscles and glands. These neurotransmitters are found in the synapses (specialised junctions), where they ensure that information is passed around the nervous system and distributed to the body's organs, in a similar way to electricity being passed around the wires in a house when the electrical equipment is switched on and off as needed. The β_2 agonists, which include salmeterol, salbutamol and terbutaline, capitalise on the way that two of these neurotransmitters, adrenaline and noradrenaline, function at the synapses of the autonomic nervous system. These neurotransmitters use two main types of adrenergic receptors; α (alpha) and β (beta). Both of these receptors are found in glands (e.g. salivary glands, lachrymal glands), cardiac muscle and smooth muscle. These β_2 bronchodilator medicines have been designed to bind selectively to only the β_2 receptors that are in the smooth muscle of the airways. Once the drug has bound to the β_2 receptors, a complicated chain of events is set in motion, which results in the smooth muscle that lines the bronchioles relaxing, leading to bronchodilation.

Although the β_2 agonist bronchodilator medicines are intended to bind selectively to the β_2 receptors in the lungs, unfortunately no available β_2 agonists are entirely selective. As a result, these drugs can bind to the sympathetic receptors in other organs, which may lead to unwanted effects, such as:

- *Heart*: Tachycardia (fast heart rate) or arrhythmia (disturbance of the heart's rhythm).
- *Skeletal muscle*: Muscle cramps and tremor (**www.bnf.org**; Downie *et al.*, 2003; Greenstein and Gould, 2004; Rang *et al.*, 2003; Simonsen *et al.*, 2006).

Salmeterol and formoterol (the other most commonly prescribed selective bronchodilator) are used for the longer-term relief of bronchospasm. They begin to work about 15-30 minutes after inhalation and are effective for up to 12 hours. Their slower onset of action and the length of time that they are effective for means that these medicines are not suitable for treating acute bronchospasm. Instead, these medicines are helpful in preventing acute exacerbations of bronchospasm and so are called preventers. Using salmeterol or formoterol means that Mr Twedell is unlikely to need to use inhalation of the short-acting β_2 agonists such as salbutamol throughout the day or at night (Tee *et al.*, 2007). This is useful for people who find it difficult to use an inhaler device because of physical difficulties (e.g. after a stroke), inability to coordinate breathing and actuation, inability to understand and follow the instructions, or, as in Mr Twedell's case, certain anatomical features making inhalation ineffective.

Pharmacokinetics Salmeterol

Absorption: Inhaled salmeterol acts locally in the lungs and so very low levels are likely to be absorbed into the plasma (**www.emc.medicines.org.uk**; Rang *et al.*, 2003).

Related knowledge Pharmacology

The inhaled β_2 agonists are available in short-acting and long-acting forms. The most common short-acting β_2 agonists are salbutamol and terbutaline. These are both used for the rapid relief of the acute symptoms of severe asthma. They begin to work within a few minutes of inhalation and are effective for 4–6 hours. The rapid onset of action of these medicines means that they are used to manage acute episodes of bronchospasm, and therefore they are known as relievers.

The short-acting β_2 agonist salbutamol is also available in oral form, both as a sustained-release form and as a syrup. If Mr Twedell were unable to use any type of inhalation device, his prescriber might consider prescribing one of these oral forms for him instead. However, because they are taken orally, these medicines take time to be absorbed, are less effective and, because high doses are needed, have a much higher incidence of adverse effects than the inhaled forms (**www.bnf.org**; Rang *et al.*, 2003).

Nursing knowledge Nursing implications

Noting that a patient is using inhaled short-acting β_2 agonists such as salbutamol or terbutaline almost continuously should ring alarm bells. This suggests that the inhaler is not effective in treating their symptoms. In such situations, it is likely that the individual has severe bronchoconstriction that needs further investigation and a different prescription. The patient needs urgent medical advice.

Although the β_2 agonists increase bronchodilation, they have little effect on the inflammatory process. In order to treat the localised inflammation in the bronchioles, the BTS and SIGN (2005) guidelines recommend that longer-acting β_2 agonists are used twice daily as prophylaxis (treatment to prevent disease) and in conjunction with an inhaled corticosteroid (step 3 in the step approach management plan shown in Figure 15.3). In his Accuhaler, Mr Twedell is using salmeterol dispensed with fluticasone, an inhaled corticosteroid.

Fluticasone

When fluticasone is given by inhalation, as it is using an Accuhaler, it has a local effect in the lungs on the small airways. Fluticasone is one of a group of glucocorticoids (corticosteroids) that are used commonly in asthma; other drugs in this group are budesonide and beclomethasone. The drugs exert an anti-inflammatory effect, resulting in a marked reduction in small airway obstruction due to localised oedema and increased and more viscous mucus. Using corticosteroids in this way helps to prevent an asthma attack, and so the Accuhaler is being used as a preventer. In severe acute attacks of asthma, glucocorticoids are administered to relieve inflammation, and so they can be viewed as both relievers and preventers, depending on the situation.

Pharmacodynamics Fluticasone

Fluticasone and the rest of the glucocorticoids inhibit the cascade of inflammatory mediators, such as leukotrienes and prostaglandins, which are released in response to cellular trauma. As a result, inflammatory changes are prevented from taking place in the bronchioles. The glucocorticoids are thought to work by changing gene transcription in the cell (Simonsen et al., 2006). Glucocorticoids also increase vasodilation and decrease the venous permeability that leads to oedema. The obstruction of smaller airways by increased production and viscosity of mucus is prevented, so allowing air to be inhaled and exhaled freely.

Pharmacokinetics Fluticasone

Distribution: Fluticasone is highly bound to plasma proteins.

Metabolism: Metabolised by the cytochrome P450 enzyme system in the liver.

Elimination: Most of the dose is excreted in the faeces, with a negligible amount being excreted in the urine (**www.emc.medicines.org.uk**; Rang et al., 2003).

Compared with the doses of glucocorticoids given when these drugs are used orally, the inhalation dose is very small and consequently the systemic (widespread throughout the body) effects are much less common. When such effects do occur, tend to be seen in individuals who regularly take high doses of corticosteroids, when they may include glaucoma, cataracts, reduced bone mineral density and adrenal suppression (**www.bnf.org**; **www.emc.medicines.org.uk**; Downie *et al.*, 2003; Greenstein and Gould, 2004; Rang *et al.*, 2003; Simonsen *et al.*, 2006).

The most common adverse effect, candidiasis or oral thrush, is a local effect as a result of the repeated fallout of the glucocorticoid on to the mucosa of the upper respiratory tract. This adverse effect may be preventable. When the patient first begins to use inhaled steroids, the nurse should advise them to wash their mouth and teeth after using the inhaler. Water is adequate for this, but some people may prefer to use a mouthwash or even a hot cup of tea. This advice would be best incorporated into Mr Twedell's asthma self-management plan. Simonsen *et al.* (2006) suggest that a large amount (75-90%) of the inhaled dose of glucocorticoids falls on the mucosa of the oropharynx and nasopharynx. Inhalation of this fallout of inhaled fluticasone results in some systemic absorption of the drug, but this varies between individuals; the manufacturer of the Accuhaler estimates systemic absorption to be 10-30% in healthy subjects (**www.emc.medicines.org.uk**). Some of the aerosols may also be swallowed, which increases systematic absorption of the drug.

> ### Personal and professional development 15.5
>
> One of the drugs in the inhaled medicine used by Mr Twedell to control his asthma is a corticosteroid, fluticasone. Identify the potential adverse effects that may result from some of this drug persistently landing on his tongue and nasopharynx. Write short notes about what the related nursing implications will be.

Self-management action plans

These written plans aim to help people with asthma recognise the early symptoms of deteriorating asthma so that they can treat it at an early stage. This prevents further deterioration, so reducing the need for emergency treatment or hospitalisation for severe or life-threatening asthma. The action plan has a number of features and can take a variety of formats depending on the needs of the patient, but it should include the following:

- Description of the maintenance medication that the person uses regularly when feeling well. This should include the name, dose, form and timing of medicine.
- How to recognise and manage early symptoms of mild airway deterioration:
  - Recognising common symptoms and increasing medication appropriately
  - How long to keep taking the increased medication
  - When help is needed and how to access help

- How to recognise and manage the early symptoms of severe airway deterioration:
  - Recognising common symptoms and increasing medication appropriately
  - How long to keep taking the increased medication.
  - When help is needed and how to access help.

Mr Twedell will be used to using a health action plan (DH, 2001). One will have been drawn up for him by the community learning disability nurse to help him use all of his medicines, including his inhaler, correctly. A written asthma management plan is an extension of this and will aid him in the future if he has another acute exacerbation.

Concordance issue with inhaled steroids

It is well known that many individuals do not adhere to their prescribed medication, with the reasons given for non-concordance being many (Vermeire *et al.*, 2001). A study exploring non-concordance in a group of people with difficult-to-treat asthma who were prescribed steroid inhalers highlights the fear of side effects (Gamble *et al.*, 2007). This was the main reason given for not using the medication as prescribed. This was a qualitative study, and so the sample used was small; this means that the results cannot be generalised but they do provide some rich data reflecting the values and beliefs of this sample of people. This study reinforces the other available evidence from a variety of studies exploring concordance and adherence in a multiplicity of disorders, which find that many people will not use medication because of a fear of adverse effects.

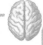

Pharmacological knowledge Other medicines used to treat asthma

A number of other medicines and groups of medicines may be prescribed to treat asthma:

Theophylline

Theophylline is recommended to be used in step 4 of the BTS and SIGN (2005) asthma management. A slow-release form of theophylline is available that can be used by patients with nocturnal (night-time) asthma. In deteriorating severe asthma in people who do not usually take theophylline, it can be administered intravenously; the drug is then known as aminophylline, as it is combined with another drug (ethylenediamine) to speed its rate of absorption. Aminophylline is given by very slow intravenous injection, usually over at least 20 minutes. This caution is because the half-life of theophylline varies considerably between individuals and it has a very narrow therapeutic range. As a result, life-threatening adverse effects such as arrhythmias can occur before any other signs of toxicity are noticeable (**www.bnf.org.uk** Rang *et al.*, 2003).

Ipratropium bromide

Ipratropium and tiotropium are antimuscarinic bronchodilators. They prevent receptors in the circular smooth muscle cells in the bronchioles from moving acetylcholine into these cells, which leads to bronchodilation. These drugs are reserved for use by inhalation in patients with acute asthma who do not respond well to the other regimes in step 4 of the BTS and SIGN (2007) guidelines or whose asthma is life-threatening. They can be given intravenously as part of the emergency treatment for severe life-threatening asthma (**www.bnf.org**; Rang *et al.*, 2003; Simonsen *et al.*, 2006).

Leukotriene antagonists

Leukotrienes are chemical mediators produced in the body's inflammatory response to disease, trauma or infection. They are produced in the lipoxygenase pathway as a response to cellular damage and induce contraction of smooth muscle. In asthma, this causes bronchoconstriction, vasoconstriction and increased vascular permeability and is chemotactic (causing cell movement). The leukotriene antagonists block the cell receptors to which leukotrienes are aiming to bind, and as a result the effects of the leukotrienes are reduced. To treat the inflammatory response in asthma, the oral leukotriene receptor antagonists montelucast or zafirlukast may be prescribed. These drugs are for the long-term prevention of asthma rather than the relief of symptoms, as they take some time to produce an effect (**www.bnf.org**; Downie *et al.*, 2003; Simonsen *et al.*, 2006).

Mr Steven Twedell

Mr Twedell has had atopic eczema almost all of his life. It has been controlled well since puberty, as long as he keeps his skin well moisturised and does not use highly perfumed products on his skin or on clothes that touch his skin. He uses aqueous cream that is prescribed for him.

THE NATURE OF ATOPIC ECZEMA

Atopic eczema is an inflammatory disorder of the skin that affects the epidermis. It is strongly associated with the other atopic disorders of hayfever and asthma. Atopic eczema usually begins in infancy and is recognised by severe itching and excoriation that results from scratching. Scratching results in skin inflammation, which then exacerbates the itching. Over a period of time, areas of the affected epidermis become

Essential terminology

Atopy

Genetic predisposition in some people to various common allergens in the everyday environment. Affected people frequently have one or two other allergic diseases as a result, such as eczema (itchy skin), allergic rhinitis (hayfever) and asthma. Although affected people do not all develop the clinical symptoms of hypersensitivity when exposed to these allergens, they do all respond by producing immunoglobulin E (IgE).

erythematous (reddened), weepy and scaly. The longer this persists, the greater is the likelihood of increased scaling and thickening of the affected epidermis (known as lichen simplex). There is then a risk of infection at the site, because the natural barrier to infection has been damaged.

PHARMACOLOGICAL INTERVENTIONS USED TO MANAGE ATOPIC ECZEMA

Aqueous cream

Aqueous cream is an emollient (soothing, softening and hydrating for the skin). It is a mixture of mineral oil and water that is applied to the skin directly; this forms a barrier, thus preventing the loss of water from the skin so that the skin stays hydrated. It may also be used to be used with water to wash the skin. Dehydration of the skin in eczema, which presents as dry skin, frequently leads to itchiness, which often results in scratching. This commonly leads into a continuous circle of itch–scratch–itch and resulting subsequent skin abrasion (**www.bnf.org**).

Related knowledge Pharmacology

Other bland emollients are available to buy over the counter and on prescription. They come in the form of creams and bath additives. Products include E45®, Aveeno® and Oilatum® (**www.bnf.org**). Topical corticosteroids are also often used.

Personal and professional development 15.6

A number of people cannot read written information. List three strategies that would be more inclusive for patients for whom written materials are difficult to comprehend or read.

Mr Steven Twedell

On his return from a holiday in Portugal with his mother and stepfather, Mr Twedell developed what he described as a 'cold'. Throughout the following day, Mr Twedell felt increasingly unwell. He developed a 'dry cough', according to his formal carer, and he was breathing much more noisily than usual. During the evening, he began to cough repeatedly, producing small amounts of greenish-yellow sputum. He felt quite warm to the touch. He contacted his formal carer, who went with him to the local walk-in centre. When Mr Twedell arrived at the centre, he was breathing fairly rapidly and very noisily. He was wheezing, coughing frequently and producing lots of mucus, which he frequently wiped away from his mouth and nose. He seemed to be frightened and distressed, from time to time grasping at the arms and hands of the staff when they stood close to him.

A staff nurse told Mr Twedell that he needed to wear an oxygen mask. The nurse attempted to put a venturi oxygen mask over Mr Twedell's mouth and nose. This made him much more agitated and distressed; he began crying, grasping at and trying to remove the mask, and pushing the staff away. Due to the difficulty in carrying out more diagnostic tests, a tentative diagnosis of acute asthma complicated by pneumonia was made. A sputum specimen was saved for culture and sensitivity. It was explained to Mr Twedell that he would be prescribed an intravenous injection of an antibiotic and some bronchodilator drugs by nebuliser, and that these medicines would continue until his breathing recovered. His formal carer pointed to Mr Twedell's MedicAlert necklace (an internationally recognised piece of jewellery that that holds medical information about the patient that may not be obvious to a healthcare professional if the patient was unable to tell them). As a result, it was recorded that Mr Twedell was allergic to penicillin. He was prescribed intravenous clarithromycin and nebulised salbutamol. A tourniquet was applied around Mr Twedell's upper arm, but as the intravenous cannula touched his skin, Mr Twedell pushed the staff away and tried to get off the trolley. He was gasping for breath, wheezing, screaming from time to time and sobbing. The staff were becoming increasingly distressed, as they felt that he was rejecting all of their best intentions.

When the results of the sputum culture and sensitivity tests were known, the infecting organism was identified as *Streptococcus pneumoniae*, sensitive to the macrolide group of antibacterials (antibiotics).

Personal and professional development 15.7

From the information given in the above scenario, do you think Mr Twedell is refusing to consent to treatment? Write short notes that will justify your decision. Using the information given in the case studies about Mr Twedell, reconsider your decision about whether he is able to consent to treatment. Do you still come to the same decision? Can you add anything to your notes that would further justify your decision?

THE NATURE OF PNEUMONIA

Pneumonia is an inflammation of the alveoli of the lungs and is usually caused by an infecting agent – a bacterium, virus or fungus. Bacterial infection is the commonest type of pneumonia. Although many people survive pneumonia today as a result of treatment with antibacterial medicines, pneumonia was still ranked fifth in the list of leading bacterial causes of mortality in England and Wales in 2005 (Wheller *et al.*, 2007). Bacterial pneumonia is usually classified as either community-acquired or hospital-acquired. This is an important distinction, as it recognises that the infecting organisms and the disease trajectories are very different.

Community-acquired bacterial pneumonia is most commonly a result of infection by *Streptococcus pneumoniae* (Bartlett *et al.*, 2000; Hoare and Lim, 2006). Infection that develops during the first 48 hours of admission to hospital is usually community-acquired pneumonia rather than hospital-acquired infection. Although anyone can develop pneumonia, a number of factors increase the individual risk of developing the condition, including:

- smoking;
- long-standing lung disorders;
- heavy drinking;
- impaired immune function;
- older age, particularly the frail older person with one or more of the other factors identified above.

The majority of people with community-acquired pneumonia are treated in the community by their GP. They are prescribed a suitable antimicrobial, if appropriate, and advised to rest and drink at least 2 litres of fluid a day. As *Streptococcus pneumoniae* is a bacterium, it is susceptible to treatment with antibacterial drugs. The drug of choice in most situations is amoxicillin, one of the penicillin-based drugs; however, Mr Twedell's MedicAlert necklace identified that he was allergic to penicillin, and therefore the prescriber must carefully consider the potential risk of anaphylaxis before prescribing any of the penicillin group of drugs for Mr Twedell. In light of this, the prescriber has chosen to prescribe clarithromycin.

PHARMACOLOGICAL INTERVENTIONS USED TO MANAGE COMMUNITY-ACQUIRED PNEUMONIA

Clarithromycin

This antibacterial drug is one of the macrolide group of antibacterial medicines and is developed from erythromycin (**www.bnf.org**; Greenstein and Gould, 2004; Rang *et al.*, 2003; Simonsen *et al.*, 2006). It is a broad-spectrum antibiotic with activity against Gram- positive and Gram-negative bacteria and aerobic and anaerobic microorganisms. It is frequently prescribed for infections of the upper and lower respiratory tract and for skin and soft tissue infections. Although clarithromycin is effective against *Streptococcus pneumoniae*, resistant strains of this bacterium are beginning to appear, and some cross-resistance is being observed between the members of the macrolide antibacterials (**www.bnf.org; www.emc.medicines.org.uk;** Greenstein and Gould, 2004; Rang *et al.*, 2003; Simonsen *et al.*, 2006). It is available in oral and intravenous forms.

Pharmacodynamics Clarithromycin

Inhibits some of the structures in the bacterial cell, primarily the ribosomes, so preventing protein synthesis.

Pharmacokinetics Clarithromycin

Absorption: Oral form of clarithromycin is well absorbed and not affected by food. Therefore, it can be taken before or after food (**www.bnf.org; www.emc.medicines.org.uk;** Simonsen *et al.*, 2006).

Distribution: Apart from those of the central nervous system, clarithromycin is distributed to all of the fluid compartments in the body (Simonsen *et al.*, 2006).

Metabolism: Clarithromycin is metabolised in the liver by one of the isoenzymes of the cytochrome P450 system. Clarithromycin inhibits the effects of other isoenzymes in this system, so it can reduce the metabolism of other drugs that use this sytem, such as warfarin. It therefore increases the serum levels of these drugs, with the potential for toxicity. This may impact on prescribing decisions related to Mr Twedell's asthma if it deteriorates further, as the P450 enzyme system is used to metabolise theophylline (**www.emc.medicines.org.uk**).

Elimination: Excreted by the liver and kidney. Poor renal function does not require the dosage to be adjusted (**www.bnf.org;** Simonsen *et al.*, 2006).

Adverse effects of clarithromycin include nausea and vomiting, diarrhoea, reversible hearing loss and jaundice, particularly with high doses (**www.bnf.org; www.emc. medicines.org.uk**).

Nursing knowledge Nursing implications

The information and advice that patients require depends on the type of pneumonia that they have. It is important to understand the rationale for different prescribing practices, as this underpins patient information and education.

From the information given in the case study, we can see that Mr Twedell's asthma is in danger of becoming more acute and must be treated urgently if it is to be prevented from becoming life-threatening. He is also unwell as a result of acquiring pneumonia. As a result of their impact on each other, Mr Twedell's asthma and pneumonia must be treated urgently. There are two alternatives for treating his acute asthma: one uses a metered dose inhaler (MDI) and a spacer device, while the other is an oxygen-driven nebuliser. We know from the case study that Mr Twedell is feeling frightened and anxious, which may affect his breathing and make him hyperventilate. We all know that feeling unwell and being feverish can make us anxious and frightened, especially if we do not understand what is happening to us. Mr Twedell is no different. It is unlikely that Mr Twedell will have used his Accuhaler device, as he knows that his inhaler is for long-term prevention rather than for relief of immediate symptoms. This is identified for him in his health action plan, which is why he sought help from his formal carer.

CONSENT TO TREATMENT

Mr Twedell's experiences in the walk-in centre raise a key medicine management concern that is relevant for all healthcare professionals – capacity to consent to treatment. The law in the UK states clearly that an adult who is mentally competent has the right to refuse treatment (DfCA, 2005). If treatment is refused by a mentally competent adult, they do not have to provide a reason for their decision and they do not need a reason for refusing treatment. Significantly, the law insists that a patient must be provided with enough information regarding both the benefits and the risks, in a form that they can understand, so that they can make an informed decision about whether or not to have the treatment (DfCA, 2005). This is commonly known as 'informed consent'. If an individual agrees to treatment and then suffers some kind of harm because of the treatment, and they believe that not enough information was given to them, they will have the right to legal redress. If the patient is mentally capable of making an informed decision and refuses treatment, but the treatment is still carried out, this can be viewed as a 'trespass to the person', which, Dimond (2003) highlights, is actionable in law. One of the questions that must be asked concerning Mr Twedell is whether he is mentally competent to make decisions about his treatment. We know that Mr Twedell has Down's syndrome with a resulting learning disability. As with every other adult in the UK, his competence to consent to treatment hinges on his mental capacity. Like many emergency situations in healthcare, the circumstances in the walk-in centre are complex and the healthcare professionals involved have limited time available in which to make decisions. Their decisions must be based on all of the information available to them at the time, rather than on their prejudices and assumptions. They are also required to act in the person's best interest.

From the information available, it could be argued that the healthcare professionals in this situation have given very little information to Mr Twedell and that the information they have given him was not in an appropriate form that he could understand easily.

Few people, whether or not they have a learning disability, are able to comprehend all the information given to them when they are dyspnoeic, frightened and anxious, as in this emergency situation. It is possible that the staff have focused on Mr Twedell's disability rather than his ability (Goodley, 2000; Rapley, 2004); they may have assumed that he is unable to consent because he cannot have the intellectual capacity to consent to treatment due to the fact that he has Down's syndrome. If this is the case, then this means that stereotyping and labelling have clouded the staff's assessment skills and clinical judgement and that Mr Twedell is being stigmatised. However, this presents an ethical dilemma. On the one hand, personal autonomy is a fundamental human right, according to the Human Rights Act 1998. The previously used personal model of disability that was firmly entrenched in the medical model and that implicitly placed a disability with the patient and their body has been replaced by the social model of ability (Oliver, 1996; Shakespeare, 1994; Shakespeare, 2000; Shakespeare and Erickson, 2000, Shakespeare and Watson, 1997), which suggests that it is the environment and society's attitudes that are disabling. On the other hand, a nurse must practise using the ethical principles of beneficence and non-malificence that underpin nursing's professional code of conduct (NMC, 2008). There is no doubt that Mr Twedell has some degree of impaired intellectual ability, but whether this is sufficient to assess Mr Twedell as not having the capacity to consent, and therefore being mentally incompetent to consent, to treatment is extremely doubtful. Assessing Mr Twedell based on the information that has been presented in the case studies, we know the following:

- Mr Twedell is able to live independently in a flat and has chosen to do so, although he does have some input from a formal carer to support him in some aspects of independent living.
- He understands that an inhaler will help to control his difficulty with breathing.
- He has learnt how to use an inhaler device in order to control his asthma relatively well.
- He is able to travel abroad to see his family.

It would seem, based on all of the information available, that Mr Twedell is able to understand that he is feeling unwell because of an infection, which is causing him to cough and making his breathing more difficult than usual. He will probably also understand that one type of medication can help to cure his infection while another type of medication can help him to breathe more easily. However, Mr Twedell will only comprehend this if the information is given to him in a manner and form that he can understand. It is clear from the last part of the case study that the information provided would be insufficient for any adult to enable them to give informed consent, let alone an adult with a learning disability. It is important that information given to all patients is expressed clearly and in an appropriate format, so that the patient understands it easily. Mr Twedell is dyspnoeic. Dyspnoea is an extremely frightening and distressing symptom, and anxiety and fear can make many people panic and hyperventilate. This makes the dyspnoea worse by fuelling their anxieties, increasing breathing difficulties and leading to increasing hyperventilation.

> ## Nursing knowledge Useful information-giving strategies
>
> - Use diagrams and pictures instead of written text.
> - Avoid conditional statements such 'Do you understand?'. These tend to be restrictive, as in order to be courteous and respectful many people acquiesce if they don't understand rather than say so. To check the patient understands, in all your communication interactions ask the patient to repeat what you have told them.

It may appear that Mr Twedell is refusing treatment. The likely reasons for his behaviour are twofold. First, all of his attention is focused on his immediate discomfort and how he can try to reduce this. Second, he is likely to be feeling that he is losing control both of the situation and of himself. A number of studies (Griffin and Rabkin, 1998; Taylor *et al.*, 1991, 2000) suggest that having a feeling of personal control is important in helping individuals to cope with the stresses that physical ill-health brings and that this helps them to adapt; thus, feeling in control is psychologically protective. An important medicines management skill for nurses is to recognise this in our assessment of a patient's abilities and concordance in managing their medicines. Although this scenario presents a person with a learning disability, the principles explored in this chapter are transferable to all situations; if we examine the situation in more detail, this will become evident.

While in the walk-in centre, Mr Twedell's anxiety, agitation and distress appear to have worsened at two distinct times: first, when someone tried to cover his mouth and nose with an oxygen mask; and second, when he saw the intravenous cannula about to enter his skin. Severe dyspnoea is usually accompanied by some degree of anxiety, and the last thing a dyspnoeic patient wants is their mouth and nose covered in any way that makes them feel as though they cannot get any air. This will make the anxiety worse and may cause the patient to panic. When attempting intravenous cannulation, there are two consecutive events: applying the tourniquet and approaching the skin with the intravenous cannula. Many people relate needles with pain and report being frightened of needles. It may well be that Mr Twedell is frightened of needles; however, he has also had a tourniquet applied – tourniquets can be extremely uncomfortable and, if a vein is not easy to find, the tourniquet may be in place for longer than anticipated, causing considerable discomfort. If the situation has not been explained adequately to Mr Twedell in a way that he understands, it may well be that the painful tourniquet has precipitated his distress. It appears that in this situation, little has been done to establish the patient's trust and confidence in the healthcare professional's caring abilities.

As with many decisions that the healthcare professional may have to take in relation to medicines management, these judgements often present not only legal dilemmas but also ethical quandaries. If a patient is reluctant to have or refuses to take medicines or other treatments, expressed either verbally or by implication, then the nurse should consider why and then query whether the individual truly understands the implications of refusing the treatment. For Mr Twedell, either the discomfort of the tourniquet or fear of a painful injection may be making him more anxious and distressed, which increases his dyspnoea, making him more anxious and distressed, thus creating a cycle of increasing dyspnoea until he is hyperventilating. The nurse must consider whether Mr Twedell is actually refusing treatment or whether his behaviour is due to him not understanding what is happening to him. The latter is more likely, as Mr Twedell may feel that the healthcare professionals are trying to harm him and that he has lost control over his life.

In emergency situations, time is not usually available for much discussion or debate. If not resolved speedily, Mr Twedell's breathing will deteriorate very quickly. In circumstances such as this, nurses and all other healthcare professionals are bound by their duty of care. Therefore, if they judge that Mr Twedell is genuinely refusing treatment and does not understand the implications that this will bring – his breathing will deteriorate quickly and he will asphyxiate (suffocate), dying in great distress as a result – then they are bound by their duty of care to act and administer the treatment that he needs. In order to do this, they may consider sedating him in some way; however, they must be sure that this does not affect his breathing and that sedation is not a knee-jerk reaction to a complex situation, such that they are using sedation as 'chemical control'. If this is their course of action, they must be sure that Mr Twedell does not have the capacity to consent and therefore is considered to be mentally incompetent. If any healthcare professional is unsure about a patient's capacity to consent and sufficient time is available, then they must seek an assessment of the patient's capacity and mental competence from a specialist. Unfortunately, time is of the essence in Mr Twedell's case and such assessment will not be possible in the time available. All NHS trusts have guidelines and procedures to be followed in these kind of situations, and all nurses should make themselves familiar with these.

The Mental Capacity Act is very clear in stating that a healthcare professional must respect the patient's views, even if these views differ greatly from those of the healthcare professional (DfCA, 2005). Therefore, if a healthcare professional believes that something is the 'right thing to do' but the patient does not have the same beliefs, then the patient is not necessarily mentally incompetent to consent to treatment; rather, they may simply think differently to the healthcare professional.

SEE CHAPTER 13

Nursing knowledge

- Consider whether an alternative treatment is available, e.g. a different form of medication such as oral rather than inhaled.

- Fear of pain is a conditioned response. It produces anxiety and may lead to aggression, particularly if the individual feels that they have no control over the situation or don't understand what is happening to them (Niven, 2006).

▶ *(continued)*

- Many nursing and medical interventions, such as venepuncture and measuring blood pressure, and even simply waiting injured or unwell in an A&E department can produce some degree of fear, and this may be communicated as aggressive behaviour.

- If procedures are essential or have to be repeated, then a psychological technique known as desensitisation could be considered (Niven, 2006).

- Mr Twedell should be given total control. The nurse should spend some time building up a relationship with him based on trust, such as allowing him to be accompanied by favourite things or carrying out the procedure according to his choice. Practitioners in an online forum discussion have carried out procedures in a variety of places, including under a table and in the garden (Foundation for People with Learning Disabilities, 2007). Having this degree of ability to fit in with the circumstances and requests of the patient maintains the patient's control. Unfortunately, building a relationship based on trust and equality takes time, and in an emergency or urgent situation, as in Mr Twedell's case, then action should be taken quickly. The patient's best interests are paramount if they do not have the capacity to consent.

Nursing knowledge Nursing implications

Assessing a patient's capacity to consent to treatment (which for nurses includes administering medicines and oxygen and taking blood pressure measurements) when they communicate in a way that is unexpected and perhaps unfamiliar can be beset with legal and ethical complexities. In the situation in this chapter, it is clearly the doctor's responsibility to assess whether Mr Twedell has the capacity to consent before administering intravenous medicines. However, a qualified nurse is required to act as the patient's advocate at all times, and so in this situation there would be an expectation for the nurse to present Mr Twedell's perspective to the doctor. In this situation, the nurse has not met Mr Twedell before; the nurse therefore does not know what his perspective actually is and so assessing his capacity to consent is imperative. This assessment of Mr Twedell's capacity to consent, the process of how the decision to treat was made, and the actions that resulted from this decision must be documented in Mr Twedell's notes (DfCA, 2007; NMC, 2008). It would be useful to consider whether using an alternative route for Mr Twedell's intravenous medicines would be appropriate here, as this would avoid using both the tourniquet and the intravenous injections. If there were an alternative route, this could be explained to Mr Twedell, along with the advantages and disadvantages. However, although these medicines are available in an oral form, there is a time delay in their mode of action when taken orally. If taken orally, the medicines must go through the pharmacokinetic process before they exert their effects, and for Mr Twedell such a delay could prove to be life-threatening.

PHARMACOLOGICAL INTERVENTIONS USED TO MANAGE PAINFUL INJECTIONS

EMLA cream

Mr Twedell needs medication urgently, which means using a route that delivers an effect quickly. A strategy to reduce the pain and discomfort associated with injections is to use a local anaesthetic such as EMLA® cream before each intravenous injection. In order to carry out certain minor procedures, treatments and investigations without causing pain or discomfort to the patient, it is possible to anaesthetise the specific area of the body concerned. This type of anaesthesia can be one of the following:

- *Local*: Injected to infiltrate the nerves. The effects (loss of sensation) are within a clearly defined area of the body.
- *Topical or surface*: A limited amount is applied directly to intact skin or mucous membranes, e.g. the eye. The effects are localised to the superficial tissue rather than penetrating the whole depth of tissue, as would happen in local anaesthesia.

In situations such as Mr Twedell's, where the individual may find a procedure such as venepuncture too distressing, the application of a topical anaesthetic such as EMLA cream before the minor procedure can help to prevent pain and discomfort. This also makes the person's experience of healthcare environments more positive, which can determine whether they will use the health service again. EMLA is a cream used for surface anaesthesia of the skin. It contains two local anaesthetics, lidocaine (ligno-caine) and prilocaine.

For venepuncture, it is recommended that EMLA cream is applied to the area to be anaesthetised in a thick layer, covered with an occlusive dressing and left in place for 1–5 hours before the venepuncture (**www.bnf.org**; Rang *et al.*, 2003; Simonsen *et al.*, 2006).

Personal and professional development 15.8

How useful would EMLA cream be in Mr Twedell's situation?

Pharmacodynamics EMLA cream

Lidocaine (lignocaine) and prilocaine block the sodium channels in neurons so that sodium ions cannot flow across the neuronal membrane. When this action is prevented, this means that the electrical activity responsible for transmitting nerve impulses within the neuron is disrupted. Nerve impulses from the skin will not be transmitted to the central nervous system, with the result that the patient will not feel uncomfortable or have painful sensations but they will still be able to move. Lidocaine is shorter-acting than prilocaine (**www.bnf.org**; Rang *et al.*, 2003; Simonsen *et al.*, 2006).

Pharmacokinetics EMLA cream

Absorption: The unbroken skin forms a watertight barrier to its underlying tissues and structures. Consequently, little of the drug content of a topically applied cream or lotion is usually absorbed from the epidermis into the dermis, where the nerve structures lie. Thus, applying EMLA cream on unbroken skin will result in very little of its constituent anaesthetic drugs being absorbed into the dermis and reaching the neuronal membranes. However, covering the applied cream with an occlusive dressing prevents sweat from evaporating and eventually macerates the epidermal layers, so losing its watertightness and allowing the drugs to be absorbed into the dermis (**www.bnf.org**; Rang *et al.*, 2003; Simonsen *et al.*, 2006).

Personal and professional development 15.9

Many people requiring medicines have special needs. Make a list of the special needs that an individual may have. Consider how equipped you feel to communicate appropriately with all of these individuals about all of their medicines. Consider using your professional portfolio to identify an area of your practice that you need to develop in order to ensure that you can communicate appropriately with everyone who needs healthcare.

In reality

It is important that EMLA cream is given time to reach its maximum effect. However, this is an emergency situation and delaying the administration of intravenous medication for Mr Twedell may have a serious impact on his condition. In emergency situations, the time factor must be considered and, if possible, explained to the patient.

OXYGEN THERAPY

Enabling Mr Twedell to understand what is happening to him and how the proposed prescription would help him utilises the same skills that are used to explain all situations to patients. Language, both verbal and non-verbal, should be tempered towards the patient's understanding and experience, with touch and distance being used appropriately. It is important to respect the patient's dignity and to establish empathy, trust and confidence. Also important is to establish alternatives, if possible, that may be less distressing for the patient. It is understandable that Mr Twedell became more distressed when an oxygen mask was applied. Covering the mouth and nose of a person who is dyspnoeic, even if they understand that its purpose is to deliver oxygen, may heighten their sense of being unable to get enough air.

Even though this is an emergency situation, nasal cannulae are a less effective way of delivering oxygen, so it may be less distressing for Mr Twedell if nasal cannulae are used, as they do not cover the mouth and nose. He will then feel more in control and that he has enough air to breathe, because his mouth and nose will not be obstructed. It is then more likely that he will tolerate oxygen administration, although it may not be at a high enough rate. There are a variety of factors that can interfere with communication in some way, and as a result healthcare professionals must consider strategies that improve their communication. The following list identifies some of the special needs that patients may have:

- Visual impairment
- Hearing impairment
- Speech impairment
- Intellectual impairment
- Illiteracy
- Non-English-speaking
- Anxiety
- Crying, hostile, angry and/or aggressive
- Under the influence of alcohol or drugs.

If time allows, the care plan used for Mr Twedell would include the following:

- Sit alongside Mr Twedell, using an open posture, leaning forward slightly, establishing eye contact and being relaxed (Egan, 2002).
- Unhurriedly and carefully explain verbally what is causing his symptoms, why oxygen is necessary and how it can be delivered.
- Draw pictures or use diagrams in addition to giving a verbal explanation.
- Explore the advantages of oxygen therapy with Mr Twedell.
- Demonstrate the equipment, and include alternatives if possible.

- Allow Mr Twedell to examine the equipment.
- Show or draw a diagram of a patient wearing a venturi mask and a patient wearing nasal cannulae.
- Demonstrate how to wear both types of equipment and talk calmly about their benefits.
- Consider the use of touch to add reassurance.
- Ask Mr Twedell if he would like to try the equipment and, if so, help him put them on.

As time is a factor in emergency situations such as this, the information that you glean from your assessment of Mr Twedell would identify the need to make an urgent clinical decision and reduce some of the steps in the care plan given above. For example, as he is in distress and has difficulty breathing, the clinical decision would probably be to use some means of delivering oxygen that would not occlude his nose and mouth. Opting to use nasal cannulae until the staff gain the confidence and trust of Mr Twedell so that he is able to use a venturi mask would be the most appropriate approach. Blood gas measurements are useful to ensure adequate oxygenation in both of these situations; however, if these measurements are unavailable as in this situation, then because he has acute severe asthma and pneumonia, Mr Twedell will need high concentrations of oxygen (35-50%) administered using a venturi mask when he is able to tolerate the mask.

If the patient with severe acute asthma also has chronic obstructive pulmonary disease (COPD), they will need lower concentrations of oxygen (24-28%) in order to maintain their hypoxic drive (**www.bnf.org**; BTS and SIGN, 2005).

Oxygen is a medical gas. It is a component of air and is essential to human life. In many illnesses it is necessary to administer oxygen as a therapy, but it must never be used indiscriminately as it can be hazardous for many people, especially those with disorders of the respiratory and cardiovascular systems that cause chronic airflow limitation, such as COPD. For this reason, when oxygen is to be administered therapeutically within the NHS, it must only be given following a prescription (**www.bnf.org**). Once the oxygen administration begins, the flow rate must be altered only following a change in the prescription. There are two reasons for this:

- Over time, individuals who have chronic airflow limitation come to rely on their chronic higher levels of CO_2 to stimulate them to breathe (hypoxic drive). Administering higher levels of oxygen than required to such patients will lower the hypoxic drive and thus reduce the driver that makes them breathe. Breathing higher levels of oxygen will cause the patient to retain more CO_2 as they hypoventilate (breathe slowly and less deeply), thus leading slowly to acidosis (build-up of carbonic acid).
- A high concentration of oxygen administered over a prolonged period of time can cause oxygen toxicity. Although oxygen is essential for life, it is not the predominant gas in inspired air. Inspired air actually contains mostly nitrogen, but this gas is not used by the body to fuel cellular activity. However, nitrogen does play a role in the respiratory system by helping to keep the alveoli open. If high concentrations of

oxygen are administered for long periods of time, the oxygen displaces nitrogen from alveolar air, so that each alveolus holds proportionately more oxygen and more oxygen diffuses into the haemoglobin to form oxyhaemoglobin. This extra oxyhaemoglobin results in increasing O_2 levels, while the reduced amounts of nitrogen are less able to keep the alveoli open. This leads eventually to alveolar collapse, damaging the alveolar-capillary membrane, and thus impairing the diffusion of gas. O_2 levels then fall, with resulting retention of CO_2 and increasing acidosis.

Oxygen is most commonly administered by one of the following methods:

- *Low-flow device*: e.g. nasal cannulae, which allow room air to mix freely with oxygen. These are more comfortable to wear, but the concentration of oxygen administered to the patient is variable, as it changes with the patient's breathing rate or depth. However, it is wasteful of oxygen.
- *High-flow device*: e.g. venturi mask, which allows a precise concentration of oxygen (24-40%) to be administered, regardless of the patient's respiratory rate or depth. Providing the mask is fitted correctly over the patient's nose and mouth, it delivers a precise ratio of oxygen to room air in relation to the flow rate per litre of oxygen set.

Precautions when using oxygen

Oxygen is a gas that supports combustion. Therefore anything that ignites or sparks will burn more efficiently and more fiercely in the presence of oxygen. There is a legal obligation for all healthcare professionals to ensure that they are mindful of the risks and act appropriately in order to not endanger the lives of patients, visitors or staff when oxygen is being used or stored.

Personal and professional development 15.10

If you are not aware of the precautions to be taken when administering oxygen, identify this in your portfolio or learning diary as a task to achieve before your clinical placement. You can check your understanding at the back of the book.

Depending on Mr Twedell's response to the treatment administered, he would be transferred to the local acute hospital trust or to the care of his GP. Whichever action results, ensuring that accurate documentation and verbal communication goes with him is paramount to ensure safe, seamless care.

BEING ACUTELY ILL AND HAVING A LEARNING DISABILITY

Down's syndrome is one of many conditions resulting in some degree of learning disability. There are thought to be approximately 1.2 million people in England with a mild to moderate learning disability, while almost a quarter of a million people are classified as having a severe learning disability (DH, 2001). Some people are born with such a disability, while others become learning-disabled through trauma or disease at some point in their life. In the UK, all adult citizens have the right to access all of the healthcare services provided by the NHS, based on clinical need and free at the point of delivery. However, Powrie (2003) suggests that people with learning disabilities increasingly access services provided by social services rather than the NHS. This, she argues, has been compounded following the movement of people with learning disability into the community from the 'old style' learning disability hospitals. Such moves have been in response to the demands for less institutional care and more support to enable people with learning disability to live in the community in the same way that most other people do. This is particularly so with regard to people with mild to moderate learning disability (DH, 2001).

Although there is evidence for some good practice in both learning disability nursing settings and adult nursing settings, this is not widespread across the UK. Many healthcare professionals working in acute services have difficulty communicating with and understanding people with learning disability (Disability Rights Commission, 2006; Mencap, 2004, 2007). Alongside this lack of communication skills, many healthcare professionals 'make some faulty assumptions about people with a learning disability' (Mencap, 2007). As a result of such attitudes, and the lack of appropriate communication and assessment skills seen in a number of healthcare professionals, many people with learning disability have to endure symptoms of acute illness for longer than non-learning-disabled people before they receive the correct treatment; people with learning disability have greatly increased mortality and morbidity rates compared with the general population as a result. Both Mencap (2004, 2007) and the Disability Rights Commission (2006) present compelling evidence that a large number of adults with learning disability receive no treatment or substandard treatment when they have problems with their physical health. These reports indicate the many difficulties that people with learning disability face in accessing and using healthcare services.

HAVING A LEARNING DISABILITY AND ACCESSING HEALTHCARE

Many people with a learning disability have difficulties in communicating their health needs and may rely upon other people, such as family, formal carers or healthcare professionals, to identify and respond to their needs. The report 'Death by Indifference' (Mencap, 2007) clearly identifies that problems arise for many people with learning disability when they present to the NHS with ill-health. The evidence that Mencap has collected indicates that many healthcare professionals are unable to assess or manage people who cannot or do not communicate in the way that they expect. These views are supported by Goldberg *et al.* (1998), who found that a large number of the health-care professionals they surveyed expected their patients to be courteous, articulate and well-informed. The Mencap (2007) report suggests that countless doctors and nurses in primary and secondary care demonstrate a woeful lack of knowledge and some extremely judgemental attitudes about people with learning disability; key areas identified include the following:

- **The signs and behaviours expressed by people with a learning disability, and in particular the clues that indicate distress in an individual**
- **The key role that carers play in interpreting distress cues**
- **The need to be more suspicious that the patient may have serious illness, and be more proactive in intervening and assessing the needs of a person with a learning disability**
- **The issues around consent and capacity to consent**
- **The difference between a professional's opinion of a patient's quality of life, and a patient's opinion of their own quality of life**
- **The professional requirement to ask for help and/or refer on when faced with a novel or puzzling clinical situation**
- **The dangers of delaying or deferring action (Mencap, 2007).**

Asthma UK acknowledged in 2007 that many people with asthma are not treated adequately and as a result need emergency hospital treatment. Currently, Mencap (2004, 2007) and the Disability Rights Commission (2006) have publicly identified that people such as Mr Twedell are frequently viewed by many healthcare professionals as what Stockwell (1984), the first nurse to identify this phenomenon in her seminal work, called 'unpopular patients'. The paternalistic model that has traditionally underpinned both medicine and nursing is being broken down by many doctors and nurses today. However, evidence such as that described above suggests that there are still many practitioners who need to examine their individual values and beliefs, change their practice in relation to 'unpopular patients' and ensure that their understanding that underpins their practice is both current and evidence-based.

The patient scenarios in this chapter have examined some medicines management issues relating to an individual with a learning disability. The principles that have been highlighted from these vignettes apply in many other situations where individuals are defined by their stereotypes, such as older people, and are consequently seen to be 'different' or 'unpopular'. Such stereotyping is usually because these individuals present some type of challenge to the skills, abilities or culture of the healthcare professional. As a number of studies (e.g. Mencap, 2007) have highlighted over the years, rather than rise to the often uncomfortable challenges that some patient present, many healthcare professionals label and stigmatise the individual and then deal with them inappropriately. Reflection as part of personal and professional development helps us to develop our understanding of medicines management issues – both the science and the art – enabling a deeper understanding of both professional practice and ourselves. This chapter has explored the understanding and skills that are needed and has applied them to medicines management in each of the patient scenarios.

Quick reminder

✔ Down's syndrome is a genetic disease. The person has an additional chromosome, which leads to intellectual disability. About 60 000 people in the UK have Down's syndrome.

✔ Some of the facial features seen in people with Down's syndrome can interfere with breathing. This may also affect the person's ability to use an inhaler.

✔ People with Down's syndrome are more prone to some disorders, e.g. chest infections, compared with the general population.

✔ Asthma is a chronic disease with acute exacerbations. It is common worldwide and its incidence is rising. In the UK, about 5 million people have asthma.

✔ The main features of asthma are due to inflammation in the smaller bronchi and bronchioles. This obstructs airflow into the lungs and increases the quality and quantity of the sputum produced.

✔ Being unable to breathe, regardless of the cause, is frightening. Anxiety can have a detrimental effect on breathlessness.

✔ Treatments for asthma are directed at relieving acute symptoms and preventing chronic inflammation.

✔ The British Thoracic Society and Scottish Intercollegiate Guidelines Network recommend a 'step approach' to the management of asthma. The first step in managing mild intermittent asthma involves an inhaled short-acting β_2 agonist such as salmeterol. If symptoms are not resolved adequately, then a further four prescribing steps may be taken by adding:

- an inhaled steroid;
- an inhaled long-acting β_2 agonist such as salbutamol;
- a leukotriene receptor agonist, or theophylline, or an oral long-acting a leukotriene receptor agonist or theophylline or oral β_2 agonist;
- a long-term continuous oral or inhaled steroid.

✔ 'Stepping-down' must also be considered regularly, so that the patient is maintained on the lowest possible amount of inhaled steroid.

✔ Consent to agree to, or to refuse, treatment is a fundamental right of all mentally competent adults in the UK. The patient must be able to make an informed decision and so must be given information in a form that they can understand.

✔ Judgemental attitudes such as stereotyping and labelling are used by some healthcare professionals and result in many people with Down's syndrome being treated inappropriately, or even fatally, when they have to access acute health services.

✔ People with asthma benefit from using a self-management action plan, which helps them to manage their asthma to fit in with their lifestyle. The plan is built on advice and support to encourage the patient's involvement in their own treatment, including using their medicines appropriately.

✔ Pneumonia may be either community- or hospital-acquired. It may be caused by a bacterium, virus or fungus. Most commonly, it is community-acquired and bacterial and therefore is treated with an appropriate antbacterial such as clarithromycin.

REFERENCES

Asthma UK (2007) *The Asthma Divide: Inequalities in Emergency Care for People with Asthma in England*. London: Asthma UK.

Bartlett J G, Dowell S E, Mandell L A, *et al.* (2000) Practice guidelines for the management of community-acquired pneumonia in adults. *Clinical Infectious Diseases* **31**, 347-382.

Boon N A, Colledge N R, Walker B R and Hunter J A A (2006) *Davidson's Principles and Practice of Medicine*, 20th edn. Edinburgh: Churchill Livingstone.

British Thoracic Society (BTS) (2006) *The Burden of Lung Disease: A Statistics Report from the British Thoracic Society*. London: British Thoracic Society.

British Thoracic Society (BTS) and Scottish Intercollegiate Guidelines Network (SIGN) (2007) *Update to the British Guideline on the Management of Asthma*. Edinburgh: Scottish Intercollegiate Guidelines Network and British Thoracic Society.

British Thoracic Society (BTS) and Scottish Intercollegiate Guidelines Network (SIGN) (2008) *British Guideline on the Management of Asthma*. Edinburgh: Scottish Intercollegiate Guidelines Network and British Thoracic Society.

Currie G and Douglas J (2007) Oxygen and inhalers. In: Currie G (ed.) *ABC of COPD*. Oxford: Blackwell.

Department for Constitutional Affairs (DfCA) (2005) *Mental Capacity Act*. London: The Stationery Office.

Department of Health (2001) *Valuing People: A New Strategy for Learning Disability for the 21st Century*. London: Department of Health.

Department of Health (DH) (2003) *Winning Ways: Working Together to Reduce Healthcare Associated Infection in England*. London: Department of Health.

Department of Health (DH) (2004) *NHS Improvement Plan*. London: Department of Health.

Dimond B (2003) Medicinal products and consent by mentally capacitated patients. *British Journal of Nursing* **12**, 1106-1107.

Disability Rights Commission (2006) *Equal Treatment: Closing the Gap – a Formal Investigation into the Physical Health Inequalities Experienced by People with Learning Disabilities and/or Mental Health Problems*. London: Disability Rights Commission.

Downie G, McKenzie J and Williams A (2003) *Pharmacology and Medicines Management for Nurses*. Edinburgh: Churchill Livingstone.

Editorial (2006) A plea to rename asthma as a disease concept. *Lancet* **368**, 705.

Egan G (2002) *The Skilled Helper: A Problem-Management and Opportunity Approach to Helping*. Pacific Grove, CA: Brooks/Cole.

Foundation for People with Learning Disabilities (2007) Discussion forum. **www.choiceforum.org/WebX?13@@.2d828455/1.**

Gamble J, Fitzsimmons D, Lynes D and Heaney L (2007) Difficult asthma: people's perspectives on taking corticosteroid therapy. *Journal of Clinical Nursing* **16**, 59–67.

Gibson P G, Powell H, Coughlan J, *et al.* (2003) Self-management education and regular practitioner review for adults with asthma. *Cochrane Database of Systematic Reviews* **1**, CD000117.

Gillissen A (2004) Managing asthma in the real world. *International Journal of Clinical Practice* **58**, 592–603.

Goldberg A I, Cohen G and Rubin A-H E (1998) Physician assessment of patient compliance with medical treatment. *Social Science and Medicine* **47**, 1873–1876.

Goodley D (2000) *Self-Advocacy in the Lives of People with Learning Difficulties*. Milton Keynes: Open University Press.

Greenstein B and Gould D (2004) *Trounce's Clinical Pharmacology for Nurses*, 17th edn. Edinburgh: Churchill Livingstone.

Griffin K W and Rabkin J G (1998) Perceived control over illness, realistic acceptance and psychological adjustment in people with AIDS. *Journal of Social and Clinical Psychology* **17**, 407–424.

Haughey J, Barnes G, Partridge M and Cleland J (2004) The Living and Breathing study: a study of patients' views of asthma and its treatment. *Primary Care Respiratory Journal* **13**, 28–35.

Hoare Z and Lim S (2006) Pneumonia: update on diagnosis and management. *British Medical Journal* **332**, 1077–1079.

Manners P J and Carruthers E (2006) Living with learning difficulties: Emma's story. *British Journal of Learning Disability* **34**, 206–210.

Martin E A (2007) *Concise Medical Dictionary*. Oxford: Oxford University Press.

McDonald V M and Gibson P G (2006) Asthma self-management education. *Chronic Respiratory Disease* **3**, 29–37.

Medicines and Healthcare Products Regulatory Agency (MHRA) (2007) *Asthma: Long-acting β_2 Agonists*. London: Medicines and Healthcare Products Regulatory Agency.

Mencap (2004) Treat me right. **www.mencap.org.uk/treatmeright**.

Mencap (2007) Death by indifference. **www.mencap.org.uk/deathbyindifference**.

Mera S L (1997) *Understanding Disease: Pathology and Prevention*, 2nd edn. Cheltenham: Stanley Thornes.

National Institute for Health and Clinical Excellence (NICE) (2007) *Appraisal Consultation Document on the Use of Corticosteroids for the Treatment of Chronic Asthma*. London: National Institute for Health and Clinical Excellence.

Niven N (2006) *The Psychology of Nursing Care*, 2nd edn. Basingstoke: BPS Books.

Nursing and Midwifery Council (2008) *The Code: Standards for conduct, performance and ethics for nurses and midwives*. London: Nursing and Midwifery Council.

O'Callaghan C and Barry P W (1997) The science of nebulised drug delivery. *Thorax* **52** (suppl. 2), 31–44.

Oliver M (1996) *Understanding Disability: From Theory to Practice*. Basingstoke: Palgrave.

Phillips J, Murray P and Kirk P (2001) *The Biology of Disease*. Oxford: Blackwell Science.

Powrie E (2003) Primary health care provision for adults with a learning disability. *Journal of Advanced Nursing* **42**, 413–423.

Rang H P, Dale M M, Ritter J M and Moore P C (2003) *Pharmacology*, 5th edn. Edinburgh: Churchill Livingstone.

Rapley M (2004) *The Social Construction of Intellectual Disability*. Cambridge: Cambridge University Press.

Reddel H K and Barnes D J (2006) Pharmacological strategies for self-management of asthma exacerbations. *European Respiratory Journal* **28**, 182–199.

Rees J and Kannabar D (2007) *ABC of Asthma*. Oxford: Blackwell.

Shakespeare T W (1994) Cultural representations of disabled people: dustbins for disavowal? *Disability and Society* **9**, 283–299.

Shakespeare T W (2000) The social relations of care. In: Lewis G, Gerwitz S and Clark J (eds) *Rethinking Social Policy*. London: The Open University and Sage Publications.

Shakespeare T W and Erickson M (2000) Different strokes: beyond biological essentialism and social constructionism. In: Rose S and Rose H (eds) *Coming to Life*. New York: Little, Brown.

Shakespeare T W and Watson N (1997) Defending the social model. *Disability and Society* **12**, 293-300.

Simonsen T, Aarbakke J, Kay I, Coleman I, Sinnott R and Lysaa R (2006) *Illustrated Pharmacology for Nurses.* London: Hodder Arnold.

St George's London University and Down's Syndrome Association (2002) Down's syndrome. **www.intellectualdisability.info/diagnosis/downs_ syndrome.htm.**

Stockwell F (1984) *The Unpopular Patient.* London: Croom Helm.

Taylor S E, Helgeson V S, Reed G M and Skokan L A (1991) Self generated feelings of control and adjustment to physical illness. *Journal of Social Issues* **47**, 91-109.

Taylor S E, Kemeny M E, Reed G M, Bower J E and Gruenewald T L (2000) Psychological resources, positive illusion and health. *American Psychologist* **55**, 99-109.

Tee A K N, Koh M S, Gibson P G, Lasserson T J, Wilson A J and Irving L B (2007) Long acting beta$_2$ agonists versus theophylline for the maintenance treatment of asthma. *Cochrane Database of Systematic Reviews* **3**, CD001281.

Tortora G J and Derrickson B (2006) *Principles of Anatomy and Physiology*, 11th edn. New York: John Wiley & Sons.

Vermeire E, Hearnshaw H, Van Royen P and Denekens J (2001) Patient adherence to treatment: three decades of research – a comprehensive review. *Journal of Clinical Pharmacy and Therapeutics* **26**, 331-342.

Wenzel S E (2006) Asthma: defining of the persistent adult phenotypes. *Lancet* **368**, 804-813.

Wheller L, Baker A, Griffiths C and Rooney C (2007) Trends in avoidable mortality in England and Wales 1993-2005. *Health Stats Quarterly* **summer**, 6-25.

World Health Organization (2006) Asthma. **www.who.int/mediacentre/factsheets/fs307/en.**

Part 5

Where next?

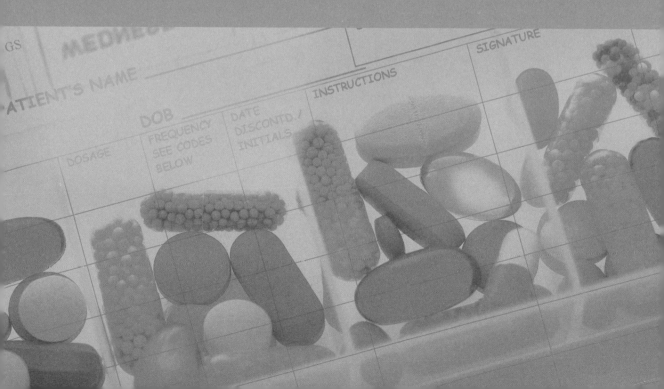

Chapter 16

Contemporary issues relating to drug and medicine development

Simonsen *et al.* (2006) suggest that 'drug therapy is playing an increasingly important role in the treatment and care of patients'. Our increasing knowledge of how the body works and disease processes has put us in a better position to develop effective medicines and rational treatments. However, patients still experience adverse effects, which contribute substantially to morbidity and mortality, and some treatment decisions are still based on 'trial and error' (Read, 2002; WHO, 2002). Read (2002) suggests that the current system for developing new medicines is 'costly and inefficient'.

Two current examples of treatments that cause adverse reactions are chemotherapy and antibiotics. As a consequence, much research is being undertaken to identify new medicines, new delivery systems for medicines and innovative approaches to treatment. One development that promises safer and more effective therapies is in the field of **pharmacogenomics** (Read, 2002).

This chapter explores new and emerging developments within pharmacology and care that have the potential to impact on the way nurses administer medicines and work with patients in the future. Some of these therapies are already in use, while others are predicted.

In 1998, the United Kingdom Central Council (UKCC) (now replaced by the NMC) document *Healthcare Futures 2010* set out to establish the health needs and wants of the general public by 2010 (Welsh Institute for Health and Social Care, 1998). Although this report is now several years old, it identified some interesting information and predicted the following epidemiological trends:

● An increase in chronic non-communicable disease, such as cancer
● A growth in mental ill-health
● An increase in overeating and obesity
● 'Emerging and resurgent' infectious diseases.

The document also suggested that the public would have greater expectations of a health care service, which may include the following:

- Faster and more accurate diagnosis
- Ability to predict future disease
- More highly targeted drugs
- The possibility of genetic therapy.

This information has been used to provide a structure for the pharmacological content of this chapter.

Learning outcomes

At the end of this chapter you should be able to:

✔ Describe a range of emerging treatments
✔ Identify some novel ways of administering medicines
✔ Identify the issues inherent in ethnopharmacology.

Chapter at a glance

Lifestyle drugs
Drug development
Genetic therapies
Ethnopharmacology
Professional issues
Quick reminder
References

LIFESTYLE DRUGS

There is much current media interest in ill-health related to modern lifestyles, such as alcohol consumption, the use of recreational drugs and overeating and obesity. Such issues have a financial cost for the NHS and considerable health costs for the patient; for example, obesity is linked to coronary heart disease, diabetes mellitus and psychological distress. Ali (2002) suggests that obesity should be seen as a chronic disease.

Anti-obesity medicines

Ideally, obesity should be tackled by the patient committing to lifestyle changes such as eating a healthy diet and exercising. However, sometimes patients find it difficult to sustain the changes required or are unable to lose sufficient weight for other reasons. A range of medicines are available that aim to help weight loss by increasing energy expenditure, suppressing appetite and reducing absorption (Ali, 2002). Two of the most recently developed and potentially most effective medicines used in this situation are orlistat and sibutramine, which were launched in 2001 and are currently recommended to treat obesity in the UK (Ali, 2002; NICE, 2006).

> **Essential terminology**
>
> **Body mass index (BMI)**
> A method used to assess the degree of obesity.
> BMI is established by dividing the person's weight (expressed in kilograms) by the square of their height (expressed in metres). This is often established using a chart that plots the patient's weight and height. A person is described as overweight if they have a BMI of 25 kg/m^2 or over and obese if they have a BMI of 30 kg/m^2 or more. (NICE, 2006)

The aims of anti-obesity medicines are to produce sustained weight loss and thus to reduce the morbidity and mortality associated with obesity. Unfortunately, drug trials to date have been limited due to high attrition rates – that is, volunteers drop out of the trial (Padwal and Majumdar, 2007). It is important to note that, in order to maintain weight loss, the patient has to be committed to changing their lifestyle. The patient also has to meet certain criteria before the treatment is prescribed.

The National Institute for Health and Clinical Excellence (NICE) (2006) has produced clinical guidelines relating to obesity. These guidelines offer criteria in relation to orlistat and sibutramine. NICE recommends that orlistat should be prescribed for the management of obesity in people with a BMI of 30 kg/m^2 or more, and in people with a BMI of 28 kg/m^2 or more with 'significant co-morbidities'. The recommendations for sibutramine are that it should be prescribed for the management of obesity in people with a BMI of 30 kg/m^2 or more, and in people with a BMI of 27 kg/m^2 or more with 'significant co-morbidities'. Other criteria relate to how much weight the patient has been able to lose and the age of the patient.

Orlistat

Orlistat helps people who have a high fat intake. It acts by inhibiting lipases (enzymes produced by the pancreas and stomach), which are responsible for converting fats to fatty acids, thus reducing the absorption of dietary fat by around 30% (Padwal and Majumdar, 2007). Because a proportion of the fat passes through the intestine without being absorbed, it can cause gastrointestinal effects such as faecal urgency and flatulence, but this might be avoided by cutting certain foods out of the diet (Simonsen *et al.*, 2006). It may also impair the absorption of fat-soluble vitamins, and so patients should be advised to make sure their diet contains plenty of fruit and vegetables; replacement vitamins are not usually required.

Pharmacokinetics Orlistat

Absorption: Minimal.

Distribution: The volume of distribution cannot be determined, as the medicine is not absorbed. It is 99% bound to plasma proteins.

Metabolism: Thought to be mainly within the gastrointestinal wall.

Elimination: Mainly (about 97%) excreted by the faecal route (www.emc.medicines.org.uk).

Sibutramine

Sibutramine helps people who cannot control their eating. It is a centrally acting appetite suppressant (a monoamine-reuptake inhibitor), originally developed as an antidepressant. It induces a sensation of fullness and maintains the basal metabolic rate, which usually reduces with weight loss. It inhibits the reuptake of noradrenaline (norepinephrine) and serotonin. It may increase the patient's blood pressure and pulse rate; other side effects include constipation, dry mouth, nausea, tachycardia and arrhythmias (Padwal and Majumdar, 2007). Sibutramine is therefore contraindicated in people with a history of cardiovascular disease. Although the side effects occur at the beginning of treatment, usually in the first 4 weeks, the patient should have their blood pressure and pulse checked at regular intervals during treatment.

Pharmacokinetics Sibutramine

Limited data are available so far.
Absorption: Well absorbed. It undergoes extensive first-pass metabolism.

Distribution: Achieves a steady state within 4 days on repeated dosing.

Metabolism: Metabolised into active metabolites. Half-life is 14–16 hours.

Elimination: Excreted in urine and faeces.

Personal and professional development 16.1
Nursing implications

Medicines that interfere with absorption are not without adverse effects and so should be prescribed only for clinically obese patients. From your reading of the text so far, identify the factors that should be considered before commencing this treatment.

Answers can be found at the back of the book.

There are other anti-obesity medicines in development related to the hormone leptin (thought to be produced by an obesity gene), appetite control and antagonists to receptors for neuropeptide Y (which increases appetite) (Ali, 2002).

DRUG DEVELOPMENT

Some of the most recent drug developments have been related to the way we administer medicines rather than the development of new drugs per se; for example, the giving of hormone replacement therapy (HRT) by patch (using the transdermal route – discussed in Chapter 4). Some of these developments include using microdoses in clinical trials, increased availability of medicines via the inhaled route, systemic treatments via the nasal mucosa and using therapies to match circadian rhythms.

Microdoses

Drug trials are under way to test treatments that contain one-hundredth of the calculated dose required (microdoses) to produce a pharmacological effect, potentially making the resulting treatment safer and more effective for the patient. Microdoses are undergoing clinical trials in the USA and Europe. They use 'high sensitivity carbon dating technology' to reduce drug doses (Bryan, 2005). An added advantage is that they may also be cheaper.

Changes in delivery

Medicines via the inhaled route

Traditionally the inhalation route has been associated with medicines that target respiratory disorders. The lungs offer a large area for absorption of medicines and the medicine is delivered to the respiratory tree, which is where it exerts its effects. There is minimal absorption of the medicine into the systemic circulation and therefore less potential for adverse reactions.

This route is now opening up for other medicines that cannot be given orally, such as insulin (Bryan, 2004a). It has been suggested that analgesics may also be given in this way. However, in order for these medicines to be absorbed into the bloodstream, they need to be delivered to the alveoli (air sacs in the lung). This therefore requires the development of a delivery device capable of doing this.

Systemic treatments via the nasal mucosa

According to Bryan (2004b), the nasal mucosa have been the subject of research for 'at least a decade'. Work is underway to develop an anti-obesity medicine to be administered via this route, which will avoid the nausea experienced with some oral medicines. The route offers the potential for bypassing the blood–brain barrier, but it will require a device that can deliver the medicine to the olfactory region.

Theoretically, the nasal mucosa should provide a fast route comparable with medicines given intravenously. Lipid-soluble molecules cross the nasal membrane with a potential bioavailability of up to 100%, but the medicine is not always able to enter the tight junctions between the nasal mucosa. This has been one of the problems in developing a form of insulin for delivery via the nasal mucosa, and so it has had limited application to date (see Chapter 4 for explanations of routes of administration and terms such as bioavailability).

Also of interest is the delivery of vaccines by this route – for example, a nasal flu vaccine to provide local immunity at the site accessed by the virus.

Transdermal drug delivery

Transdermal delivery refers to medicines being absorbed into the bloodstream via application to the skin. Transdermal patches are used for a variety of replacement treatments, such as nicotine and hormone replacement, and for prophylaxis, such as glyceryl trinitrate for angina. Research is being undertaken to explore the potential for transdermal delivery using electricity, ultrasound, radiofrequencies and microneedles (Bryan, 2004c).

Medicine delivery patterns that match circadian rhythms

The term 'circadian rhythm' describes the 24-hour day/night cycle (from Latin: *circa*, 'about', *dies*, 'day') and refers to the cycle of rest and activity that has an importance for normal body functioning. Sleep is associated with 'restorative functions', such as tissue restoration (Wickens, 2005). It is proposed that physiological and biochemical activity has a 'unique circadian rhythm' (Wickens, 2005). We know, for example, that body temperature varies over the course of the 24-hour period, information that is important for the nurse to acknowledge when assessing a patient's health. Likewise, we identified in Chapter 10 that simvastatin is usually taken in the evening, as it is believed that the liver's production of cholesterol takes place mainly during the night.

It has been a goal of research for some time to discover a way of targeting the release of a medication to the 'maximum clinical manifestation of a disease' rather than delivering a constant blood level, for example in relation to cancer cell division (Bryan, 2005). To date, this has not been possible for more than a handful of medicines, due to the problem in designing products that are resistant to breakdown in the gastrointestinal tract. A number of systems are now being produced that enable 'timed delivery', possibly many hours after taking the medicine, based on the use of polymers attached to medicines and osmosis. On balance, however, there is little evidence available to support these claims, and inevitably such developments will be expensive (Bryan, 2005).

GENETIC THERAPIES

Genetic variations in individuals can account for up to 95% of the differences in effects of medicines seen within the general population (Lanfear and McLeod, 2007). Hopkins Tanne (1998) suggests that half these variations can be 'exploited to develop safer, more effective drugs', whilst Read (2002) suggests that ultimately it will be possible to produce 'customised treatments' associated with specific cancers, as all cancers involve some type of abnormal gene function.

Medicines do not always produce a response and in some situations the 'adverse effect' is that there is *no* effect – that is, the medicine doesn't work. For example, according to WHO (2002), 30% of patients show no response to statins.

The **Human Genome Project** has opened up the potential for the development of 'genetic testing, therapy and prevention' (Skirton and Patch, 2000), with pharmacokinetics being one of the first objectives. This, together with genetically modified viruses and developments in **cloning**, offer the promise for the development of a range of gene therapies with the potential to treat an extensive range of diseases (Wiffen *et al.*, 2007). The Department of Health (DoH) (2003) has suggested that future management of disease will be based upon correcting genetic mutations or the protein product that provides the code for the faulty gene.

Pharmacogenetics, the interaction between genetics and drugs/medicines, is defined by Brice and Sanderson (2006) as 'the application of genetic analysis to predict drug response, efficacy and toxicity' based upon an understanding of how an individual's genetic structure influences their reaction to drug treatment. The terms 'pharmacogenetics' and 'pharmacogenomics' are often used interchangeably, but pharmacogenomics implies a broader understanding of genes and gene products 'that may be suitable targets for new drug discovery or that interact with other genes and environmental factors in determining drug response' in relation to genome approaches rather than focusing on one or two genes (Brice and Sanderson, 2006; Lanfear and McLeod, 2007). Pharmacogenomics therefore is 'a significant opportunity for the development and delivery of safe and effective medicines' by considering, for example, medicine dosage (**www.dxsgenotyping.com**).

Related knowledge Applied physiology

Humans have 46 chromosomes arranged in 23 homologous pairs. Chromosomes are made of deoxyribonucleic acid (DNA), which contains all of an individual's genetic information on the genes.

A gene is the basic unit of genetic material. Genes occur at specific places on a chromosome, rather like stations on a railway line. Genes produce all of the body's proteins through a code in the DNA.

An allele is an alternative form of the same gene occupying corresponding sites on homologous chromosomes, e.g. in human blood groups, the alleles are A, B and O.

The genome is the total genetic material of an organism. The human genome consists of 20 000–25 000 genes arranged on 23 pairs of chromosomes. The mutation (changes in the amount or structure) of these genes accounts for

▶ *(continued)*

human individuality. These genes provide the code for the production of proteins; because of this, they can also generate the individual's normal function in relation to transport mechanisms, drug receptors and metabolic activity, all of which affect the efficacy of medicines. The mutation can vary from determining individual traits (different normal variations) to affecting whole sections of chromosomes. The cell can repair some mutations, but if not corrected the protein coding and DNA can be seriously disrupted, resulting in disease. If this mutation occurs in sperm or ovum cells, it can be passed on to future generations.

Genetic disorders are the result of changes in DNA mutation that can be inherited. They may be single-gene disorders (these can usually be traced through generations of families, e.g. cystic fibrosis) or multifactorial (combination of several environmental factors and a number of genes, e.g. diabetes mellitus, coronary heart disease).

Genetics can mean the study of biological inheritance, the function of genes in normal and abnormal body functions, or a special application such as genetic engineering or gene therapy (Brice and Sanderson, 2006; Burton and Shuttleworth, 2003; James *et al.*, 2002).

Most medicines in use today are based upon how the 'average' patient will respond. The Human Genome Project offers us 'high expectations for dramatic improvements in treatment and prevention of disease' (McLeod and Marsh, 2001). Thus, we may have the opportunity to make 'individual treatments', as it is thought that patients' reactions, including adverse reactions, to medicines are determined genetically (Long, 2004).

It has been suggested that up to 95% of patients' response to medicines is genetic. Therefore, increasing our understanding of the genetic mechanisms involved in the response or lack of response to a medicine, and its toxicity, will improve patients' quality of life. It will also allow us to identify the best treatment for the individual patient based upon their polymorphism map (see below).

These mechanisms may impact in three ways, producing differences in:

- the biotransformation and transport of drugs, due to genetic polymorphisms;
- varied concentrations of the medicine at the site of action due to differences in drug-metabolising enzymes (see Chapter 4);
- mutations in drug targets such as receptors, proteins and enzymes (Robertson *et al.*, 2002; WHO, 2002).

Polymorphisms

Mutations occur continuously during DNA and cell replication (Brice and Sanderson, 2006). The term 'polymorphism' refers to the several types of a single gene in a species that explain individual differences such as eye colour (Galbraith *et al.*, 2007). Such individual genetic polymorphisms (differences) can also explain the way in which drugs and medicines exert different effects in different people.

More than one gene can alter the person's response to a drug/medicine. Studying the variations in DNA within the genes can identify differences in the drug target and improve the efficacy of the treatment (Lanfear and McLeod, 2007; Long, 2004).

Most adverse drug reactions (ADRs) are caused by genetic variations in the way that individuals metabolise drugs (Read, 2002). It is thought that nearly all the drug-metabolising enzymes are polymorphic (Lanfear and McLeod, 2007). For example, polymorphisms in the enzyme CYP2C9, involved in warfarin metabolism, are responsible for adverse drug reactions to warfarin (an anticoagulant).

Burton and Shuttleworth (2003) suggest that diagnostic kits will eventually be available in pharmacies to help identify the most appropriate medicine for each patient, but such technology is in its infancy. It may also be possible to adjust doses related to drug metabolism, thus improving the safety and efficacy of treatments.

> **Personal and professional development 16.2**
> **Explaining responses to medicines**
>
> Can you identify some other reasons to explain why prescribed medicines may exert no appreciable effect?
> Some answers can be found at the back of the book.

Current therapies that use genetic information

The use of genes in therapy is not new. We have been using 'human' insulin since the 1980s, the production of which involves a process that uses genetic engineering to produce a human insulin cell. One method involves incorporating human insulin DNA into the genetic material of the bacterium *Escherichia coli* (Galbraith *et al.*, 2007).

Another example is alteplase, a naturally occurring human protease produced in response to the formation of a thrombus (see Chapter 10). This is used in acute clinical situations to dissolve clots.

Gene therapy

According to the DH (2003), there are about 10 000 single-gene disorders, such as cystic fibrosis. The study of genes holds the promise for treating or even curing genetic and acquired diseases. Chester and Hull (2002) describe gene therapy as 'the transfer of selected genes into a host with the hope of ameliorating or curing a disease state'.

Wiffen *et al.* (2007) describe two approaches to gene therapy: gene replacement and gene addition. Gene replacement is used where the disease is caused by a single faulty gene, such as cystic fibrosis, in which the faulty gene is replaced with a normal gene. Gene addition involves 'adding' a gene or genes to a cell in order to provide a new function to the cell. An example of this is adding a tumour suppressor gene to cancer cells (tumour suppressor genes are discussed in Chapter 7). This involves delivering the gene to its target site, the DNA of the target cell. This is called 'gene transfer' (Wiffen *et al.*, 2007) and can involve a non-viral or viral system.

A major problem associated with gene therapy is the lack of a delivery system that is both effective and safe. Viral vectors have the potential to cause infection and toxicity, and the size of the viral genome limits the amount of other genetic material that can be accommodated.

Non-viral systems such as liposomes are less toxic and produced more easily, but they are not as efficient as viral vectors and enable only low levels of gene transfer (Wiffen *et al.*, 2007).

Viral vectors have an innate ability to place genetic material into (i.e. infect) an identified host cell. Viruses are virulent causes of infection and so they are genetically modified to reduce their ability to infect the host cells; these viruses are described as 'replication-deficient', indicating that they cannot replicate. Common viruses used for this purpose are the adenovirus, retroviruses and herpes virus (Chester and Hull, 2002).

There has been some success with gene therapies for cystic fibrosis. James *et al.* (2002) describe the process of inserting cloned copies of normal genes into an inactivated adenovirus (vector) that normally would infect the respiratory system. The vector is inhaled and then delivers the corrected gene to the epithelial cells. Unfortunately, the cell ultimately dies (due to the normal cell cycle) and so the treatment needs to be repeated frequently.

Coile (2001) suggests that we may see the following interesting developments in relation to 'the genetic revolution':

- Patients will carry their unique genetic risk profile on a microchip.
- Drug-development cycles will be quicker.
- Universal stem cells will be used to generate cells and tissues.
- 'Designer genes' will be used to develop new treatments.
- Nanotechnology will be utilised.
  - Tiny nanosensors will be used to carry information about the health of a patient.
  - Nanobots will be used to clear plaque.
  - A 'camera in a pill' to be swallowed will provide information about the patient's gastrointestinal tract.

- Xenotransplantation: the use of genetically modified animal tissue.
- Individualised treatments will be used.
- Gene-based diagnostics will identify the most appropriate medicine for the individual.
- There will be a move from treatment to prediction.
- Genetic therapies will cost more than current treatments and so will need financial investment.

Nursing implications of genetic therapies

Chester and Hull (2002) suggest that 'gene therapy is a new and rapidly evolving area with promising applications', but they also note that nurses' responsibilities in this area should be very clear, as, due to the contemporary nature of such therapies, our knowledge base in this area is still evolving.

Issues for nurses in relation to gene therapy may relate to cost, research, education and patient care, although it could be argued that these areas are inextricably linked:

- The cost, initially at least, will be considerable:
  - The implications of this are that drug companies may be reluctant to embrace these developments.
  - The cost will have to be met from existing purses.
  - Staff and patients may find the decisions taken in relation to how the money is spent difficult to understand and justify.
- A great deal of medical and pharmacological research is being undertaken in this area. Nurses with specialist knowledge and skills may be involved in this and must at least be able to understand and use research-based evidence in their practice.
- Nurses will need to widen their knowledge to include a greater understanding of genetics, causes of disease, drug actions and the risks to the patient.
- The nurse-patient relationship will be affected as more screening becomes available. Patients' increasing needs for support, information and confidentiality should be considered.
- Nurses are often the first point of contact for patients and so will need to be able to provide information and answer questions.
- Nurses will also need to reassure patients receiving 'novel' therapies.

Genetic technology has the potential to affect many aspects of healthcare, including diagnosis, treatments, relationships with patients and government policies (Reiger, 2001). In June 2003 the UK government produced a White Paper 'Our Inheritance, Our Future' (DH, 2003), which was concerned with the 'safe, effective and ethical application' of genetic therapies. This paper identifies the potential for:

- more accurate diagnosis;

- prediction of risk;

- new treatments;

- individualised prevention and treatment.

The DH's stated aims in setting out the paper were to:

- strengthen specialist genetics services;

- incorporate genetic advances into mainstream care delivery;

- disseminate knowledge in order to build the confidence of healthcare professionals;

- explore the benefits of genetic knowledge;

- realise the benefits of genetic research;

- promote public understanding, acceptance and confidence in such therapies.

This paper clearly identifies the support and education required by all healthcare staff and acknowledges that there will need to be a strong regulatory framework in order to address potential public concerns.

Personal and professional development 16.3
Ethical considerations

Can you identify what these 'public concerns' might relate to?
Some answers can be found at the back of the book.

ETHNOPHARMACOLOGY

There are well-documented differences in illness patterns across communities. For example, there is a suggestion that black and minority ethnic groups in the UK generally have poorer health than other groups in the population (Parliamentary Office of Science and Technology, 2007). It is difficult to say how much these differences can be explained by factors such as lifestyle, socioeconomic status and environment, either individually or collectively. Many researchers believe that there are biological differences between certain ethnic groups. Brice and Sanderson (2006) suggest that ethnic differences can be explained by genetic differences and therefore used as 'markers of genetic differences'. We know, for example, that Chinese people metabolise alcohol differently from caucasians, producing a higher plasma concentration of acetaldehyde. Chinese people are also more sensitive to propranolol (a beta-blocker). Afro-Caribbean people, on the other hand, are less sensitive to beta-blockers (Rang *et al.*, 2003).

There are also genetic variations across racial and ethnic groups, and differences between ethnic groups that might be due to non-genetic factors such as diet.

Rahemtulla and Bhopal (2005) argue that to classify such differences as 'ethnic' simply 'reinforces existing social differences', which may result in inequalities. Brice and Sanderson (2006) note the controversy surrounding the development of BiDiL® (isosorbide dinitrate plus hydralazine), hailed as an 'ethnic drug' when it was marketed in America for the treatment of heart failure in African Americans because it has been demonstrated to be more effective in this ethnic group. However, a study undertaken by McDowell *et al.* (2006) demonstrated on a small scale that adverse reactions to cardiovascular medicines could be predicted in some ethnic groups. Ethnicity may therefore be a predictor of risk in relation to specific treatments.

In fact, genetic differences within specific groups are inconsistent (Rahemtulla and Bhopal, 2005), although these same authors acknowledge the potential that exists if such genetic variations are proven.

PROFESSIONAL ISSUES

In Chapter 5 we identified some of the changes to the administration of medicines as a consequence of developments in information technology (IT) services. Such developments will enable us to use:

- electronic patient records;
- computerised prescribing;
- ward-based electronic medicine cupboards;
- barcodes to check a patient's identity (Timbs and Pike, 2006).

The DH (2007) has produced a document recommending and supporting the use of 'bar-coding and similar technologies' in order to improve patient safety. The document includes an action plan designed to promote the use of technology in the NHS and to encourage manufacturers to code medicines and devices appropriately. The DH suggests that the use of such IT strategies will minimise the risk of medication errors, reduce wrong-site surgery, provide a more accurate 'track and trace of surgical instruments, equipment and other devices' and improve record-keeping, thus reducing costs and improving efficiency. Such strategies are voluntary at the time of writing.

Quick reminder

✔ Growing technology is increasing the rate of potential new therapeutics.
✔ Novel therapies are not always related to medicine actions and effects but may relate to delivery systems.
✔ Genetic therapies offer the potential for innovative, specific and individualised treatments.

✔ There is a growing body of research related to predicting the risk of adverse drug reactions associated with genetic and ethnic differences.

✔ Information technology offers the potential for the safer administration of medicines.

✔ Nurses need to be able to maintain their knowledge base and possibly work in new ways.

REFERENCES

Ali O (2002) Pharmacotherapy. *Pharmaceutical Journal* **268**, 687-689.

Brice P and Sanderson S (2006) Genetics, health and medicine. *Pharmaceutical Journal* **277**, 53-56.

Bryan J (2004a) Inhaled products of the modern era: drugs for non-respiratory conditions. *Pharmaceutical Journal* **273**, 161-162.

Bryan J (2004b) Getting systemic treatments into the bloodstream via the nasal mucosa. *Pharmaceutical Journal* **273**, 649-650.

Bryan J (2004c) Transdermal drug delivery may be a common technique in the future. *Pharmaceutical Journal* **273**, 292-293.

Bryan J (2005) Microdoses open new horizons for trials. *Pharmaceutical Journal* **275**, 54.

Burton H and Shuttleworth A (2003) Genetics education for pharmacists. *Pharmaceutical Journal* **270**, 84-85.

Chester M and Hull D (2002) The role of the gene therapy nurse in cancer care. *Cancer Nursing Practice* **1**, 25-29.

Coile Jr R C (2001) Impact of the 'new science' of genomics. *Journal of Healthcare Management* **46**, 365.

Department of Health (2003) *Our Inheritance, Our Future: Realising the Potential of Genetics in the NHS*. London: Department of Health.

Department of Health (2007) *Coding for Success: Simple Technology for Safer Patient Care*. London: Department of Health.

Galbraith A, Bullock S, Manias E, Hunt B and Richards A (2007) *Fundamentals of Pharmacology: An Applied Approach for Nursing and Health*, 2nd edn. Harlow: Pearson Education.

Hopkins Tanne J (1998) The new word in designer drugs. *British Medical Journal* **316**, 1930-1931.

James J, Baker C and Swain H L (2002) *Principles of Science for Nurses*. Oxford: Blackwell.

Lanfear D E and McLeod H L (2007) Pharmacogenetics: using DNA to optimize drug therapy. *American Family Physician* **76**, 1179-1183.

Long P (2004) What pharmacists need to know about pharmacogenomics. *Pharmaceutical Journal* **273**, 756.

McDowell S E, Coleman J J and Ferner R E (2006) Systematic review and meta-analysis of ethnic differences in risks of adverse reactions to drugs used in cardiovascular medicine. *British Medical Journal* **332**, 1177-1181.

McLeod H L and Marsh S (2001) Using the genome to improve therapeutics. *Lancet* **358**, 1559.

National Institute for Health and Clinical Excellence (NICE) (2006) *Clinical Guideline 43: Obesity - The Prevention, Identification, Assessment and Management of Overweight and Obesity in Adults and Children*. London: National Institute for Health and Clinical Excellence.

Padwal R S and Majumdar S R (2007) Drug treatments for obesity: orlistat, sibutramine, and rimonabant. *Lancet* **369**, 71-78.

Parliamentary Office of Science and Technology (2007) Ethnicity and health. *Postnote* **276**, 1-4.

Rahemtulla T and Bhopal R (2005) Pharmacogenetics and ethnically targeted therapies. *British Medical Journal* **330**, 1036-1037.

Rang H P, Dale M M, Ritter J M and Moore P K (2003) *Pharmacology*, 5th edn. Edinburgh: Churchill Livingstone.

Read C Y (2002) Pharmacogenomics: an evolving paradigm for drug therapy. *Medsurg Nursing* **11**, 122–125.

Reiger P (2001) The role of oncology nurses in gene therapy. *Lancet* **341**, 85–87.

Robertson J A, Brody B, Buchanan A, Kahn J and McPherson E (2002) Pharmacogenetic challenges for the health care system. *Health Affairs* **21**, 155–166.

Simonsen T (2005) In Simonsen T, Aarbakke J, Kay I, Coleman I, Sinnott P and Lysaa R (2006) *Illustrated Pharmacology for Nurses*. London: Hodder Arnold.

Skirton H and Patch C (2000) The 'new genetics' and nursing: what does it have to do with me? *Nursing Standard* **14**, 42–46.

Timbs O and Pike H (2006) Technology in the health care arena. *Pharmaceutical Journal* (suppl. 277) B22.

Welsh Institute for Health and Social Care (1998) *Healthcare Futures 2010*. London: UKCC Education Commission.

Wickens A (2005) *Foundations of Biopsychology*. Halow: Pearson Education.

Wiffen P, Mitchell M, Snelling M and Stoner N (2007) *Oxford Handbook of Clinical Pharmacy*. Oxford: Oxford University Press.

World Health Organization (WHO) (2002) Progress in pharmacokinetics and pharmacogenomics. *WHO Drug Information* **1**, 17–20.

Chapter 17

Contemporary issues in medicines management for nurses

This chapter examines two contemporary issues related to medicines management for nurses: nurse prescribing and medication errors. Exploring these two themes highlights not only that adult nursing has changed but also that the role of adult nurses is still evolving. Implementing the government's drive for the modernisation and improvement of the NHS has utilised nurses' skills and exploited the 24 hours/7 days a week/365 days a year availability of nurses to bring about a number of the major service developments seen throughout the NHS over the past few years. One of the improvements to the service is seen to be extending the number of professionals who are able to prescribe medication. In addition to administering medication, many nurses are now able to prescribe medication; this increases the risk of problems occurring. As with any nursing procedure, prescribing and administering medicines is not without risk; strategies for recognising and managing this risk are suggested in this chapter.

✔ Learning outcomes

At the end of this chapter you should be able to:

✔ Give an overview of the historical development of nurse prescribing

✔ Discuss the tensions that have arisen as a result of nurse prescribing

✔ Explain how common the incidence of medication errors is in the NHS

✔ Discuss the practices that can lead to medication errors

✔ Discuss tactics that would minimise the risk of medication errors occuring.

Chapter at a glance

SETTING THE SCENE

Looking back through the history of nursing in the UK, it is easy to see that there have been some considerable changes in the role of the adult nurse over time. Although these changes can be more easily seen in the differing knowledge and skills that adult nurses now have compared with nurses in earlier times, their attitudes, beliefs and values have altered too (Hallett, 2007). Many nurses today use skills that were once purely within the domain of the doctor. Not too long ago, assessment of the pulse and blood pressure were highly respected skills that were very much the remit of the doctor. Doctors had the ability to undertake such assessments and they knew what they were looking for and how to interpret their findings, seek further information, reach a diagnosis and prescribe treatment. For a number of years, skills that were previously perceived as highly skilled medical tasks have been passed on to nurses, changing both nursing and medicine. Our society has also changed over time, so that the attitudes, values and beliefs of healthcare professionals have evolved to reflect this. As a result, the expectations that the public have of health, the NHS and healthcare professionals have also altered with time. Alongside all of these changes, science and technology have developed too but now seem to be advancing more and more quickly. Although nursing has altered considerably and many nurses have been influential in its development over the years, many recent drivers for change in nursing have been political. Challenged with meeting changing public expectations, improving the health of the population and keeping in check escalating healthcare costs, successive governments have confronted the power of medicine and tried to develop an NHS that delivers what they believe voters want. There is no doubt that this central political control of the NHS has been and remains a major influence today in developing the role of the nurse.

DEVELOPMENTS INFLUENCING MEDICINES MANAGEMENT

Many of the major changes in nursing over the past two decades have altered the way in which many of the NHS services are delivered and also created new roles and responsibilities, such as nurse consultants. Implicit in developing the skills to perform many of these new roles are medicines management and non-medical prescribing. Midwives have long had the right to prescribe a limited number of medications for labouring women, including the opioid analgesics diamorphine, morphine, pethidine and pentazocine. Until 1992, the only professionals who could legally prescribe a full range of medicines in the UK were doctors, dentists and vets for animal use. In 1992, the NHS introduced nurse prescribing, which permitted certain nurses, health visitors and midwives to prescribe a number of medicines. More recently, the right to prescribe medicines has been widened further to include a variety of other healthcare professionals and is now termed 'non-medical prescribing'. People who are now able to prescribe a variety of medicines are vets, dentists, medical doctors and independent non-medical prescribers, the latter including nurses, midwives, health visitors, physiotherapists and pharmacists.

Many adult nurses have developed their roles in order to become specialist nurses and consultant nurses. In such roles, independent and supplementary prescribing have enabled them to help patients manage their own conditions more effectively. At the same time, information technology (IT) has enabled the NHS to collect more information, with some of these data clearly demonstrating the risks that are inherent in hospitals. In relation to medicines management and nursing, many of the threats for both patients and nurses arise from using a medicine trolley to carry out medicine administration on a ward or a part of a ward of patients – that is, a medicine round. Another major key area that has been identified to increase the risks to patients is patient identification. The National Patient Safety Agency (NPSA) (2007) mounted a major national campaign to ensure that every hospitalised patient is issued with, and wears, an accurate and readable identity bracelet. Identification is a fundamental issue in the administration of medicines to patients in all health care institutions and is one of the factors that make medicine administration a risky activity that can result in a medication error. Developments in healthcare technologies may well help to make medicine administration and all prescribing much safer for both patients and staff in the future.

Although the administration of medicines is a key skill for many nurses, it is not the only skill inherent in medicines management for nurses. Having an understanding of anatomy, physiology, pharmacodynamics and pharmacokinetics, along with communication skills and teaching ability, are also imperative. Such knowledge and understanding do not stand still; rather they change and develop and so the skills of lifelong learning are also essential. The prevention and treatment of disease in the Western world seems to be at a crossroads, with new technologies promising much, although the delivery of this promise has been extremely slow. When it does deliver, adult nurses could be at the forefront of these advances by capitalising on technological developments. One aspect of developing technologies that will give nurses much improved medicines management skills is that arising from some of the areas of knowledge and understanding coming from genetics and the work related to genetics – that is, proteomics (Cole, 2001; Jenkins and Calzone, 2007; Pierce *et al.*, 2007). Nurses could capitalise on this to develop a further role in relation to medicines management, managing adverse drug reactions and increasing concordance.

Drivers of contemporary changes in adult nursing

As we highlighted in Chapter 1, a number of political and social drivers, including the legal requirement to reduce the hours worked by junior doctors and the redevelopment of medical staff training as a result of the Calman report (DH, 1993) have been part of a wave of influences that have changed the face of adult nursing over the past two decades. Adult nursing has changed in a way that many of the previous generations of nurses may only have dreamed of. The way in which healthcare is delivered in the UK has also evolved. These influences that have had such a major impact come from a variety of sources and suggest that change and development of the nurse's role will be ongoing. Just as the scientific discoveries of microbiology and infection control influenced nursing activity in the nineteenth century, so the newer sciences such as genetics, proteomics, nanotechnology, psychoneuroimmunology and information technology are likely to lead to developments that are currently seen only in science-fiction films. Some of these predicted developments are nearer to being adopted in mainstream nurses' work than others; however, history tells us that there is little doubt that some of these predictions and promises will 'die on the vine' while others will 'ripen and bear fruit'. This suggests that there will be some exciting developments in the future, just as there have been in the past, although the process of change seems to happen more quickly now. However, groundbreaking ideas that may impact positively on many people do not always become mainstream or can take many years to do so (Rogers, 2003). The following example from the discipline of medicine demonstrates this quite clearly. The example is a well-known story from the medical specialty of gastrointestinal surgery.

In reality Recognising *Helicobacter pylori*

This example highlights the ten or more years that it took for medicine to accept that *Helicobacter pylori* (*H. pylori*) is a bacterium that can grow freely in the extremely acidic medium of gastric juice, leading to peptic ulcers and gastric carcinoma in a large number of people. Previously there was a strong belief that because gastric juice is a strong acid (pH 1-2), the environment in the stomach was too hostile for microorganisms to grow. In the early 1980s, Drs Marshall and Warren discovered a new bacterial species and

▷

▶ *(continued)*

found that this organism grows in the stomach's gastric juice. This species appeared to be responsible for producing gastric ulcers and gastric carcinoma. (The World Health Organization has since classified *H. pylori* as a class 1 carcinogen.) When Marshall and Warren disseminated their study results to their colleagues, they met with considered indifference. Medicine eventually recognised that this perceived wisdom was incorrect, and the Drs Marshall and Warren were eventually awarded the Nobel Prize for Medicine and Physiology in 2005.

The recognition of the organism *H. pylori* and its link to peptic ulceration has had a major impact both for people with peptic ulcers and their families and for the medical specialty of gastrointestinal surgery and nursing. Previous to the discovery, many people were admitted with life-threatening haemorrhage following peptic ulceration, needed emergency gastrointestinal surgery and then required high dependency nursing care for a number of days following surgery. The advent of triple therapy (treatment with two types of antibacterial and a proton pump inhibitor) has revolutionised the lives of patients infected with *H. pylori* and changed the face of gastrointestinal surgery and nursing. Now, people describing the symptoms of peptic ulcer have a non-invasive test for *H. pylori*. Those who are infected are prescribed triple therapy, following which they are retested to confirm that the infection has been eradicated.

The acceptance that *H. pylori* was able to populate the stomach in many individuals was ignored by most influential gastrointestinal physicians and surgeons in Western medicine for many years. Since, the recognition that microorganisms can grow in gastric juice, the development of an antibiotic regime has led to much less morbidity and mortality and also a revolution in the use of surgical facilities, as comparatively few people now need emergency surgery or after-care for gastrointestinal haemorrhage as a result of peptic ulcers. This reduction in theatre time, bed occupancy and resources such as blood for transfusion has had a major impact on the roles of theatre nurses and general surgical nurses, who have seen their workload and their role change. Many general surgical beds across the UK have been lost as a result.

NURSE PRESCRIBING: HISTORICAL PERSPECTIVE

In the UK, at around the same time that Marshall and Warren were reporting the results of their experiments in Australia that led to the discovery of *Helicobacter pylori*, a report was produced in the UK investigating the role of the district nurse. This report, *Neighbourhood Nursing: A Focus for Care*, produced by a team headed by Baroness Cumberlege (DHSS, 1986), was instrumental in laying the foundations for nurse prescribing.

One of the many traditional practices that had grown up in district nursing since the inception of the NHS concerned writing and signing prescriptions. Commonly, the district nurse returned to the surgery or health centre, after seeing patients with long-term conditions in their home and requiring medication for many such patients. Frequently, it seemed to the nurse that the patient's need for medicines was urgent. A routine became established whereby the nurse returned to the surgery, wrote out a prescription, dated the prescription and left the prescription on the doctor's desk for their signature. The doctor then signed and dated the prescription. The district nurse then took the prescription to the patient's home or directly to the pharmacy. This practice begs the question, which the Cumberlege Report asked: who is actually prescribing the medication in instances such as these – the doctor or the nurse?

In reality

This practice demonstrates clearly that the doctor's signature is valuable. The nurse's experience and their understanding of the patient, condition, circumstances and possible suitable treatments are seen to be less valuable, as the nurse is able to do everything but sign the prescription. This demonstrates the power that was, and often still is, demonstrated in many interprofessional teams (medical hegemony). Examining this behaviour in more detail highlights that the legal need for a doctor to sign a prescription could be considered a means of professional protectionism used by doctors. The two discrete key skills that have always distinguished medical doctors from other health professionals is their ability to diagnose and prescribe. The ability to prescribe rests on the ability to diagnose. This, along with doctors' perceived control over life and death, is what has made doctors distinct as a profession and led society to reward them with money, power and status. Interestingly, other people probably have more control over the life and death of most people than do doctors. If you travel by car or public transport regularly, ask yourself who maintains the brakes on the vehicle. Does the mechanic have your life and death in their hands much more often than a medical doctor? Are such people rewarded by society in the same way as doctors, whether with money, power or status? This issue is raised here not to debate it but to flag up the issue of medical hegemony in the NHS that recent UK governments have attempted to challenge.

Allowing others to prescribe medicines and other treatments means doctors giving other professionals the skill of prescribing. However, if others can prescribe, does that mean that doctors are also giving away the skill of diagnosis; are the two inextricably linked (Duffin and Yu, 2002; Kmietowicz, 2003)? This begs the question that if other healthcare professionals are allowed to prescribe and therefore diagnose, then how is medicine a distinct profession and therefore worthy of higher reward in terms of money, status or power?

As a result of this enquiry into the role of the district nurse, Baroness Cumberlege (DHSS, 1986) suggested that if nurses in secondary care had the ability to prescribe medicines, then the quality of the healthcare many people received would be improved considerably. Much has been written in journals and books about the historical development of nurse prescribing, and interested readers are directed to Green (2002), Jones (1999) and McCartney and Tyner (1999). Here, we present only an overview of nurse prescribing sufficient to provide the reader with enough understanding to appreciate the context, challenges and opportunities that such a change has presented and the dilemmas and tensions that have resulted. The drivers that were influential in moving non-medical prescribing forward are summarised in Figure 17.1.

Nurse prescribing has attracted considerable interest and debate. The Home Office opened up a public consultation early in 2007 that questioned whether the range of controlled drugs that can be prescribed independently by nurse independent prescribers should be expanded and whether pharmacist independent prescribers should be permitted to independently prescribe controlled drugs (**www.homeoffice.gov.uk**). This consultation proposed to open the current restriction that allows nurse independent prescribers to prescribe 12 controlled drugs (including morphine and diamorphine), but only for specified medical conditions, primarily in palliative care. It is proposed that

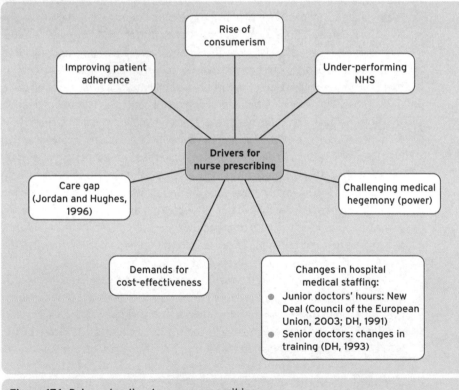

Figure 17.1 Drivers leading to nurse prescribing

nurse independent prescribers and pharmacist independent prescribers will be 'considered in the same way as doctors' (**www.homeoffice.gov.uk**). Until such a change in the law is enacted, the previous changes to the law and NHS regulations that followed the 2005 Medicines and Healthcare Regulatory Agency (MHRA) consultation (**www.mhra.gov.uk**) still stand. These allow nurse independent prescribers to prescribe any licensed medicine for any medical condition within their competence, other than controlled drugs, which are subject to the restrictions identified earlier. Following the granting of public approval to the latest consultation, nurse independent prescribers will, for the first time, be able to prescribe from the whole of the BNF. This decision has been a long time coming. The need to address the requirements of patients who fell through what Jordan and Hughes (1996) called the 'Care Gap' was first recognised officially in 1986 with the publication of the Cumberlege report (DHSS, 1986). In acute hospitals, patients frequently waited for junior doctors to prescribe medicines that were often suggested by the nurse (Stein, 1967; Stein *et al.*, 1990; Sweet and Norman, 1995). When the first trials of nurse prescribing went ahead, however, nurse prescribers in the community were prescribing mostly products that nurses in acute hospitals gave to patients without the need for a prescription and that patients could buy over the counter. In their survey of nurse prescribers prescribing from the original Nurse Prescribers Formulary, While and Biggs (2004) highlighted the dissatisfaction of these prescribers with this formulary because it did not meet their prescribing needs.

When the British Labour government came to power in 1997, it had a clear strategy to modernise the way in which the NHS delivered services to patients. Developing the roles of the nurse and nurse prescribing were part of this strategy. Nurse prescribing is inherent in the Modernising Medicine Management initiative introduced by the Audit Commission (2001) in its report *A Spoonful of Sugar*, which highlighted an increasing number of medication errors and adverse reactions and the low rate of compliance of many patients with NHS prescriptions. In order to ensure better use of medicines, the report recommended using nurse prescribing. A number of other reports and white papers that address the issue of managing long-term conditions more effectively also recommend nurse prescribing, including *The NHS Plan* (DH, 2000b), *Liberating the Talents* (DH, 2002a) and *Our Health, Our Care, Our Say: A New Direction for Community Services* (DH, 2006b). Nurse prescribing also became part of the Chief Nursing Officer's ten key roles for adult nurses.

The necessity for nurse prescribing to enable a variety of unmet patient needs for access to medicines to be tackled was given official recognition in 1986, with the publication of the Cumberlege Report. Despite a number of pilot sites demonstrating the success of nurse prescribing, there was little political will to allow the development of this role until legislation was first passed in 1992. This legislation, amended in 1994, allowed nurses to prescribe for the first time, under the Medicinal Products: Prescription by Nurses Act (1992 and amended 1994). There was much resistance from medical staff to the introduction of nurse prescribing. However, the Department of Health had to meet the new European Union directives enforcing a reduction in the working hours of junior doctors. This was a major driver in moving nurse prescribing forward more quickly, despite the opposition of many of the medical staff, and 2002 saw the introduction of independent nurse prescribing (DH, 2002b). Since the original legislation to allow nurse prescribing from the original nurse prescriber's formulary, there has been some further legislation; the changes are summarised below:

- *2002*: What was known previously as extended formulary nurse prescribing was termed nurse independent prescribing. Following the necessary training, these nurse independent prescribers could prescribe from the Nurse Prescribers Extended Formulary, which allowed the extended nurse prescriber to use certain medicines to treat a limited list of medical conditions. The medicines included:
  - all prescribable general sales list (GSL) medicines;
  - all prescribable pharmacy (P) medicines;
  - a selected list of prescription-only medicines (POM) to allow the management of:
    - minor ailments;
    - minor injuries;
    - health promotion and maintenance;
    - palliative care.
- *2003*: A list of six controlled drugs was added to the Nurse Prescribers Extended Formulary, which could be prescribed mostly for palliative care situations but also in emergency situations for myocardial infarction and trauma.
- *February 2004*: Following a change to the Misuse of Drugs Regulations 2001, the Extended Nurse Prescribers Formulary now contained a list of about 180 POMs (prescription only medicines) (plus all relevant P and GSL medicines) to treat around 80 medical conditions, including six controlled drugs for pain relief in the management of palliative care, myocardial infarction and trauma.
- *May 2006*: The formulary was extended further so that 12 controlled drugs (including diamorphine and morphine) solely for specified medical conditions could be prescribed by these nurses. Since May 2006, suitably qualified nurse independent prescribers are able to prescribe these 12 controlled drugs and any other licensed medicine for any medical condition from the rest of the BNF.

  N.B. As well as working within the law, all prescribers, both medical and non-medical, have to work within the new governance arrangements of Safer Management of Controlled Drugs (2007) (the fourth report of the Shipman Inquiry).

REQUIREMENTS FOR NURSE INDEPENDENT PRESCRIBING

In order to become a nurse independent prescriber, the nurse must be qualified in the area in which they are expected to prescribe and be an expert in their current role. The nurse must then become appropriately qualified as an independent non-medical prescriber. Once qualified, the nurse has to integrate this new area of practice into their existing role. The nursing code of conduct (NMC, 2008) encourages nurses to develop their skills and expertise in relation to their own situation. In order for a nurse to become a nurse independent prescriber, some rigid criteria have been laid down; the nurse must be a first-level registered nurse or midwife who:

- holds valid registration on the NMC professional register;
- has at least three years' post-qualification clinical experience;
- has successfully completed the nurse independent prescribing preparation programme at level 6 (degree level);
- is registered with the NMC as a nurse independent prescriber;
- has a doctor's agreement to contribute to practice preparation and post-qualifying supervision;
- has their employer's agreement for course completion, supervised practice and continuing professional development;
- has access to a prescribing budget;
- holds a post in an NHS organisation or GP practice.

To complete the programme successfully, nurse independent prescribers have to achieve the proficiencies laid down in the NMC (2006) Standards of Proficiency for Nurse and Midwife Prescribers.

SUPPLEMENTARY PRESCRIBING

From 1994, in addition to the original nurse prescribers there was a type of nurse prescriber known as 'dependent prescriber'. Working with the doctor, the two prescribers drew up a clinical management plan for the patient. This plan identifed what medicines could be prescribed, how and when dosages could be altered, and what changes in the patient's condition should lead the dependent prescriber to refer the patient to a doctor. In April 2003, however, dependent prescribing saw its name change to 'supplementary prescribing'; at the same time; the legislation permitted pharmacists to become supplementary prescribers too. Since 2005, this type of prescribing has been extended further and allows supplementary prescribers, including nurses, pharmacists, physiotherapists, podiatrists, optometrists or radiographers, to work with individual patients; however, it sets limits on their decision-making skills, as they must work in partnership with a doctor. The main principles of supplementary prescribing are as follows:

- Supplementary precribing is a voluntary partnership between an independent prescriber, who must be a doctor, and a first-level nurse or other specified healthcare professional.

- The two prescribers work together with the patient to draw up and implement a clinical management plan. (Examples of such plans are available at **www.dh.gov.uk/en/Policyandguidance/Medicinespharmacyandindustry/ Prescriptions/TheNon-MedicalPrescribingProgramme/Supplementaryprescribing/ DH_4123030.**)

- The clinical management plan sets out what medicines can be prescribed, dose changes and when the patient should be referred on.

- As long as the medicine can be legally prescribed by a doctor on the NHS there are no legal restrictions as to which drugs can be prescribed on the clinical management plan. This therefore includes unlicensed medicines and controlled drugs.

- The DH expects the scheme to be used in both primary care and the acute hospital sector of the NHS for the management of a range of long-term conditions, such as diabetes.

Further information about supplementary prescribing is available at **www.dh.gov.uk/ en/Policyandguidance/Medicinespharmacyandindustry/Prescriptions/ TheNon-MedicalPrescribingProgramme/Supplementaryprescribing/DH_4123025.**

The original nurse prescribers are still permitted to prescribe from a limited list of medicines and products contained in what was originally called the Nurse Prescribers' Formulary. This name has changed and it is now known as the Nurse Practitioners' Formulary for Community Practitioners. However, if they wish or are required to become nurse independent prescribers, these prescribers require further training. All community specialist practice preparation programmes now include the opportunity to achieve the NMC proficiencies to enable the practitioner to prescribe from this formulary.

PATIENT-SPECIFIC DIRECTIONS AND PATIENT GROUP DIRECTIONS

New terminology is being used in an attempt to clarify what has become a messy area. Department of Health and Nursing and Midwifery Council literature in relation to the supply and administration of medicines now refers to patient-specific directions (PSD), patient group directions (PGD) or medicine administration charts (DH, 2006a; NMC, 2007). The term 'patient-specific direction' refers to an instruction written for an individual patient following a consultation by an independent prescriber for a medicine or medicines to be supplied; that is, a patient-specific direction describes what was previously known as a prescription. The independent prescriber may be a doctor, nurse independent prescriber or pharmacist independent prescriber. For nurses who are administering medicines in a hospital or other institution, the instructions, written by an independent prescriber (usually a doctor) are for administration only and so are referred to as 'patient medicines administration charts' (DH, 2006a; NMC, 2007). When nurses who are not prescribers are required to supply and administer medicines to individuals from a group of patients with the same diagnosis, this is known as 'administration following patient group directions'. The DH expects patient group directions to be used in acute care to manage a different range of conditions and situations compared with those managed by non-medical prescribing. The main features of patient group directions are as follows:

- Written directions compiled by medical staff to enable nurses to give specific medication to an individual belonging to a particular patient group.
- Nurses, pharmacists and a variety of almost all qualified healthcare professionals, including ambulance paramedics and speech and language therapists, who are not prescribers, are permitted to sell, supply and administer medicines using a PGD.
- No specific training is required.
- Over the years, the legality of this form of administration has been questioned, clarified under Crown and further clarified by the DH (2000a).
- PGDs are defined as the 'supply and administration of a named medicine in identified clinical situations' for the diagnostic group of patients identified.
- The PGD requires local agreement and is only for local use.
- Each PGD must be drawn up by senior medical staff and pharmacists.
- The PGD must be approved by the appropriate NHS trust board (NMC, 2007).
- Settings where PGDs are commonly used include emergency situations, minor injury clinics, out-of-hours services, family planning clinics and immunisation clinics.

Comprehensive information about all aspects of non-medical prescribing is available in *Medicines Matters* (DH, 2006a). This presents the position related to 'the prescribing, supply and administration of medicines to support the development of new roles or service redesign' as well as the development that is being proposed around non-medical prescribing.

BENEFITS OF NURSE PRESCRIBING

A number of benefits have been ascribed to nurse prescribing since its implementation. Benefits include the following:

- It offers greater continuity of care for many patients.
- It ensures that a service user is more likely to be involved in their own care management.
- Not having to wait for a doctor means faster access to care.
- Opportunistic health promotions are taken advantage of more frequently.
- Increased patient satisfaction is noted.
- There is increased concordance.
- Improved communication is found (Luker *et al.*, 1997).

Nurses can be rightly proud that many positives have accrued from nurse prescribing for patients, but it is important to recognise that not all of the evidence that has supported its continued development is particularly robust. Non-medical prescribing is an important challenge to the role of the doctor and consequently the power of the medical profession. It is interesting to note that the evidence that the Department of Health has used to support the implementation and continuing rollout of non-medical prescribing is based on so few research studies, many of which use a qualitative methodology. In addition, much of this evidence is from the qualitative end of the research spectrum and is not generalisable. This was the very same reason that held back the widespread implementation of nurse prescribing in the early days of the nurse prescribing pilots following the Cumberlege report in 1986. Perhaps this illustrates that often nurses and their roles are very much at the mercy of their political masters.

The evidence that is readily available is limited and not robust. A survey that was part of a study into the effectiveness of nurse prescribing (Luker *et al.*, 1998) explored patients' experiences of nurse prescribing. The authors reported that the patients were very positive about nurse prescribing, but the study was qualitative and consequently the researchers used a very small convenience sample to collect their data. The patients in this sample were both frequent users of the nursing services that were examined in these studies and regular users of the nurse prescribers who were under observation. Thus, although it is a useful study that highlights user experiences, by its nature its data are not generalisable. Another study frequently cited in support of nurse prescribing is that of Brooks *et al.* (2001), whose study used an even smaller sample than that of Luker *et al.*, (1998); in addition, all of the patients were chosen by the nurse prescribers. However, Luker *et al.* (1998) identified that some patients had limited expectations of nurse prescribers, whereas a later survey by Latter and Courtenay (2004) highlighted that some patients had unmet information needs about their medicines following their interaction with a nurse prescriber. This is a somewhat surprising finding, given that the DH suggests that the opposite is true and that nurse prescribers are better than doctors at meeting patients' information needs about their medicines.

PRINCIPLES TO GUIDE NURSE PRESCRIBERS

In order to help nurse independent prescribers to develop their new skills a number of support mechanisms are available, not least of which is supervision and mentorship from a doctor. Exploring this support is not appropriate to the readership that this book is aimed at; however, the National Prescribing Centre has identified a set of seven principles to follow to assist nurse prescribers' decision-making skills (**www.npc.co.uk/nurse_bulletins/sign1.2.htm**). These principles are discussed here as they can be used as a framework to aid your thinking and help you to develop your medicines management skills.

Related knowledge Patient education

Herxheimer (1976) presented a questionnaire for patients to use in their consulations with doctors so that patients could find out as much as possible about their medicines. Although the questionnaire was designed for patients three decades ago it is still relevant to nurses, nurse prescribers, other healthcare professionals and patients. It is useful to develop the habit of using the questions when you are involved in medicines management. This helps you to reflect on the knowledge that a patient needs when taking medication and also acts as a guide to identify your learning needs. The questionnaire asks the following questions:

- What is it for and for how long?
- What kind of tablets are they? How do you expect them to help? How should they be taken? Will the patient be able to tell if they are working? If so, how?
- How important are they?
- How important is it for the patient to take them?
- What is likely to happen if he/she doesn't take them?
- Any adverse effects?
- Do the medicines have any other effects that the patient should look out for?
- Do they ever cause any trouble?
- Can he/she drive whilst taking them?
- Are they all right with other medicines that they take?

The seven principles of good prescribing follow a step-pyramid model (Figure 17.2), which demonstrates the hierarchical order of thinking that nurse prescribers should use. By using this pyramid to guide their decision-making, the nurse prescriber can be certain that any prescription they write is not only effective and safe but also acceptable to the patient.

The Audit Commission (2001) report *A Spoonful of Sugar* was groundbreaking at the time, as it was the first national audit of the medicines service in the NHS. As a result, it was the first national report to highlight the need for nurse prescribing to promote the better use of medicines in the NHS. The report proposed that nurse prescribing would help to both increase patient concordance and reduce the NHS medicines bill. The report was also the first in the UK to bring to attention the large amount of public money spent by the NHS on medicines that were prescribed and dispensed but not actually used by large numbers of patients. It also made public that, as in other Western heathcare systems, adverse drug reactions not only were very common but also had a substantial impact on concordance. The likelihood of medication errors being much more common than was previously understood was also raised publicly in this report for the first time.

In reality Nurse prescribing: deskilling doctors or 'upskilling' nurses

For a considerable number of years, there has been an ongoing debate about how nursing should be developed. Nurse prescribing is a good example to demonstrate how this debate is polarised. One argument is that the nursing profession should expand the role of the nurse by developing nursing skills, while the other is that nursing should be extended to incorporate other skills that may have been considered to be part of the role of other healthcare professionals. So, is nurse prescribing really about expanding the role of the nurse and consequently providing a greater understanding of the profession/discipline that is nursing, which is how other professions develop? Or is it about taking on the work of other healthcare professionals in an attempt to meet political targets? Looking at nurse prescribing from an historical perspective tells us that it reflects the experiences of many of the developments of nursing roles, as these have often been as a result of passing on the work of junior hospital doctors to nurses. For example, measuring and recording blood pressure and pulse was once a key diagnostic skill of a doctor, and nurses were not allowed to do this. Today, such assessment is often the role of a healthcare assistant. However, what has been lost along the way in this delegation of tasks is the skill of interpretation. Measuring and recording blood pressure and pulse cannot be seen as isolated tasks, as they are part of the skill of diagnosis. If the healthcare professional taking these measurements does not know how to interpret the readings because they have no understanding of disease processes or homeostasis, then this puts the patient at risk, and so much so that the National Institute for Health and Clinical Excellence now recommends that NHS trusts use variable scoring systems so that staff can see when a patient's condition is deteriorating. Is nurse independent prescribing comparable to this scenario? Prescribing is not an isolated task either, needing the ability to diagnose along with a sound understanding of physiology, pathophysiology and pharmacology (McGavock, 2000). The question that must be asked is whether independent prescribers are truly adequately prepared for their new role or whether a number of problems will come to light in the future, as we have seen with the delegating of measuring and recording blood pressure and pulse. In relation to nursing, this leaves us with a number of tensions, including:

- Nurse prescribing is often seen to be of a higher status or value than many of the other roles that nurses have always fulfilled.

- While experienced nurses are taking on doctors' roles with less training and remuneration, who is carrying out the work that these nurses are unavailable to do or no longer have time for?

- If nurses can diagnose and prescribe following minimal extra training, why train doctors?

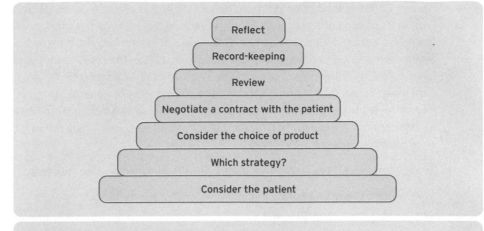

Figure 17.2 Prescribing pyramid (after Anon, 1999)

MEDICATION ERRORS

> ## Personal and professional development 17.1
>
> If you are a driver, take a few minutes to think about a journey that you drive regularly, for example from home to work every morning. Now think about the last time you drove this journey. How much of this trip did you remember when you arrived? Did you arrive and then later have little or no recollection of how you got there?

Incidence and types of medication errors

Medication error has been identified as the most common threat to patient safety in healthcare today (Neale *et al.*, 2001). A number of studies have indicated that medication error is a patient safety issue in all hospitals. To highlight how common this safety issue appears to be, two research studies will be used as examples in this chapter. These studies reveal the frequency of medication errors and the form that these errors take. One of the studies is that by Bruce and Wong (2001) (see **www.saferhealthcare.org.uk**), which found a 25% error rate when they observed nurses preparing and administering intravenous medicines in a medical admissions ward. This result is quite alarming, as it means that a quarter of all of the medicines drawn up and administered intravenously, while the researchers were observing, were wrong for some reason. Bruce and Wong (2001) observed that 15% of the administrations were wrong because the medicines were injected at the wrong time. The second study concluded that, in a hospital of 400 beds, at least one patient experiences a potentially serious drug error every day (Taxis and

Barber, 2003). In their observational study of 113 nurses and one doctor in the intensive care units of two London hospitals, one a teaching hospital and the other non-teaching, Taxis and Barber found that of the 1042 doses of prescribed intravenous medicines administered to 106 patients, there was an error in 49% of the cases observed. This is not what members of the public, users of the NHS or healthcare professionals expect of the care given in any clinical area. Although the studies are not generalisable, because the samples used were too small, they do pinpoint the possibility that mistakes around medications are much more common than was once supposed, which may prevent the public from having confidence in the service.

Typical errors found in Taxis and Barber's (2003) study include the following:

- Preparing the wrong drug
- Selecting the wrong solvent
- Giving a bolus injection too quickly
- Giving up to five times the prescribed dose of an anticoagulant
- Failing to have spare supplies of adrenaline (epinephrine) to hand when intravenous medicines are administered.

Personal and professional development 17.2

Nursing has long had a set of 'rules' to guide nurses when they administer medicines, often referred to as 'rights'. To ensure that no medication errors ever happen and that medicine administration is safe, the recommendation is that nurses follow these rules or rights. Can you list these rules or rights?

Just before Bruce and Wong (2001) and Taxis and Barber (2003) published their studies, the DH (2000a) commissioned a report that used computer modelling to estimate how often a medication error would occur. This report estimated that in an average-size NHS teaching hospital of 600 beds that had a 99% error-free ordering, dispensing and administration system for medicines delivery, some 4000 drug errors would happen every year. To put this into perspective that means 6.666 medication errors per hospital bed per year (or one error every 2 months). If medication errors are potentially so common even with a virtually error-free ordering, dispensing and administration system, then it behoves us to ask two questions: what must the incidence be in the real world? And, as a nurse working in a hospital ward, when will an error happen to you? After all, how many organisations anywhere in the world operate systems that are 99% error-free?

The Audit Commission (2001) identified errors in prescribing and administration as a major preventable cause of death and illness in UK hospitals. The financial costs of the medication errors made in NHS hospitals were estimated to be between £200 million and £400 million a year (DH, 2004). However, there are other costs to be mindful of too: those borne by the patient and their family and friends; sadly, some patients pay the ultimate cost – with their life. Medication errors can also affect the staff involved and may have a large impact on the healthcare professional implicated, leading to guilt, lowered self-esteem and confidence, the possibility of losing their job and the possibility of legal prosecution.

The National Patient Safety Agency was set up to raise awareness of and make improvements to patient safety as a whole in the NHS. It established the National Reporting and Learning System (NRLS) database so that accurate data could be collected nationally. This has enabled a number of NHS trusts to add their experiences of patient safety issues to the national database, so, for the first time, helping to identify the common patterns and contributing factors (NPSA, 2005). Although a large number of NHS trusts did not contribute any information when the first data-collection exercise took place, more trusts subsequently contributed to the following year's collection, which was being analysed at the time of writing. The majority of incidents reported to the NRLS are from acute NHS hospitals rather than primary or secondary care, and no data have been sought from private healthcare establishments. A more detailed analysis of these incidents is presented in Table 17.1. It is important to note that the NPSA states that these data come from only a small number of acute hospitals. The reported medication errors are shown as being involved in 8.6% of patient safety incidents. This is much more frequent than infection control incidents, identified as compromising 0.9% of the total. On the basis of these data, it is much more likely that a patient will suffer a medication error than develop a healthcare-acquired infection, and yet much of the adverse publicity about safety issues in the NHS is focused primarily on infection.

Rather than blame individuals ('operator error'), the NPSA looked for other causes. In the ongoing analysis of the data reported to the NRLS to establish the cause of medication errors, the NPSA is trying to establish the systems that must be changed in order to prevent future occurrences. One of the possible causes that is relevant to both nurses and medication administration is that of automatic behaviour.

Behaviour can become automatic in both our personal life and our professional life. Think back to the earlier activity that asked you to consider driving. Driving is very much taken for granted, but it is a risky activity, just like medicines management. Most people remember very little of a familiar journey because behaviours such as driving a very familiar route encourage what Schon (1991) calls 'over learning'. We become locked into the routine of everyday activities and do not engage fully in the thinking process. When we transfer this type of thinking to our professional life, we can become insensitive to a situation because it is so familiar. Many nurses in acute hospitals still use a medicine or drug round to administer medicines to patients, using a medicine trolley. In nursing, this type of medicine administration is an example of 'over learning' and it is reinforced by the culture of nursing, which frequently empha-

Table 17.1 Reported incident types in acute hospitals

	Number	% of total
Patient accident	30063	44.6
Medication	5797	8.6
Documentation (e.g. records, identification)	3746	5.6
Consent, communication, confidentiality	2894	4.3
Access, admission, transfer, discharge	3863	5.7
Clinical assessment (e.g. diagnosis, scans, tests)	3065	4.6
Infrastructure (e.g. staffing, facilities, environment)	4526	6.7
Medical device/equipment	2709	4.0
Treatment, procedure	6632	9.8
Implementation of care and ongoing monitoring/review	1352	2.0
Disruptive, aggressive behaviour	440	0.7
Infection control	624	0.9
Patient abuse (by staff/third party)	129	0.2
Other	1504	2.2
Total	**67344**	**100.0**

Source: reports in the NRLS database up to 31 March 2005,
www.npsa.nhs.uk/site/media/documents/1269_PSO_Report_FINAL.pdf

sises medicine administration to be a task or procedure. Many nursing textbooks focus on the correct procedure that ensures, for example, that the correct dose of prescribed tablets is dispensed into a container and given to the correct patient at the correct time. These are often referred to as the 'five rights' of medicine administration, but they omit much of the process that should be taking place. The 'five rights' are as follows:

- Right patient
- Right medicine
- Right dose
- Right route
- Right time.

Advantages and disadvantages of the 'five rights' of medicine administration

For several decades, student nurses have been taught to follow the five 'golden rules' or 'rights' of medicine administration in a bid to ensure safe practice. In addition, many qualified nurses use the same mantra to help them practise safely. These five rights are still found in many nursing textbooks today. However, using these 'rights' can lull one into Schon's 'over learning' situation described earlier. So, instead of providing safe medicines management practice for patients and nurses, it actually offers only a sense of protection. Using the 'rights' can encourage automatic behaviour and lead many nurses to believe that their practice must be safe simply because they have followed the procedure.

Rules such as the 'five rights' were originally established in nursing help overcome operator error. Introducing rules such as these and encouraging people to use them was thought to enable anyone to do their job properly – in other words, for a nurse to become proficient. Baker and Napthine (1994), among others, have long argued that such rules can lead to ritualistic behaviour – that is, Schon's (1991) 'over learning', which can then lead to error. However, there is a need for the individual to go beyond this kind of behaviour. Creating an understanding in all nurses that all that medication administration consists of is the five simple rules instils in many nurses a reliance on only the motor skills of 'giving out the tablets'. The administration of medicines is a psychomotor skill (a 'doing skill'), but, as with other psychomotor skills, in nursing the 'psycho' ('of the mind') part is frequently overlooked. Medicine administration is both a 'psycho' and a 'motor' skill – that is, a thinking and a doing skill. Cognitive skills such as observation, listening, analysis, critical judgement, clinical judgement, decision-making, teaching and interpersonal skills are often unrecognised and consequently undervalued (Figure 17.3). But these are all skills needed to help the patient under-stand the purpose of the medication, why the medication has been prescribed, why they should take it, what the adverse effects are and how long they will have to take it for. Sadly, even today, after a number of years of communication skills being a key part of the pre-registration nursing curriculum, users of NHS services often complain of a lack of good communication. It seems that interpersonal skills are still interpreted as simply talking to people rather than listening and then responding appropriately; sometimes, talking is inappropriate. Recognising this enables nurses to acknowledge that medicine administration is, as the NMC (2007) emphasises, more than the task. Schon (1991) suggests that reflective practice is the ideal way to manage 'over learn-ing' and to help professionals be more conscious of the cognitive skills that are often not acknowledged.

Many nurses seem to engage in task-oriented, ritualistic behaviour. Ritualistic practice is often reinforced unconsciously by our nursing culture, which values the nurse who is seen to be proficient (the 'good nurse') over the nurse who, at times, seems unable to meet the demands of task-focused practice; the latter nurse is then seen as ineffi-cient (the 'bad nurse') (Alavi and Cattoni, 1995). As a result, nursing culture in the NHS still classifies nurses who make medication errors as 'bad nurses', as their ineffi-ciency led to an error. The DH (2000a, 2004) and the Audit Commission (2001) suggest that the systems approach to error management has replaced the system of blame culture and disciplinary actions that the NHS previously used when a medica-tion error occurred. Traditionally, in the NHS when medicine errors have occurred, nurse managers supported by much of the nursing literature have put the blame

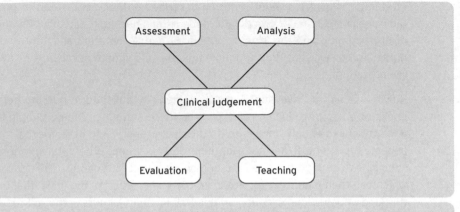

Figure 17.3 Key skills in medicine administration

squarely on the shoulders of the nurse who administered the medications. This is known as a person-centred approach to managing risk, or a blame culture, and it means admonishing, disciplining and possibly dismissing the nurse for making the mistake, regardless of the circumstances when the mistake occurred. However, the DH (2000a) and the NPSA (2005) state that in hospitals the administration of medicines is a multisystem, multiprofessional process: doctors write the majority of prescriptions, pharmacists and pharmacy technicians dispense the medications, and portering staff deliver the medicines to the clinical areas. Blaming the nurse involved acknowledges only that the nurse made a mistake (operator error), but the picture is usually wider and more complex than that. Many nurses work in wards or units where they perform complex tasks, and they are seldom able to carry out a medicine round uninterrupted; they often have to multi-task and use inadequate equipment. A standard-issue medicine trolley is often too small to hold all of the medicines and related equipment needed, and its poor design fails to help the nurse identify the contents. Medicine bottles and packs look very similar and are all identified with white labels. In addition, many medicines have similar names, for example:

- penicillin (an antibiotic) and penicillamine (an anti-inflammatory);
- tramadol (an analgesic) and trazodone (an antidepressant/anxiolytic);
- co-codamol (an analgesic) and co-dydramol (another analgesic).

The NHS is moving away from a blame culture to a systems approach of managing safety (DH, 2000a, 2004; NPSA, 2005). The DH (2000a) and Anderson and Webster (2001) suggest that medication errors are most likely to happen because of systems failure. An often-cited example of an organisation that has a different approach to dealing with errors or near-errors is that of the airline industry. This industry works on the principle of the 'law of large numbers'; that is, if we perform even a low-risk behaviour often enough, eventually something will go wrong and an accident or mistake will result. Consequently, the systems in place in any organisation should be those that reduce this risk of error to the minimum. In order to examine risky work environments in any organisation, it is recommended that the systems in place in all organisations should be reviewed regularly.

Anderson and Webster (2001) remind us that systems are a combination of:

- design;
- equipment;
- procedures;
- operators;
- supplies;
- environment.

Personal and professional development 17.3

Identify a clinical area that you have worked in where medicine administration was undertaken by nurses. In relation to the medicines administration practice that you have observed, consider all of the factors highlighted by Anderson and Webster (2001). From your observations in this clinical area, list how safe you consider each of the relevant factors to be for the administration of medicines. In relation to the medicines administration observed, list some alternative practices that could be used in order to reduce these risks and make a safer environment.

MAINTAINING PATIENT SAFETY

Ensuring patient safety is a key role in the administration of medicines. However, evidence from the UK and other Western healthcare systems suggests that the nature of the healthcare environment and the fact that healthcare professionals are human beings and therefore fallible means that medicine administration has the potential to be a very risky activity.

There are a number of practices that improve patient safety in general and medication errors in particular, such as ensuring that each patient wears a correctly completed identification bracelet. The NPSA (2005) and Vincent (2006) have demonstrated clearly that other practices help to reduce the risk of medication errors for patients and healthcare professionals, including the following:

- Patient self-administration
- Uninterrupted medicine administration to individual patients

- Colour-coding of packaging
- Standardised packaging
- Prefilled syringes and prefilled individualised tablet containers
- Using barcodes, scanners and Wi-Fi.

Building a Safer NHS (DH, 2004) gives a variety of recommendations to ensure a safe environment for users of the NHS. In relation to medicines, it offers the following suggestions for good practice by nurses:

- When a syringe is used to administer liquid medicine, an oral syringe rather than a syringe designed for injection use should be used.
- Never take oral medicine in a syringe and intravenous medicines to the patient's bedside at the same time.
- The distal end of all lines should be labelled in order to ensure that the site of access for medicine administration can be identified.
- Staff must ensure that they receive training to use infusion devices.
- Use infusion devices only for the purpose for which they are designed.
- Always confirm the route of administration during the checking process (DH, 2004).

The NPSA also provides a series of aids and resources to help healthcare professionals to improve patient safety, particularly with regard to the areas of medicine administration that they have identified as high risk, such as anticoagulant medicines and liquid medicines (**www.npsa.nhs.uk/health/alerts**).

CONCLUSION

Exploring two of the key contemporary issues influencing medicine management for nurses has shown that a number of changes have taken place in the NHS since its inception. These changes have included major developments in the role of the nurse. Perhaps the most contentious of these developments has been that of non-medical prescribing, which has resulted in nurse independent prescribers being permitted to prescribe the widest range of medicines of all non-medical prescribers. As well as increased accountability, this role brings with it an increased risk of medication error. Until recently, the risks of medication error for nurses were as a result of their involvement with medication administration; however, for the small number of nurses who are able to prescribe independently, there are now added risks. This chapter has identified that patient safety is an important part of the nurse's role and clearly identified that ensuring a patient's safety while administrating medicines means not only having a sound understanding of the medicines used but also having systems in place that support a safe working environment.

Quick reminder

✔ Many of the changes in the roles of nurses are implemented by the government of the day in an attempt to deliver its healthcare agenda.

✔ Medicines management is a key skill that nurses need in order to help people use their medicines safely and effectively.

✔ Since 1992 a central government driver has been to increase the number of prescribers in order to cope with this need for effective medicines management.

✔ The introduction of non-medical prescribers (independent or supplementary) has been the mainstay of this policy.

✔ Nurses who are not prescribers may supply and administer medicines to particular categories of patients by following a distinct set of instructions - patient group directions.

✔ Nurses still administer medicines to individual patients following written instructions - patient-specific directions (previously known as prescriptions).

✔ There has been increasing concern about the risk of medication errors.

✔ The National Patient Safety Agency's analysis of the data reported by NHS trusts highlights clearly that medication errors can occur at any point in the process and therefore can happen when prescribing, dispensing or administering medicines.

✔ In order to ensure patient safety, nurses should be uninterrupted when preparing and administering medicines.

✔ The administration of medicines is much more than just the task; it also includes assessment, analysis, evaluation and teaching.

✔ Encouraging more patient self-administration of medicines would ensure greater patient safety.

REFERENCES

Alavi C and Cattoni J (1995) Good nurse, bad nurse. *Journal of Advanced Nursing* **21**, 344-349.

Anderson D J and Webster C S (2001) A systems approach to the reduction of medication error on the hospital ward. *Journal of Advanced Nursing* **35**, 34-41.

Anon (1999) *Nurse Precsribing Bulletin* **1**, 1. Liverpool: National Prescribing Centre.

Audit Commission (2001) *A Spoonful of Sugar: Medicines Management in NHS Hospitals.* Wetherby: Audit Commission Publications.

Baker H and Napthine R (1994) Nurse and medication. Part 6: rituals and workloads - medication errors. *Australian Journal of Nursing* **2**, 34-36.

Brooks N, Otway C and Rashid C (2001) Nurse prescribing: what do patients think? *Nursing Standard* **15**, 33-38.

Bruce J and Wong I (2001) Parenteral drug administration errors by nursing staff in an acute medical admission ward during day duty. *Drug Safety* **24**, 855-862.

Cole R C, Jr (2001) Impact of the 'new science' of genomics. *Healthcare Quarterly* **5**, 87-90.

Council of the European Union (2003) Directive 2003/88/EC of the European Parliament and of the Council of 4 November 2003.

Department of Health (DH) (1991) *Hours of Work of Doctors in Training: the New Deal*. London: The Stationery Office.

Department of Health (DH) (1993) *Hospital Doctors: Training for the Future*. London: The Stationery Office.

Department of Health (1998) *Review of the Prescribing, Supply and Administration of Medicines: Second Crown Report*. London: The Stationery Office.

Department of Health (DH) (2000a) *An Organization With a Memory*. London: The Stationery Office.

Department of Health (2002b) *The NHS Plan: A Plan for Investment, a Plan for Reform*. London: The Stationery Office.

Department of Health (2002a) *Liberating the Talents: Helping Primary Care Trusts and Nurses Deliver the NHS Plan*. London: The Stationery Office.

Department of Health (2002b) *Developing Key Roles for Nurses and Midwifes: A Guide for Managers*. London: The Stationery Office.

Department of Health (DH) (2004) *Building a Safer NHS for Patients: Improving Medication Safety*. London: The Stationery Office.

Department of Health (DH) (2006a) *Medicines Matters: A Guide to Mechanisms for the Prescribing, Supply and Administration of Medicines*. London: The Stationery Office.

Department of Health (DH) (2006b) *Our Health, Our Care, Our Say: A New Direction for Community Services*. London: The Stationery Office.

Department of Health and Social Security (DHSS) (1986) *Neighbourhood Nursing: A Focus for Care – Report of the Community Nursing Review*. London: Her Majesty's Stationery Office.

Duffin C and Yu R (2002) Doctor's dissent. *Nursing Standard* **16**, 2212-2213.

Green J (2002) Development of the nurse prescribing initiative. In: Humphries J and Green J (eds) *Nurse Prescribing*. Basingstoke: Palgrave.

Hallett C (2007) Editorial: a gallop through history – nursing in social context. *Journal of Clinical Nursing* **16**, 429-430.

Herxheimer A (1976) Sharing the responsibility for treatment. *Lancet* **308**, 1294.

Jenkins J and Calzone K A (2007) Establishing the essential nursing competencies for genetics and genomics. *Journal of Nursing Scholarship* **39**, 10-16.

Jones M (1999) *Nurse Prescribing: Politics to Practice*. Edinburgh: Baillière Tindall/RCN.

Jordan S and Hughes D (1996) Bioscience knowledge and the health professions: has professional monopoly created a care gap. *Social Sciences in Health* **2**, 80-84.

Kmietowicz Z (2003) Doctors struggle to define the essence of being doctors. *British Medical Journal* **326**, 1352.

Latter S and Courtenay M (2004) Effectiveness of nurse prescribing: a review of the literature. *Journal of Clinical Nursing* **13**, 26-32.

Luker K, Austin L, Hogg C, *et al*. (1997) *Evaluation of Nurse Prescribing: Final Report*. Liverpool and York: University of Liverpool and University of York.

Luker K, Austin L and Hogg C (1998) Nurse patient relationships: the context of nurse prescribing. *Journal of Advanced Nursing* **27**, 235-242.

McCartney W and Tyner S (1999) Nurse prescribing: radicalism or tokenism. *Journal of Advanced Nursing* **29**, 348-354.

McGavock H (2000) My grave concern over nurse prescribing. *Prescriber* **11**, 45.

National Patient Safety Agency (NPSA) (2007) Standardising wristbands improves patient safety. Safer practice notice no. 24. London: National Patient Safety Agency.

National Patient Safety Agency (NPSA) (2005) *Building a Memory: Preventing Harm, Reducing Risks and Improving Patient Safety*. London: National Patient Safety Agency.

Nursing and Midwifery Council (NMC) (2006) *Standards of Proficiency for Nurse and Midwife Prescribers*. London: Nursing and Midwifery Council.

Nursing and Midwifery Council (NMC) (2007) *Standards for Medicines Management*. London: Nursing and Midwifery Council.

Nursing and Midwidery Council (NMC) (2008) *The Code: Standards of conduct, performance and ethics for nurses and midwives*. London: Nursing and Midwifery Council.

Neale G, Woloshynowych M and Vincent C (2001) Exploring the cause of adverse events in NHS hospital practice. *Journal of the Royal Society of Medicine* **94**, 322-330.

Pierce J D, Fakhari M, Works K V and Pierce J T (2007) Understanding proteomics. *Nursing and Health Sciences* **9**, 54-60.

Rogers E (2003) *Diffusion of Innovations*, 5th edn. New York: Free Press.

Schon D A (1991) *The Reflective Practitioner: How Professionals Think in Action*. Aldershot: Avebury.

Stein L I (1967) The doctor-nurse game. *Archives of General Psychiatry* **16**, 669-703.

Stein L I, Watts D T and Howell T (1990) The doctor-nurse game revisited. *New England Journal of Medicine* **322**, 546-549.

Sweet S J and Norman I J (1995) The nurse-doctor relationship: a selective literature review. *Journal of Advanced Nursing* **22**, 165-169.

Taxis K and Barber N (2003) Ethnographic study of incidence and severity of intravenous drug errors. *British Medical Journal* **326**, 684-686.

Vincent C (2006) *Patient Safety*. Edinburgh: Elsevier Churchill Livingstone.

While A E and Biggs K S M (2004) Benefits and challenges of nurse prescribing. *Journal of Advanced Nursing* **45**, 559-567.

Using medicines to relieve pain

ANALGESIC AGENTS USED

Type of pain		Examples of pain	Analgesia	Uses and effects
Short-term	Mild	Headache Dysmenorrhoea	Non-narcotics	Available over the counter, or may be prescribed by nurse or doctor
			Aspirin, ibuprofen	Inhibit prostaglandin production
			Paracetamol	Acts centrally on CNS
	Severe	Postoperative pain	NSAIDs (e.g. diclofenac)	Where risk of respiratory problems or addiction
		Trauma Myocardial infarction Renal colic	Morphine, diamorphine, pethidine (artificial), pentazocine, dihydrocodeine	Opioids (controlled drugs) act centrally on CNS Problems: tolerance/addiction, may cloud consciousness, drowsiness, nausea, vomiting, constipation, depression of respiratory function
Long-term	Mild	Frozen shoulder Chronic degenerative disease, e.g. arthritis	NSAIDs (mainly paracetamol and combination of paracetamol and another, e.g. co-codamol)	
	Severe	Chronic degenerative disease, e.g. arthritis	Sustained-release morphine	Symptom relief
		Life-threatening illness such as cancer or progressive neurological disease	Adjuvants, e.g. tricyclic antidepressants	Frequency and pattern of dosage according to WHO analgesic ladder Hospice care – Macmillan nurse Syringe driver or intravenous minibag PCA

CNS, central nervous system; NSAID, non-steroidal anti-inflammatory drug; PCA, patient-controlled analgesia.

OTHER MEDICINES USED

Type of medicine	Examples	Notes
Amnesics	Diazepam – minor surgical procedures, endoscopy	May need cooperative patient
	Nitrous oxide (Entonox®) before painful procedures	
Specific	Trigeminal neuralgia – carbamazepine	Anticonvulsant, but also blocks the trigeminal nerve pathways
	Angina – GTN	Symptom relief only
	Migraine – sumatriptan	Specific antimigraine drug
Steroid	Where pain is caused by inflammatory process, e.g. arthritis, shingles	
	Terminal illness – beneficial effects, e.g. wellbeing, increased appetite	
Local anaesthetics	EMLA cream Throat lozenges Nerve block for dental work	Careful timing for maximum effect before procedures
Phenol	Severe cancer pain	Destroys nerve and therefore prevents pain transmission
		Used when other methods are ineffective
NSAIDs used for local effect	Aspirin used as gargle Throat lozenges	To relieve sore throats
	Ibuprofen in creams	Muscle pain

GTN, glyceryl trinitrate; NSAID, non-steroidal anti-inflammatory drug.

Infection

Antibiotics and antibacterials are used very commonly in the UK today. There are probably very few readers of this book who have never been prescribed one of these types of medicine. It seems pertinent to explore these drug groups here, because although they are commonly used they are not without their problems.

THE NATURE OF INFECTION

Mera (1997) writes that humans probably have more microorganisms than cells in and on their bodies. Every one of us is a host to a whole range of microorganisms, most of which are bacteria. These bacteria are commonly found in the oropharynx, in the gastrointestinal tract and on the skin. Other microorganisms that can inhabit the human body include viruses, fungi, protozoa and prions. Microorganisms that live in or on the human body are known as normal flora or commensals. Under normal conditions, commensals present little risk to the host. However, if the commensals move or are moved from their preferred site to another site in or on the body, and the individual is immunocompromised, the microorganism is extremely virulent or the microorganisms are present in great numbers, then the risk of developing an infectious disease is highly likely. The consequences of this can be fatal, and even in the twenty-first century in the UK infection is still an important cause of morbidity and mortality (Wickens and Wade, 2004).

Antibacterial agents are commonly prescribed to treat infections that are acquired in hospitals and the community. However, overzealous use of antibacterials is implicated in the current growth of a number of highly publicised healthcare-acquired infections (HCAIs), including methicillin-resistant *Staphylococcus aureus* (MRSA), a bacterium that is resistant to (unaffected by) the antibacterial drug methicillin. Plowman *et al.* (2001) suggest that some 15–30% of all HCAIs in the NHS could be prevented.

Since 2001, when an Audit Commission (2000) report (cited in Plowman *et al.*, 2001) highlighted that HCAIs were of grave concern, a number of guidelines and reports have been published that attempt to improve the situation (CHAI, 2005, 2006; DH, 2002, 2003, 2005, 2006a, b, c; Pratt *et al.*, 2007). However, at the time of writing, although there is some evidence of a small amount of improvement in the MRSA morbidity and mortality statistics, little seems to have changed (HIS and ICNA, 2006), despite the best efforts of many NHS staff. It should be noted that HCAIs affect all healthcare institutions, although to date the only robust national statistics that have been collected and made public are those for NHS institutions.

There has also been a rise in the number of antimicrobial-resistant microorganisms. This makes HCAIs much more difficult to treat effectively and efficiently and also results in higher costs to the taxpayer because of longer hospital stays and greater patient morbidity and mortality. The reasons for this are many, but they are rarely articulated clearly. The morbidity and mortality rate of HCAIs in the NHS is much higher than that in other Western countries and is still rising (Crowcroft *et al.*, 2004; Pellowe, 2007). This increasing rate is due to organisational, staff and patient factors.

Organisational factors include:

- high pace of patient throughput (the NHS regularly boasts about treating more patients more quickly);
- high bed occupancy rates (NHS nurses joke about beds never getting a chance to cool before the next patient is ensconced);
- large numbers of patients being 'boarded out' and moved between wards;
- multiple occupancy patient rooms/areas (there is a long-held belief by many DH and NHS staff that patients like sharing a bedroom, living room and washing and toilet facilities with a number of strangers, often of both sexes, and that it provides much-needed support);
- inadequate ventilation systems;
- lack of sufficient and adequate isolation areas;
- insufficient and/or poorly sited handwashing facilities;
- lack of sufficient high-quality cleaning staff and systems (Pellowe, 2007).

Staff factors include:

- poor hygiene practices, such as poor handwashing and person–person transmission;
- inadequately understood infection-prevention behaviours, particularly in relation to insertion and handling of invasive medical devices;
- strong beliefs in the ability of antimicrobials to effectively treat all infections;
- high standards of infection control practices being given low priority (Pellowe, 2007).

Patient factors include:

- large numbers of very ill people who are to a greater or lesser degree immunocompromised being cared for;
- frequent usage of invasive medical devices, such as urinary catheters and intravenous cannulae, ensures easy access for many infecting organisms, such as *Staphylococcus epidermis*, whose ability to colonise plastic leads to localised and systemic infection following insertion (Pellowe, 2007).

DEFINING ANTIBIOTICS AND ANTIBACTERIALS

Although we commonly refer to all drugs used to prevent or treat infection as 'antibiotics', this is technically inaccurate. Strictly speaking, antibiotics are 'substances produced by some micro-organisms that kill or inhibit the growth of other micro-organisms' (Rang *et al.*, 2003). An antibiotic is thus a naturally occurring substance, and this reflects the history of the development of this group of drugs. However, many of the medicines that are referred to as antibiotics in clinical practice should actually be called 'antibacterials' because they are produced synthetically rather than occurring naturally. All antibiotics are antibacterial drugs, but not all antibacterials are antibiotics.

The term 'antimicrobial' is used to include; the antibiotics, antibacterials, antiviral drugs and antifungal agents (SMAC, 1998). Antibiotics and antibacterials are suitable only if the patient has a bacterial infection. If an infection is caused by a virus, an antiviral medication may be required and prescribed.

Antibacterial drugs can assert their effects in one of two ways: they may be bacteriostatic (e.g. sulphonamides, tetracyclines), or they may be bactericidal (e.g. penicillins, cephalosporins). Bacteriostatic medicines rely upon the body's defence mechanisms: they inhibit the growth and development of bacteria but do not totally destroy the bacteria, and therefore the patient needs a sound immune system in order to eliminate the weakened bacteria. Bactericidals, on the other hand, actually kill the bacteria; therefore, a patient with a very weakened immune system can still be treated successfully, as the immune system does not need to deal with the resulting dead bacteria in any way. Bactericidal drugs act most effectively on rapidly dividing organisms.

> ### Essential terminology
>
> **Antibiotic**
> A drug produced by some microorganisms that destroys or interferes with the development of a living organism.
>
> **Antibacterial**
> A substance that destroys or inhibits the growth of bacteria.
>
> **Antiviral**
> A substance that destroys or inhibits the growth of a virus.
>
> **Antifungal**
> A substance that destroys or inhibits the growth of a fungus.

ANTIMICROBIAL USE

About 80% of all UK human prescribing of antibiotics is in the community, with only 20% being prescribed in hospitals (McNulty *et al.*, 2007; SMAC, 1998). However, antibiotics are also prescribed and administered to many farm animals, and by eating their meat we take in their antibiotic history.

Of the community prescribing, 50% is for respiratory tract infection (RTI) and 15% for urinary tract infection (UTI) (McNulty *et al.*, 2007; SMAC, 1998). Although hospital prescribing accounts for only approximately 20% of the human use of antibacterial drugs in the UK, this actually accounts for 10-30% of the annual medicines budget (McNulty *et al.*, 2007). The reasons for this include the following:

- The infections seen in hospital inpatients are often more complex and the responsible organism(s) more virulent compared with those in the community.

- In wards and clinics, people are often crowded together, with little personal space and poor ventilation.

- Hospital beds are rarely left empty for long, and many wards are encouraged to 'hot-bed' patients.

- A large number of hospital inpatients are immunocompromised in some way due to their illness, and so infection tends to be concentrated in this population. These patients present an ideal opening for opportunistic bacteria that are adept at accumulating resistance to antibiotic (antibacterial) drugs.

Our antibacterial history, along with poor practice in both community and hospital pre-scribing contribute to the increasing problem of antibacterial drug resistance. Probably the most well-known example of antibacterial drug resistance is that of MRSA. It has been well understood for many years that indiscriminate prescribing and the unnecessary use of antibacterials leads to antibacterial (antibiotic) resistance. For example, the prescribing that takes place for upper respiratory tract infection (URTI) is mostly for sore throat, otitis media (inflammation of the middle ear), sinusitis (inflammation of the nasal sinuses), coughs and wheezes (McNulty *et al.*, 2007). However, the infecting organisms in the majority of these instances are viruses, and so the antibacterials given are actually ineffective; to treat a virus, an antiviral drug, if available, is required.

Antimicrobial resistance

Some microorgansims are resistant to antimicrobials for one of two reasons. First, many microorgansims develop a resistance following the use of an antimicrobial to treat an infection; this is known as acquired resistance. Second, the nature of their metabolism or structure means that other microorgansims are naturally resistant to some antimicrobials; this is known as inherent resistance. MRSA and *Clostridium diffi-cile* are two well-known microorganisms. Many healthy individuals have *Staphylococcus aureus* in their normal body flora. *Staphylococcus aureus* becomes resistant to treatment by many antimicrobials because it is capable of passing on resistance factors (R factors). Although originally *Staphylococcus aureus* seemed to be resistant only to methicillin, one of the penicillin group of antibiotics, these R factors can actually produce resistance to a wide variety of antibiotics. Previously, vancomycin and teicoplanin were held in reserve so that they could be used to treat MRSA, but vancomycin-resistant *Staphylococcus aureus* (VRSA) is becoming much more common and now of all the antimicrobials listed in the BNF only very few are available to effectively treat MRSA.

As a result of the widespread misuse of antimicrobials (antibiotics) over the past half-century, about one-third of the UK population now has MRSA as part of their body flora, usually on their skin or in their nose (DH, 2007). MRSA is very difficult to treat and its presence influences public confidence in the NHS in relation to the cleanliness of NHS premises and the skill, efficiency and professionalism of NHS staff.

FACTORS INFLUENCING PRESCRIBING DECISIONS

Infections can pose problems for the prescriber. A decision has to be made either to prescribe an antibacterial with a broad action against a range of infecting organisms and therefore the potential to add to the problem of antibacterial resistance, or to wait for culture and sensitivity results to come from the pathology department, which will indicate the infecting organism and which antimicrobial it is sensitive to. The major disadvantage of the latter course of action is that the onset of treatment is delayed by at least 24 hours, and possibly longer if sensitivity is requested; such a wait could mean the patient's condition deteriorating, perhaps fatally.

Infection/colonisation

When pathogenic microorganisms are present in body tissues but are not causing disease with clinical signs and symptoms, this is known as colonisation. Pathogenic microorganisms invading body tissues and causing disease are known as infection. It is important, therefore, for the prescriber to identify whether the patient is infected or colonised (Wickens and Wade, 2004). For example, it can be catastrophic for an ill patient to develop a wound infected with MRSA, with the resulting fever, pain, inflammation and purulent discharge. It is also possible for someone to have MRSA bacteria in a wound, but not in sufficient quantity to produce an infection, in other words the wound is colonised with MRSA.

Superinfection

According to Wickens and Wade (2004), the gold standard in treating infection is to choose the most appropriate antimicrobial for the infection, which is established by sending a specimen (e.g. swab, urine or sputum, depending on what is most appropriate) for microbiological examination – that is, culture and sensitivity. An added advantage of individualising the treatment to the specific infecting organism in this way is that unwanted effects such as infection by opportunistic microorganisms (superinfections) are minimised. Superinfections occur due to destruction of the body's normal flora by antibiotics. Normal body flora has an important function in maintaining health; if the normal body flora is destroyed by antibiotics, then areas of the body become vulnerable to opportunistic organisms via a process that is still not clearly understood (Navarini et al., 2006). In patients who are already very ill, this puts extra demand on the body's metabolism and immune system, and may shift the balance for the patient from morbidity to mortality.

Bacterial classification

Bacteria can be classified using a number of different systems (Mera, 1997). The main classification systems that the nurse should be familiar with are those used in pathology reports, such as culture and sensitivity results, which guide antimicrobial prescribing. Three of these systems consider (i) the shape of the bacteria, (ii) whether the bacteria take up a crystal violet stain (Gram stain) and (iii) whether the bacteria are aerobes or anaerobes. The prescriber considers these classifications when deciding which type of antibacterial would be most useful in a given situation.

Antimicrobial drugs act at different sites in the organism that they are targeting. They either:

- act on the cell wall of the microorganism, e.g. the cephalosporins and penicillins; or
- slow down protein production (synthesis), within the cell itself, e.g. chloramphenicol and erythromycin. They do this by interfering with the build-up of the peptide chains on the ribosome of the organism (Greenstein and Gould, 2004; Rang *et al.*, 2003).

Unless the situation is an emergency and the patient's condition will be compromised, there are two fundamental principles in antibacterial prescribing:

1. Identify the infecting organism (if practicable).
2. Determine its susceptibility to a particular drug.

Personal and professional development A2.1

Name the test that the nurse should carry out in most situations when an infection is suspected.
The answer can be found at the back of the book.

THE ROLE OF THE NURSE IN ANTIBACTERIAL PRESCRIBING

Whether the nurse is administering or prescribing antibacterials (antibiotics), they play an important part in preventing antibacterial resistance by:

- Being familiar with the prescribing protocols (antibiotic policy) of the NHS trust that they work in.
- Help patients and or their carers to understand the nature of their illness as well as the actions and side effects of their medication.
- Prevent and control infection especially in hospitals and other long term care facilities.

(Ashurst, 1994)

PROBIOTICS

People in the UK are increasingly being advised to take responsibility for their own health and to adopt a healthy lifestyle. One aspect of this that is gaining in popularity is to encourage a healthy immune system by increasing the amount and types of bacteria that an individual has in their gastrointestinal system. There are thought to be some 400–500 different strains of bacteria in the gastrointestinal system.

Probiotics are live microorganisms that are added in considerable numbers to certain drinks and yoghurts and are also available as dry powders and in capsules. Probiotics are said to increase the normal flora of the gastrointestinal tract, which it is claimed has a beneficial effect on the health of the individual. The health improvements that are claimed are rather general: probiotics are often said to improve vitality, wellbeing and energy. They were first marketed following a researcher's observations of some long-living Russian people. It was noticed that those people ate large quantities of a type of natural yoghurt that contained large numbers of naturally occurring bacteria. It was concluded that consuming these bacteria made these people long-livers. Following the publication of these observations, a variety of products containing probiotics have been introduced.

Probiotics are marketed in rather a 'grey' area: on the one hand they are considered to be a food product and therefore not subject to scrutiny of the claims made by the manufacturer; on the other hand, they could be considered as pharmaceuticals because they are often promoted as a 'cure' for a variety of gastrointestinal diseases. Probiotics may well play an important role in the protection of the gastrointestinal tract against infection. Many people claim that taking probiotics has improved gastrointestinal symptoms such as diarrhoea and abdominal bloating after a course of antibiotics, but there is currently little reliable or valid evidence available for the role of probiotics either in the maintenance of health or in the prevention of disease.

Probiotics are one of a number of 'nutraceuticals' – food products that are promoted as having a beneficial effect on health. The healthcare claims made about probiotics suggest that they:

● reduce the frequency of antibiotic-induced diarrhoea in children;

● are an effective treatment for inflammatory disorders of the bowel;

● support and improve the function of the immune system.

A variety of strains of microorganisms are claimed to produce a beneficial effect. The numbers of microorganisms that have to be taken in order to produce an effect are unknown, and the kind of outcome that they produce is unknown. No large reliable studies have provided robust evidence to support the claims listed above, and so there is a real need for further research in this area. Wickens and Wade (2004) suggest that such research would be able to:

● explore whether there are any relevant physiological **biomarkers**;

● confirm whether these biomarkers would be useful to assess the function of probiotics;

● follow up the preliminary studies with confirmatory studies;

● clearly establish any mechanisms of action of probiotics;

● study the dose–response relationship in probiotics;

● define the active ingredients in probiotics.

PREBIOTICS

Prebiotics are found in a number of different foods. They are the complex carbohydrates in a particular food that provide nourishment to sustain the normal flora of the gastrointestinal tract (Parkes, 2007). Eating a diet rich in prebiotics is thought to ensure the variety and quantity of flora needed in the gastrointestinal system.

As yet, little is known about the role of bacteria in and on the human gastrointestinal system. There is also still much to learn about how the bacterial population of the gut is influenced by dietary intake, particularly by complex carbohydrates such as the oligosaccharides: fructose, galactose and isomaltose. Early work suggests that certain types of food may increase the quantity and variety of bacteria in the colon. These studies seem to suggest that prebiotics not only have some positive influence on the immune system but also affect the health of the gastrointestinal mucosa (Macfarlane *et al.*, 2006; Woodmansey, 2007). However, these studies must be viewed from the perspective that there is very little understanding about, for example, how many, what types of, and in what combination bacteria reside in the gastrointestinal tract, and the effects of bacteria on the gut wall and the body in general.

REFERENCES

Ashurst A (1994) The role of nurses in antibiotic therapy. *British Journal of Nursing* **3**, 864–865.

Audit Commission (2000) *The Management and Control of Hospital Acquired Infection in Acute NHS Trusts in England*. London: National Audit Office.

Commission for Healthcare Audit and Inspection (CHAI) (2005) *Management, Prevention and Surveillance of* Clostridium difficile. London: Healthcare Commission.

Commission for Healthcare Audit and Inspection (CHAI) (2006) *Investigation into Outbreaks of* Clostridium difficile *at Stoke Mandeville Hospital, Buckinghamshire Hospitals NHS Trust*. London: Healthcare Commission.

Crowcroft N S, Duckworth G, Griffiths C, Lamagni T L and Rooney C (2004) Trends in MRSA in England and Wales: analysis of morbidity and mortality data for 1993–2002. *Health Statistics Quarterly* **21**, 15–22.

Department of Health (DH) (2002) *Getting Ahead of the Curve: A Strategy for Combating Infectious Diseases*. Report by the Chief Medical Officer. London: Department of Health.

Department of Health (DH) (2003) *Winning Ways: Working Together to Reduce Healthcare Associated Infection in England*. Report by the Chief Medical Officer. London: Department of Health.

Department of Health (DH) (2004) *NHS Improvement Plan*. London: Department of Health.

Department of Health (DH) (2005) *Saving Lives: A Delivery Programme to Reduce Healthcare Associated Infection (HCAI) Including MRSA*. London: Department of Health.

Department of Health (DH) (2006a) *The Health Act 2007: Code of Practice for the Prevention and Control of Healthcare Associated Infections*. London: Department of Health.

Department of Health (DH) (2006b) *Essential Steps to Safe, Clean Care*. London: Department of Health.

Department of Health (DH) (2006c) *Going Further Faster: Implementing the Saving Lives Delivery Programme – Sustainable Change for Clearer, Safer Care*. London: Department of Health.

Department of Health (DH) (2007) *On the State of the Public Health: Annual Report of the Chief Medical Officer 2006*. London: Department of Health.

Greenstein B and Gould D (2004) *Trounce's Clinical Pharmacology for Nurses*. Edinburgh: Churchill Livingstone.

Hospital Infection Society (HIS) and Infection Control Nurses Association (ICNA) (2006). *The Third Prevalence Survey of Healthcare-associated Infections in Acute Hospitals*. Press release 27 October 2006. **www.his.org.uk/_db_documents/ press_informationdoc.**

Macfarlane S, Macfarlane G T and Cummings J H (2006) Prebiotics in the gastro-intestinal tract. *Alimentary Pharmacology and Therapeutics* **24**, 701–714.

McNulty C A M, Boyle P, Nichols T, Clappison P and Davey P (2007) The public's attitudes to and compliance with antibiotics. *Journal of Antimicrobial Chemotherapy* **60** (suppl 1), i63–i68.

Mera S (1997) *Understanding Disease: Pathology and Prevention*. Cheltenham: Stanley Thornes.

Navarini A A, Recher M, Lang K S, *et al.* (2006) Increased susceptibility to bacterial superinfection as a consequence of innate antiviral responses. *Proceedings of the National Academy of Sciences of the United States of America* **103**, 15535–15539.

Parkes G C (2007) An overview of probiotics and prebiotics. *Nursing Standard* **21**, 43–47.

Pellowe C (2007) Managing and leading the infection prevention initiative. *Journal of Nursing Management* **15**, 567–573.

Plowman R, Graves N, Griffin M, *et al.* (2001) The rate and cost of hospital acquired infections occurring in patients admitted to selected specialties of a district general hospital in England and the national burden imposed. *Journal of Hospital Infection* **47**, 198–209.

Pratt R J, Pellowe C M, Wilson J A, *et al.* (2007) Epic 2: national evidence-based guidelines for preventing healthcare associated infections in NHS hospitals in England. *Journal of Hospital Infection* **65** (suppl 1), S1–S59.

Rang H P, Dale M M, Ritter J M and Moore P K (2003) *Pharmacology*, 5th edn. Edinburgh: Churchill Livingstone.

Standing Medical Advisory Committee (SMAC) (1998) *The Path of Least Resistance*. London: Department of Health.

Wickens H and Wade P (2004) The right drug for the right bug. *Pharmaceutical Journal* **274**, 365–368.

Woodmansey E J (2007) Intestinal bacteria and ageing. *Journal of Applied Microbiology* **102**, 1178–1186.

Answers

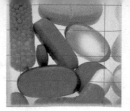

2.1

- Uses
- Indications
- Cautions
- Contraindications
- Side effects
- Dosages
- Costs.

2.5

Non-selective beta-blockers have an effect on bronchial and peripheral blood vessel receptors, which may result in bronchospasm (narrowing of the bronchi). The consequences of this could be:

- reduced airflow through the bronchi;
- dyspnoea (difficulty in breathing);
- interference with the treatments that the patient is already receiving; e.g. bronchodilators such as salbutamol selectively stimulate β_2 receptors in the bronchi to relax smooth muscle, so that the airway is opened (dilated).

2.9

- Anatomy and physiology/disordered physiology
- Disease processes
- Research process
- Professional responsibilities, e.g. NMC
- Government publications.

2.12

- *Drink plenty of fluids*: One potential effect of diuretics, particularly potent medicines such as furosemide, is dehydration, and so nurses need to make sure that patients' intake of fluid is appropriate. This can be established by maintaining a fluid balance chart.
- *Weigh the patient weekly*: Weighing the patient helps to establish how much fluid has been lost.

4.2

Patient/public perception, e.g.

- *Drug*: Hard drug, illegal, heroin, addictive.
- *Medicine*: Soft, legal, curative, liquid.

4.3

- Alcohol
- Tobacco
- Caffeine.

4.4

- *Maintenance therapy*: For chronic conditions that need to be maintained, such as hypertension (high blood pressure), e.g. beta-blockers.
- *Replacement therapy*: For people who cannot produce essential substances, e.g. insulin.
- *Health maintenance*: Not essential but will improve the quality of life of the patient, e.g. hormone replacement therapy (HRT).
- *Palliative therapy*: Aimed at improving quality of life rather than effecting a cure, e.g. salbutamol used in chronic obstructive pulmonary disease to maintain open airways, or analgesia for cancer-related pain.
- *Emergency medicines*: For patients who are acutely ill and need acute interventions, e.g. adrenaline (epinephrine) for the treatment of anaphylactic shock.
- *Complementary therapies*: 'Alternative' or less conventional therapies, e.g. herbal and homeopathic therapies. St John's wort is a herbal remedy that has been shown to have some efficacy in treating depression.
- *Lifestyle drugs*: Treatments for clinical obesity, nicotine replacement, erectile dysfunction.
- *Supportive therapies*: 'Covering' important drugs to prevent the unwanted effects of essential drugs, e.g. anti-emetics for patients receiving cancer treatment or pain relief for chronic conditions.
- *Recreational drugs*: Ecstasy, cocaine, alcohol.

Diagnosis: Fluorescein sodium is used in eye drops by optometrists to highlight damage to the cornea. There are other examples of substances used in diagnostic tests such as barium used in X-ray investigations.

Nursing implications: using information about medicines

- *Reduction in plasma proteins*: Change in the drug concentration, and therefore a potential for adverse effects for mother and baby. The dose of the medicine needs to be considered.
- *Increased liver enzyme activity*: Faster elimination of some medicines. There will be a need for good control, e.g. in epilepsy, with a potential need for an increase in the dose.
- *Increased renal blood flow*: Potential for increased elimination of medicines; however, the only group of medicines this actually affects is the penicillins. The dose should be increased.

4.6

- Familiar
- Convenient
- Does not require sterile preparation or aseptic technique
- Safest method of medicine delivery
- Overdoses can be dealt with before absorption is complete (e.g. by gastric washout)
- Cheap.

4.8

- Aspirin gargles for a sore throat
- Gels for infants who are teething
- Loperamide used in the treatment of diarrhoea. This drug slows bowel activity and reduces the loss of water and salts, thus producing firmer stools and reducing frequency
- Omeprazole, which reduces acid production to relieve gastritis. This medicine is also used to relieve the symptoms and promote healing of gastric ulcers.

4.9

- The patient should be sitting up and take the medication with a glass of water, otherwise tablets may become lodged in the oesophagus and cause erosion and ulceration (Downie *et al.*, 2003).
- Taking a drink before the medication can help.
- Medicines should be taken separately.
- Placing the medicine as far back as possible on the tongue may help.

4.11

- Contact with body fluids
- Needle-stick injuries
- Sensitivity to the medication if the medication is squirted into the atmosphere.

4.12

- Apply to unbroken skin.
- Apply to hair-free skin.
- Change the site each time a new patch is applied, in order to avoid irritation.

4.13

Pessaries, enemas, syrups, emulsions, linctuses, mixtures, elixirs, capsules, creams, lotions, ointments.

5.1

- Treatment of mental illness
- To promote sleep.

5.4

There are said to be five key pieces of labelling information:

- Name
- Strength
- Route of administration
- Dose
- Warnings.

We also need to consider the following:

- Expiry date
- Storage instructions, such as ideal temperature.

Professionals and patients need to be able to identify at a glance the information required to use medicines safely. The size and colour of the font can be important for people with visual problems or dyslexia.

5.5

A correct prescription should:

- be based on patient consent;
- be legible;
- clearly identify the patient;
- identify the medicine (generic name), form, dose, route, timing, and start and finish times;
- be signed and dated by an authorised prescriber.

Controlled drugs should be stated in dosage and number of doses or course.

5.6

- Patients on complex medication regimes, e.g. taking several medicines
- Patients who have experienced adverse effects of medicines
- Patients with chronic conditions
- Older adults
- Patients who are having problems with adherence to their treatment.

5.7

- Name and purpose of the medication
- Dose and route of administration
- Frequency of dose
- Length of treatment
- Adverse effects, including the implications of stopping and starting medication without medical advice
- Storage of the medicines and information on how to obtain more supplies
- A contact number for queries or concerns.

- *Cognitive skills*: Sound knowledge and understanding.
- *Interpersonal skills*: Such as listening, choice of language, verbal and written skills, and positive reinforcement of purpose of treatment.
- *Professional skills*: Such as assessment, problem-solving and decision-making skills.

5.9

- *Intravenous*: Via a vein.
- *Intraosseous*: Within a bone, usually the tibia; needs a wide-bore needle to deliver the medicine into the bone marrow. Used when no other route is available.
- *Tracheal*: Via the endotracheal tube.

6.4

Grapefruit juice is thought to increase the plasma concentration of many cardiovascular drugs, including nifedipine LA and the statins (Committee on the Safety of Medicines, 2004; Miscellaneous, 2005). The active drug is the drug carried dissolved in the plasma rather than that which is bound to plasma proteins; this means that there is thought to be more of the calcium channel blocker drug dissolved in the plasma and therefore more active drug. Grapefruit juice is thought to potentiate the action of this group of medicines.

Actions:
- Measure and record Ms Small's blood pressure, both lying down and standing, to check for hypotension following an interaction between nifedipine LA and grapefruit juice.
- Explain about drug–food interactions and suggest an action plan to help Ms Small lower her blood cholesterol by means of diet and exercise. Remember that such a plan will have to consider Ms Small's rehabilitation needs following her hip replacement. Therefore, liaison with the physiotherapist will be necessary.
- Suggest to Ms Small that she refrains from eating grapefruit and drinking its juice while she is taking antihypertensive medication.
- Point out to Ms Small that alcohol may also enhance the hypotensive effect. Encourage and explore with her how she can also incorporate this into her action plan.
- Document your discussion.

6.5

- Talk to Mr Robson and find out whether he is taking the St John's wort, why and for how long.
- Recommend that he stop taking the St John's wort, and explain why: Using St John's wort causes reduced blood levels of digoxin, with resulting loss of control of heart rhythm and/or heart failure. Interventions: arrange for blood levels of digoxin to be checked.
- St John's wort causes decreased blood levels of warfarin and a need for an increased dosage of warfarin. Interventions: arrange for international normalised ratio (INR) levels to be checked and then monitor them closely, as blood levels may increase on stopping St John's wort (rebound action). Warfarin dosage may need to be adjusted.
- Discuss drug interactions with Mr Robson and draw up an action plan.
- Document your discussion.

For advice for healthcare professionals about St John's wort, see Breckenridge (2000) and **www.mhra.gov.uk**.

6.6

Echinacea has been associated with hypersensitivity (allergic) reactions, including anaphylaxis. Acknowledge that he is correct in thinking that it is used for the prophylaxis and treatment of viral, bacterial and fungal infections (Ang-Lee *et al.*, 2001) and that it may be effective in preventing and reducing the effects of the common cold (Shah *et al.*, 2007). However, he is asthmatic and therefore is more than likely to have some sensitivity to common allergens. He should be advised that if he does decide to use echinacea, he should consider using it only with extreme caution. Document your discussion.

7.4

- *Visual analogue scale (VAS)*: Measures pain intensity, using a scale from no pain to worst possible pain.
- *Numerical rating scale (NRS)*: Patient rates their pain between 1 and 10.
- *Verbal rating scale (VRS)*: Uses words to describe the pain; each word has a score.
- *McGill pain questionnaire (MPQ)*: Multidimensional; combines a list of questions about the nature of the pain with a body map to identify location.
- *Non-verbal pain scale (NVPS)*: For patients unable to use verbal or numerical scales.

Nursing implications: management of problems

- Good mouth care, including brushing teeth with a small brush and rinsing frequently
- Providing ice to suck
- Antiseptic or saline mouthwashes.

7.6

- Transcutaneous electrical nerve simulation (TENS)
- Cognitive-behavioural therapies, such as relaxation, imagery and distraction (MacLellan, 2006)
- Applications of heat and cold
- Acupuncture
- Providing information
- Relief of pressure
- Careful moving and positioning.

7.7

- Painful injection site
- Setting the syringe driver incorrectly
- Patient may have misperceptions about the use of syringe drivers and therefore refuse this method of treatment
- Most adjuvants are not available via this route.

Nursing knowledge: health education related to medicines

- Do not stop taking the aspirin unless directed by the doctor.
- Adverse effects include allergy (runny nose, itchy skin, swelling), stomach irritation, pain, black tarry stools (indicating bleeding), and ringing or buzzing in the ears.
- Aspirin is contraindicated in patients with asthma, as they might be allergic to aspirin.
- Avoid taking other medicines such as warfarin, diuretics, antacids and other NSAIDs, unless directed by the doctor.
- Alcohol may increase the risk of adverse effects, such as gastro irritation.
- Inform other health professionals, e.g. dentist and surgeon, about the treatment.

10.4

- Recent major surgery
- Recent trauma
- Severe and uncontrolled hypertension.

10.6

Diet:
- Explain the links between saturated fat in the diet and the build-up of atheroma.
- Check labels on food for fat and salt content; provide advice about recommended daily intake of both.
- Give examples of how to cut down fat within existing meal plans, e.g. substitute low-fat spread for butter, use wholemeal instead of white bread, use oven chips instead of fried chips.
- Encourage him to eat five portions of fruit and vegetables a day.
- Encourage him to eat more oily fish such as mackerel.
- Advise on what is meant by a 'beneficial' level of alcohol intake.
- Advise him to maintain his weight within current guidelines for his weight and height.

Activity:
- Advise him to consult his doctor before commencing any exercise programme.
- Advise him to build up exercise and activity gradually.
- Advise him to stop exercise immediately if he experiences chest pain.

Health:
- Advise him to attend for regular blood pressure measurements at his GP's surgery.
- Advise him to maintain his weight within the guidelines.

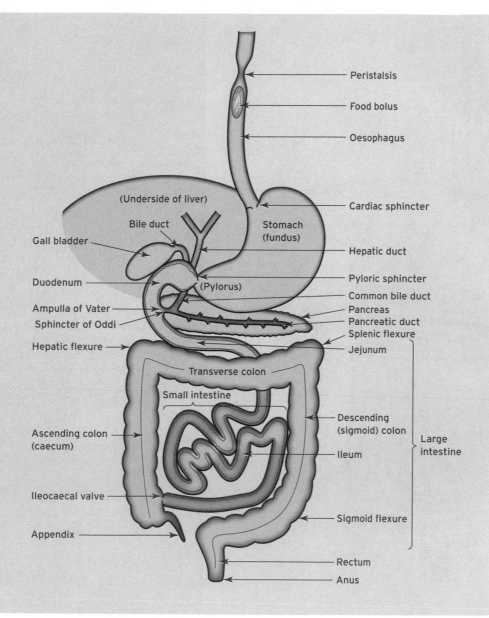

Peristalsis

Food bolus

Oesophagus

(Underside of liver)

Bile duct

Gall bladder

Stomach
(fundus)

Cardiac sphincter

Hepatic duct

Duodenum

(Pylorus)

Pyloric sphincter

Common bile duct

Ampulla of Vater

Pancreas

Sphincter of Oddi

Pancreatic duct

Splenic flexure

Hepatic flexure

Jejunum

Transverse colon

Small intestine

Descending
(sigmoid) colon

Ascending colon
(caecum)

Ileum

Large
intestine

Ileocaecal valve

Sigmoid flexure

Appendix

Rectum

Anus

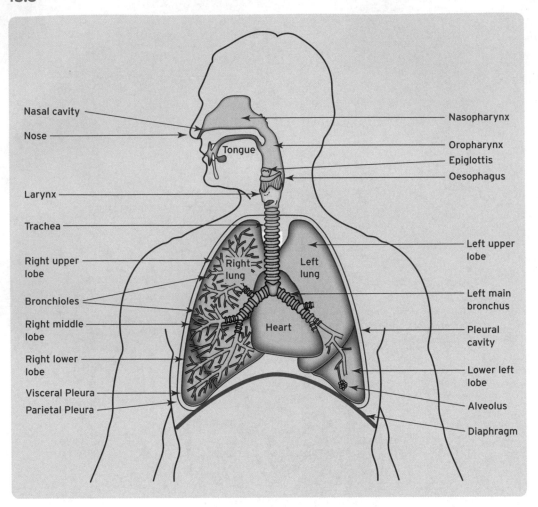

Nasal cavity

Nose

Tongue

Larynx

Trachea

Right upper
lobe

Bronchioles

Right middle
lobe

Right lower
lobe

Visceral Pleura

Parietal Pleura

Right
lung

Left
lung

Heart

Nasopharynx

Oropharynx

Epiglottis

Oesophagus

Left upper
lobe

Left main
bronchus

Pleural
cavity

Lower left
lobe

Alveolus

Diaphragm

15.10

The following precautions should be implemented when using oxygen:

- Oxygen is an increased danger if there is a fire, as it makes anything that is burning burn more quickly and fiercely. Always ensure that you know where the fire extinguishers are located and that you are familiar with the local fire procedures.
- Ensure that flammable items are kept well away from oxygen supplies. Such items include aerosol sprays, solvents and oil.
- Smoking should never be allowed near any oxygen supply. As smoking is no longer permitted on NHS trust premises, the risk of this has been reduced.
- Facemasks and nasal cannulae are for single use so must be disposed of after use in each patient.
- Using oxygen dehydrates the oronasal mucous membranes. This is why oxygen is humidified when it is administered to patients. The patient may complain of a dry mouth or you may observe this. Only water-based lubricants such as KY Jelly® should be used to lubricate the patient's lips and anterior nares when they are using oxygen. Advice for a patient being discharged home on oxygen therapy, especially if they smoke, should highlight that petroleum jelly lip salves are best avoided as these are oil-based products. Although burns to the face as a result of fire and oxygen therapy are rare, oil-based products do encourage any flames to burn at higher temperatures.

- Oral hygiene is particularly important because of the dehydrating effect of oxygen. If the patient is able to drink, encourage them to take regular sips of fluid.

16.1

- Medicines should be accompanied by lifestyle changes in diet and exercise.
- The patient's ability to adhere to the associated lifestyle changes should be assessed.
- The age of the patient should be considered.

16.2

- Patients may be reluctant to make lifestyle changes, e.g. altering their diet.
- Patients may not take their medication as prescribed.

16.3

Designer babies:

- The selection of fertilised embryos as a match for siblings with disease processes.
- The eradication of 'undesirable' traits.

A2.1

A wound swab would be taken for culture and sensitivity.

Glossary

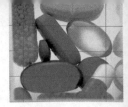

Abscess Cavity full of pus, usually as a result of an infection.

ACE inhibitors Group of medicines used in the treatment of high blood pressure and heart failure.

Acidosis Increased acidity of blood resulting from an increased number of hydrogen ions dissolved in the blood.

Adherence Ability of an individual to continue to follow a prescribed plan of treatment supported by a health professional. This prescription may include taking medicines or other treatments such as exercise, dietary changes or smoking cessation.

Adjuvant Describes a medicine used in combination with another medicine to enhance its effects.

Adverse effects Undesirable, often harmful medicine actions.

Advocacy Acting to promote and safeguard the wellbeing of the patient.

Aerobic Describes microorganisms that need oxygen in order to live and grow.

Aetiology Study of the causes of a medical condition.

Agenda for Change National policy that governs salary scales and working conditions for all NHS staff.

Aggregation Clumping together of blood cells.

Agonist Substance that produces a response.

Allopathic medicine Conventional Western medicine.

Amitriptyline Antidepressant medicine.

Anaerobic Describes microorganisms that thrive in environments that have little or no oxygen.

Analgesic Medicine taken to relieve pain. Medicines used for this purpose can range from those used to treat mild pain to those used to treat severe pain.

Analogue Medicine that varies in its molecular structure from its parent medicine.

Anaphylaxis Abnormal and immediate response to, for example, a medicine.

Androgens Hormones (steroids) secreted by the testes and cortex of the adrenal gland that produce secondary male characteristics. These hormones also build up protein tissues, which is one reason why this group of steroids is used by body-builders.

Angina Pain that occurs when the myocardium (heart muscle) is deprived of oxygen (myocardial ischaemia).

Angioplasty Technique employed to reopen an occluded coronary artery.

Antacid Medicine used to relieve digestive discomfort by neutralising the hydrochloric acid secreted by the stomach.

Antagonist Substance that prevents a response.

Antibiotic Medicine used to treat bacterial infections.

Anticoagulant Medicine that prevents blood from clotting.

Anticonvulsant Medicine used to reduce the severity of convulsions/seizures.

Anti-emetic Medicine used to relieve vomiting.

Antihypertensive Medicine used to reduce high blood pressure.

Anti-inflammatory Medicine that reduces inflammation.

Antiplatelet Medicine that prevents platelet aggregation.

Antipyretic Medicine taken to reduce body temperature.

Anxiolytic Medicine that relieves anxiety and calms the patient.

Apical pulse Another way of describing the heart rate; recorded by placing a stethoscope over the apex of the heart.

Arrhythmia Abnormal heart rhythm.

Arthroplasty Surgical reconstruction of a joint.

Asthma Condition associated with bronchospasm (narrowing of the airways) and inflammation, which result in the patient experiencing difficulty in respiration, particularly expiration (breathing out), and often associated with an expiratory wheeze.

Ataxia Unsteady gait.

Atheroma Formation of fatty plaques in the walls of the arteries.

Atria The smaller chambers of the heart that receive blood.

Attrition Reduction in the number of volunteers in a clinical trial.

Aura Forewarning of a convulsion.

Autoimmune Destruction of tissues by the body's own immune response.

Bacillus Rod-shaped (straight) microorganisms.

Barbiturates Group of medicines that depress the activity of the central nervous system.

Beneficence Moral principle that requires nurses to act for the benefit of others.

Beta-adrenoceptor blocker Medicine that prevents the stimulation of specific (beta-adrenergic) receptors at the nerve endings of the central nervous system. As a consequence, the activity of the heart is reduced.

Beta-blocker An alternative name for a beta-adrenoceptor blocker.

Binge drinking Drinking large amounts of alcohol at one time in order to get drunk.

Bioavailability Proportion of a medicine that enters the bloodstream in an active form.

Biomarker A biochemical molecule that may indicate the presence or absence of a particular cellular process.

Biphasic Having two different parts. In relation to insulin this usually refers to a premixed medicine containing both intermediate- and long-acting insulin.

Blood–brain barrier Mechanism that regulates which molecules enter the cerebrospinal fluid and tissue spaces/cells of the brain.

BMI Body mass index; the weight of an individual expressed in kilograms divided by the square of the height expressed in metres.

Bolus Whole dose of a medicine given intravenously in a larger amount than a standard intravenous injection. Given according to manufacturer's instructions, e.g. over 2–3 minutes.

Bradycardia Slow heart rate, often related to age.

Bronchospasm Narrowing of the bronchi by muscular contraction.

Calcium channel blocker Medicine that prevents the entry of calcium into cardiac and smooth muscle cells.

Cancer Overall term used to describe malignant cell growth.

Cannulation Insertion of a cannula (flexible, hollow tube) into a blood vessel, body cavity or duct and used to administer medicines or drain body fluids. A cannula may have a stiff, sharp, pointed inner known as a trocar to ease cannula insertion. Once in place, the trocar is removed, leaving only the cannula in place.

Carbohydrate Compound containing carbon, hydrogen and oxygen (CHO). Carbohydrates are an important food group; examples include sugar and starch.

Carcinogen Any substance that may predispose to cancer.

Cardiac cycle Sequence of events between one heart beat and the next.

Catalyst Substance that alters the rate of a chemical reaction without itself being changed.

Chemotherapy Term commonly used to describe some anticancer treatments but meaning the prevention or treatment of disease by chemical substances.

Chronological Information about time events classified in some sort of order or sequence.

Clinical governance Quality assurance strategy. The local health service is responsible for maintaining standards in clinical practice.

Cloning Production of identical genes by genetic engineering.

Coccus Round or oval-shaped microorganism.

Cognitive Describes 'mental processes'.

Commensal One of two different species that live together in a non-harmful or beneficial manner.

Co-morbidity Condition in a patient with another condition.

Compliance Extent to which a patient follows the instructions or advice of a healthcare professional relating to, for example, medicines and nutrition.

Concordance Partnership between the patient and prescriber. The patient's preferences and beliefs are respected in order to enable the patient to take their treatment effectively.

Contraindication Factor in the individual's condition that indicates that the medicine is inappropriate.

Covert administration Disguising medicines in food or drink.

Culture Shared values and beliefs.

Culture and sensitivity Specific microbiological test frequently ordered by nurses in order to determine whether a wound is infected, which type of microorganism is present and which antimicrobial it is sensitive to. The test comprises two parts carried out at the same time. The first part of the test (culture) is carried out by growing microorganisms in a sterile container filled with a sterile growing medium. The second part of the test (sensitivity) is carried out by impregnating the growing medium with small amounts of antimicrobial drugs.

Cyanosis Blueish tinge to the skin and mucous membranes (e.g. lips) as a result of poor oxygenation of the blood.

Cystic fibrosis Hereditary disease affecting cells of the exocrine glands. Features include the production of thick mucus, which affects the lungs and intestines.

Dehydration Reduction of fluid.

Delphi study Research technique (methodology) named after the Ancient Greek oracle. The methodology seeks the anonymous opinions of experts, who are then invited to present their opinions on a given topic. These opinions are combined and the consensus of expert opinion is fed back to the same panel of experts a number of times, and refined further each time, until a total agreement is reached about the topic under study.

Demographics Characteristics of a population, e.g. age.

Dependence Replaced the term 'addiction'.

Dermis Layer of skin that lies below the epidermis (surface layer) of the skin. Contains nerve endings, blood vessels, sweat glands and lymph vessels.

Differentiation Degree of similarity of cancer cells to the body tissue they are invading.

Diffusion Random movement of molecules from an area of high concentration to an area of low concentration.

Dilate Widen.

Diuretic Medicine used to increase the production of urine.

Drug Any substance that affects the structure or functioning of a living organism.

Drug tolerance Situation that occurs when increasing doses of a medicine are required in order to achieve the same effect.

Dysmenorrhoea Painful menstrual periods.

Dyspepsia Burning, boring feeling in the upper abdomen that many people describe as heartburn, acid stomach or upset stomach.

Dyspnoea Difficult or laboured breathing.

Endocrine Arising from within the body. Usually refers to the endocrine system or ductless glands that secrete hormones directly into extracellular spaces to enter the blood or lymph.

Enteral Relating to the intestinal tract.

Enuresis Bed-wetting (usually by children).

Enzyme Protein catalyst responsible for metabolic processes.

Epithelium Tissue that forms a thin protective layer on exposed bodily surfaces and forms the lining of internal cavities, ducts and organs.

Erectile dysfunction Inability to achieve a satisfactory erection for the purposes of sexual intercourse.

Evacuant Removal of the contents of a cavity.

Excipient Substance, usually inactive, that is added to a medicine to assist in the delivery of the medicine.

Extravasation Escape of fluid from a cannula into the surrounding tissues.

First pass effect Metabolism of a drug during its first pass through the liver.

Fusion Joining together of the articular surfaces of a joint.

Gene Basic unit of genetic material (a sequence of DNA or RNA) carried at a specific point on a chromosome.

Generic name Name of a medicine that is not protected as a trade name.

Genetic engineering Inserting genetic material from one source into the DNA of another organism; e.g. the human gene for insulin is inserted into bacterial DNA – this altered DNA is then described as recombinant DNA.

Glucagon Hormone secreted by the pancreas that lowers blood sugar.

Gluconeogenesis Synthesis (creation) of glucose from non-carbohydrate sources such as protein in the absence of carbohydrate.

Glycogenesis Process by which glucose is converted into glycogen in the liver.

Glycogenolysis Process by which glycogen is converted into glucose in the liver.

Gram stain Purple stain used in bacteriology laboratories to identify bacteria by the type of material in their cell wall. If the bacteria pick up the Gram stain and turn purple, they are described as being Gram-positive. If they do not pick up any Gram stain, they are Gram-negative. Prescribing decisions can be based on whether infecting bacteria are Gram-positive or -negative.

Granuloma Granulation tissue that forms into a small tumour, frequently after an infection.

Half-life Calculation of the time taken for a medicine to reach half of its dose within the body. This is thought to be a more accurate way of calculating dose intervals than using the full time it takes for a medicine to clear (be eliminated) from the body.

Heart failure Condition in which the output from the ventricles is unable to meet the needs of the body, ultimately resulting in circulatory failure.

Hereditary Transmission of genetic characteristics from parents to children that persists through generations.

Heterogeneous Composed of unrelated parts. In this context, it relates to a condition that has a disease range of predisposing and unconnected factors, rather than one cause.

Homeostasis Physiological process that maintains the equilibrium of body systems.

Hormone Protein that modifies the structure or function of a tissue.

Human Genome Project International research project that identified for the first time the entire sequence of genes on all the human chromosomes. This has enabled the identification of genes associated with many hereditary disorders, including identifying a genetic basis for diseases not previously thought to have a genetic basis.

Hyperglycaemia Raised levels of glucose in the bloodstream.

Hyperlipidaemia High levels of lipoproteins in the bloodstream.

Hypersensitivity Intensified sensitivity. Exaggerated response to a particular cause.

Hypertension Abnormally high blood pressure.

Hypnotic Sleep-inducing.

Hypoglycaemia Reduced level of glucose in the bloodstream.

Hyponatraemia Low levels of sodium in the bloodstream.

Hypotension Low blood pressure.

Hypoventilate Breathe slowly and shallowly.

Hypovolaemia Low circulating blood volume.

Iatrogenesis Treatment-induced disease.

Idiopathic Of unknown cause.

Ileocaecal valve One-way valve at the junction of the ileum and caecum, the purpose of which is to prevent bowel content backflowing from the caecum into the ileum.

Immunocompromise Inefficient functioning of the immune system, leaving the patient at increased risk of infection. The more immunocompromised the patient, the greater the chance of them developing an infection.

Incidence Epidemiological term that uses numbers to describe the chances of a disease occurring in a population. New cases are frequently expressed as a proportion of the population, i.e. number of cases per 1 million per year, but they can also be expressed as total numbers.

Inhibitor Substance that prevents an action.

Inotrope Agent that affects the contraction of the heart muscle.

Invasive Surgical or diagnostic procedure that involves penetration of the skin by a knife or needle.

Ischaemia Reduced blood supply to a part of the body.

Ketoacidosis Life-threatening condition in which acidosis occurs as a result of the accumulation of ketone bodies, which are products of fat metabolism. This occurs when the body cannot utilise glucose for energy and so seeks an alternative source.

Knowledge and Skills Framework Tool used by managers in the NHS to determine salary bands. The framework lists the key knowledge and skills necessary for an individual's job.

Lactic acidosis Accumulation of lactic acid in the bloodstream.

Laxative Medicine given to relieve constipation or empty the rectum.

Licence Required in order for a medicine to be marketed. Issued by the Medicines and Healthcare products Regulatory Agency (MHRA).

Localised Restricted to one part of the body.

Lumen Space inside any of the body's tubes, i.e. arteries, veins and bowel.

Macerate Soften the epidermis (skin surface) by soaking it in liquid for a period of time.

Macrovascular Relating to the large blood vessels.

Medicines management Process involving the selection, procurement, delivery, prescription, administration and review of medicines.

Metabolic syndrome Collection of symptoms that includes hypertension (high blood pressure), obesity, hypertriglyceridaemia (high blood levels of triglycerides), increased insulin resistance and hyperinsulinaemia (high blood levels of insulin). Also known as syndrome X.

Metabolism 1. Transformation of a medicine within the body to make it more hydrophilic. 2. Chemical activity that takes place in body cells in order to provide essential energy and nutrients. It consists of two processes; Anabolism – the building-up in cells of simple substances into more complex compounds – and catabolism – the breakdown of complex compounds into more simple substances. Catabolism produces energy, carbon dioxide and water.

Metastases Secondary cancers that occur as a consequence of cancer cells being transferred from their primary source, e.g. by blood or lymph.

Micturition Release of urine from the urinary bladder.

Mitosis Cell division in which a single cell generates two identical cells.

Monoclonal antibody Antigen produced by a bioengineering process. First discovered over 30 years ago, they were thought to be elusive 'magic bullets', but they have been limited in their clinical application. Until recently, they have been used mainly for diagnosis. However, rather then using mouse cells to produce monoclonal antibodies, scientists can now grow human B-cells in mice so the cells are mostly human in composition. As a result, many of the previous problems of the human immune system recognising foreign protein have been overcome. These newer monoclonal antibodies are known as recombinant monoclonal antibodies.

Monocyte Type of white blood cell

Monosaccharide Simple sugar, such as glucose.

Monotherapy Single medicine treatment.

Morbidity Incidence of disease in a population.

Mortality Incidence of death in a population.

Myocardium Heart muscle.

Necrosis Death of tissue.

Neoplasm New growth.

Neuroleptic Also known as an antipsychotic, i.e. a medicine that acts upon the nervous system and is used in the management of depression and schizophrenia.

Neuropathy Degeneration of the peripheral nerves.

Nociceptor Receptor at the end of a sensory neuron that is sensitive to pain.

Nocturnal enuresis Night-time bed-wetting.

Non-malificence Moral principle that requires that nurses should prevent harm being done to others.

NSAID Non-steroidal anti-inflammatory drug, described in this way to differentiate from corticosteroids, naturally occurring substances within the body that reduce inflammation.

Oedema Excessive accumulation of fluid in body tissues.

Oral hypoglycaemics Group of medicines that reduce the level of glucose in the blood.

Palliative Treatment that provides relief from symptoms but does not cure the underlying condition.

Parenteral Route other than oral.

Partial antagonist Substance that produces a limited response; may also block an action.

Pathophysiology Altered physiology.

Persistence Ability of an individual to continue following a prescribed plan of treatment for as long as is necessary, perhaps for the rest of their life.

pH Term from chemistry that describes the degree of acidity or alkalinity of a substance by measurement. It uses a scale of 1-14, with 1 being highly acid and 14 being extremely alkaline. Seven, the centre of the scale, is neutral, neither acid nor alkali.

Phagocytosis Process whereby cells engulf material such as bacteria.

Pharmacodynamics Effect of a drug on the body.

Pharmacogenetics Individual's response to medicines based upon their genetic makeup.

Pharmacogenomics Study of genes and their implication for new medicine development.

Pharmacokinetics Study of medicine action within the body; absorption, distribution, metabolism and excretion (ADME).

Pharmacology Science of the properties of drugs.

Pharmacotherapeutics Use of pharmacological agents (drugs) to treat diseases and disorders.

Placebo Substance with no pharmacological effect.

Polydipsia Excessive thirst.

Polypharmacy Concurrent treatment of a patient with more than one medicine.

Polyuria Passing large volumes of urine.

Postprandial Occurring after eating.

Prescription-only medicine Medicine that requires a written prescription, except in emergency situations.

Prevalence Frequency of an event in the general population.

Proliferative Divides rapidly.

Prophylaxis Prevention.

Psychosis Form of mental ill-health in which the patient experiences a loss of contact with reality.

Pulmonary embolism Part of a venous thrombus that breaks away and lodges in the pulmonary circulation.

Recreational drugs Psychoactive (alter the processes of the mind) drugs such as cannabis, ecstasy and heroin used for non-medical purposes.

Remission Reprieve from, or a lessening of severity of, the problems and symptoms of an illness.

Resection Surgical removal of diseased or damaged parts of the body.

Resistant Term used in microbiology and pharmacology to describe an organism that is unaffected by a particular drug.

Reticulo-endothelial system Collection of phagocyctic cells found mostly in the liver, spleen and bone marrow.

Reye's syndrome Rare condition occurring in childhood that results in encephalitis (inflammation of the brain).

Rhinitis Inflammation of the nasal mucous membranes. As a result of this inflammation, there is usually an increased amount of accompanying nasal mucus.

Ribosomes Parts of a cell that collect the correct sequence of amino acids to make the proteins found in the intracellular fluid (cytosol).

Self-administration Administration of a prescribed medication by the patient to themselves.

Sensitivity Response of a patient or organism to a substance such as an external agent (e.g. pollen) or a drug (e.g. an antibacterial).

Side effect Unwanted but predictable effect produced by a medicine.

Social phobia Shyness, extreme self-consciousness and overwhelming anxiety when in social situations.

Spirochaete Corkscrew or curve-shaped microorganisms.

Statin Medicine that reduces the action of an enzyme in the liver, resulting in a decreased production of cholesterol.

Steady state Concentration of a medicine achieved by regular administration.

Stem cell Undifferentiated cell.

Steroids Group of naturally occurring substances (hormones), some of which may be used therapeutically, e.g. to reduce inflammation.

Sublingual Route of administration in which the medicine is placed under the tongue for rapid absorption.

Synovectomy Surgical procedure that removes the synovial membrane from damaged joints.

Systemic Widespread throughout the body, as opposed to local, which means in a very small, contained area of the body.

Teratogenesis Potential of a medicine to cause foetal abnormalities.

Therapeutic effect Beneficial effect of a medicine.

Therapeutic range Ratio between the desired effect and the toxic effect of a medicine. A medicine with a wide therapeutic range exerts its effect at a dose substantially lower than its toxic dose.

Therapeutics 'Best' use of medicines to ensure that patients receive the maximum benefit from them.

Thrombus Blood clot.

Toxicity Potential of a substance for poisoning.

Tranquilliser Medicine used to relieve anxiety and tension.

Vaccine Products of infectious agents used to stimulate the development of antibodies to confer immunity.

Vasoconstrictor Substance that causes a narrowing of the lumen of blood vessels.

Vasodilation Increase in the diameter of the walls of veins, which increases the blood volume within the venous circulation.

Vasodilator Substance that produces widening of the blood vessels and so increases blood flow.

Venous thromboembolism Blood clot that forms within the venous system and travels within the bloodstream.

Ventricles The chambers of the heart that contract to expel blood into the circulation.

Vibrio Curved, rod-shaped microorganism.

Visceral Relating to the organs.

Yellow card scheme Scheme that involves the reporting of previously unreported adverse reactions that a patient may experience when taking a medicine.

Index

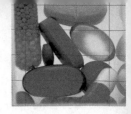

Note: Figures and Tables are indicated by *italic page numbers*, and glossary terms by **emboldened numbers**